Springer Series in Pharmaceutical Statistics

Series Editors

Thomas Permutt, Walnut Creek, CA, USA

José Pinheiro, Raritan, RJ, USA

Frank Bretz, Basel, Switzerland

Peter Müller, Austin, TX, USA

Recent advances in statistics have led to new concepts and solutions in different areas of pharmaceutical research and development. "Springer Series in Pharmaceutical Statistics" focuses on developments in pharmaceutical statistics and their practical applications in the industry. The main target groups are researchers in the pharmaceutical industry, regulatory agencies and members of the academic community working in the field of pharmaceutical statistics. In order to encourage exchanges between experts in the pharma industry working on the same problems from different perspectives, an additional goal of the series is to provide reference material for non-statisticians. The volumes will include the results of recent research conducted by the authors and adhere to high scholarly standards. Volumes focusing on software implementation (e.g. in SAS or R) are especially welcome. The book series covers different aspects of pharmaceutical research, such as drug discovery, development and production.

More information about this series at http://www.springer.com/series/15122

Christy Chuang-Stein · Simon Kirby

Quantitative Decisions in Drug Development

Second Edition

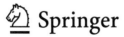 Springer

Christy Chuang-Stein
Kalamazoo, MI, USA

Simon Kirby
Ramsgate, UK

ISSN 2366-8695   ISSN 2366-8709 (electronic)
Springer Series in Pharmaceutical Statistics
ISBN 978-3-030-79733-1   ISBN 978-3-030-79731-7 (eBook)
https://doi.org/10.1007/978-3-030-79731-7

This Springer imprint is published by the registered company Springer Nature Switzerland AG
The registered company address is: Gewerbestrasse 11, 6330 Cham, Switzerland

To Parents, Bruce, Terresa and Isaac

Christy Chuang-Stein

To Dad, Mum, Katie, Theo, Helen, Rob and Andy

Simon Kirby

Preface

By all counts, 2020 was an unusual year. COVID-19 lockdowns and pandemic-related travel restrictions had placed huge limits on our mobility. Many clinical trials were adversely impacted, and some were placed on hold due to uncertainties surrounding patient recruitment and care delivery. On the other hand, the unprecedented speed with which COVID-19 vaccines were developed and approved for emergency use was truly breathtaking. For the first time in modern product development history, the identification and the commercialization of a game-changing innovative medicine occurred in less than one year. Who would have thought this to be possible before 2020?

Confined to our respective locations and deprived of frequent family outings, we have decided to use the time wisely and revise the first edition of our book. The timing was good since a lot of new advances have been made since the publication of our first edition. The revision also allowed us to correct a few errors that went undetected when the first edition was published and a mistake spotted by an observant reader.

By and large, the second edition follows the structure of the first edition. We have decided to devote an entire chapter (Chap. 13) to the topic of adaptive designs, resulting in 14 chapters in the revision.

Chapter 1 offers a high-level overview of clinical testing and regulatory review of a pharmaceutical product. Chapter 2 reviews the Frequentist approach to the testing of hypotheses and in particular the two-action decision problem. In the context of drug development, the two actions correspond to progressing or not progressing a drug for further development. We discuss multiplicity and selective inference as well as how their indiscriminate uses have contributed to the replication crisis and the P-value controversy. Chapter 3 discusses the metrics commonly used to characterize the performance of a diagnostic test. Chapter 4 draws an analogy between successive trials conducted during the clinical testing of an investigational product and a series of diagnostic tests. Under this analogy, the condition to diagnose by a clinical trial is the existence of a clinically meaningful effect for the investigational product. We have found this analogy particularly useful to explain to our clinical colleagues why replication is such an important concept in drug development and to show why replication is not as easy as many people might hope.

The predictive power of a diagnostic test depends on the existing information concerning the prevalence of the condition to be diagnosed in a relevant population. Similarly, the predictive power of a clinical trial depends on available prior knowledge concerning the investigational product. Articulating such prior knowledge is the topic of Chap. 5. In the past 10 years, we have witnessed an increasing use of historical control data in the design and analysis of clinical trials, both when concurrent control data are available and when they are completely absent. We expanded Chap. 5 to include this topic and include an example on the challenge and use of historical control data when the trial providing evidential basis for an orphan drug approval included no concurrent control. In Chap. 6, we describe metrics that are useful to evaluate designs and associated decision rules for efficacy assessment at the various stages of pre-marketing development. The focus on efficacy is due to the generally well-defined endpoints to decide upon the beneficial effect of a new drug. Chapter 7 covers the proof-of-concept stage, while Chaps. 8 and 9 cover the dose–response and confirmatory stage, respectively. Throughout Chaps. 7–9, we have added new examples where the primary endpoint is binary.

Chapter 10 focuses on assessing the design of a trial for comparative effectiveness assessment. By comparative effectiveness, we mean the comparison of different active treatments to determine which treatment works best. This focus reflects the increasing importance of these comparisons in the market place due to the need to justify the price and to qualify for reimbursement.

The metrics used in Chaps. 7–10 do not include any cost consideration explicitly. But, cost is an integral part of drug development strategy optimization. Incorporating cost into design consideration is the topic of Chap. 11 with two example approaches. The first one optimizes a benefit–cost efficiency score that measures the cost-effectiveness of a proof-of-concept trial design. The second approach combines costs and potential commercial returns to assess drug development options. The chapter includes a detailed discussion on the calculation of the expected net present value which could be of interest to readers without much exposure to product valuation.

In Chap. 12, we examine the bias that can be produced by use of Phase 2 results that have been selected because of a favorable outcome. We have hinted at this source of bias in earlier chapters and have dedicated Chap. 12 to this issue. We have expanded this chapter to include an approach based on the maximum likelihood estimation of a truncated Normal distributions and new approaches we published in the literature in recent times. We compared different adjustment methods with respect to bias and other measures such as the probability of launching a Phase 3 trial and the average statistical power of the launched trial. We offer some recommendations based on the comparative results.

Chapter 13 is new, starting with classes of adaptive designs discussed in the finalized guidance on adaptive design issued by the Food and Drug Administration (FDA) in the United States (USA). We have included four examples of adaptive designs for, a group sequential trial with an interim analysis for futility, an adaptive dose–response study, a Phase 3 trial with a pre-planned sample size re-estimation plus population enrichment and a seamless Phase 2/3 trial.

In the final chapter of the book, we include selected topics that affect design and decision choices at all stages of drug development. Examples include sequences of trials with a correlated treatment effect, benefit–risk and economic assessment. These are all active research areas. Even though we offer some references, it is not our intent to cover these areas in detail in this book.

While the majority of the book is dedicated to trial planning and setting up decision rules, we have also included the analyses of completed trials to share insight and lessons learned. Examples with this objective include two dose–response studies of tofacitinib for moderate and severe rheumatoid arthritis in Chap. 8 and three adaptive designs in Chap. 13.

We have included numerous guidances published by the US FDA, the European Medicines Agency (EMA) and the International Council for Harmonisation (ICH). Instead of providing URL links to these guidances which could become obsolete over time, we are offering paths to locate these guidances. For guidances issued by the US FDA, readers can use the "Search All FDA Guidance" option at the path of www.fda.gov -> Drugs -> Guidance, Compliance and Regulatory Information. Guidances issued by the ICH could be reached by selecting the "Work Products" tab followed by "All Guidelines" option at the ICH home page www.ich.org. As for the EMA guidelines, readers can use the "Search for scientific guidelines" link in the middle of the page reached by paging through www.ema.europa.eu -> Human Regulatory -> Research and Development -> Scientific Guidelines.

As we stated in the Preface for the first edition, developing a new drug is a high-risk and high-reward enterprise. The high risk is reflected by the generally low success rate of turning a new molecular entity into an approved drug. The success rate has fluctuated over time and has also varied across therapeutic areas. While the success rate has improved in recent years for cancer drugs due to the advent of targeted therapies, the rate has been disappointingly low for certain disorders such as Alzheimer's disease.

In addition to the high risk, the cost of developing a new drug has increased at a pace faster than inflation. Tuft's Center for the Study of Drug Development has published a series of reports examining the average pre-tax industry cost to bring a new medicine to market. The most recent report, published in 2016, estimated an average cost around $2.56 billion USD in 2013 money. By comparison, in 2003, the cost was about $1.04 billion in 2013 dollars, based on the same method of calculation. While some researchers have questioned these figures, these reports nevertheless show a substantial increase in the cost of drug development over a few decades.

The low success rate and the high cost have motivated many pharmaceutical companies to look for better methods to make portfolio decisions including whether to invest in a particular new molecular entity and how to make Go/No-Go decisions. Since the majority of development programs are likely to fail, it is important to be able to terminate a program with a low probability of success as early as possible.

At Pfizer, where both of us worked for many years, the journey to quantitative decisions began during the first decade of the twenty-first century. The implementation began with proof-of-concept studies. Teams designing these early studies were required to present, to a technical review committee, the operating characteristics of their trials/decision rules with respect to the target product profile. The move to assess the probability of success in the late-stage trials was firmly in place by the year 2010 with the establishment of a Probability of Technical and Regulatory Success (PTRS) Council.

Many statisticians and scientists played a critical role in the above journey. The input from commercial colleagues helped solidify the need to quantitatively incorporate the target product profile when designing a trial and setting up the subsequent decision rule. We have learned a great deal from the early pioneer advocates at Pfizer. Their work inspired us to write this book. We are particularly indebted to Mike Brown, Alan Clucas, Vlad Dragalin, Wayne Ewy, Bradley Marchant, Ken Kowalski, Mike K. Smith, Jonathan French, Cyrus Hoseyni, Richard Lalonde, Scott Marshall, Peter Milligan, Mohan Beltangady, Phil Woodward, Joanna Burke, Neal Thomas and Liam Ratcliffe for their scientific and organizational leadership.

The book is written for readers with a broad range of responsibilities in drug development. While the book contains a lot of technical details for quantitative scientists, it also contains plenty of concepts presented in a unified framework which, we believe, can help less quantitative readers make more quantitative decisions.

We hope you will enjoy reading the book as much as we did writing and revising it. Try as we may to ensure that the contents of the book are correct, there is always the possibility that some mistakes have gone undetected. If you spot one of these mistakes, we would be grateful if you could let us know by mailing us at christyazo@gmail.com (Christy Chuang-Stein) or s.kirby1.kirby@btinternet.com (Simon Kirby). Alternatively, we can be reached at www.linkedIn.com.

To close, we hope that we will all come out of the pandemic with new insights on trial conduct and what public–private partnerships could accomplish in expediting the development of life-saving medicines.

Kalamazoo, USA   Christy Chuang-Stein
Ramsgate, UK   Simon Kirby
March 2021

About This Book

Quantitative Decisions in Drug Development, 2nd edition, focuses on important decision points and evidence needed for making decisions at these points during the development of a new drug. It takes a holistic approach toward drug development by incorporating explicitly the knowledge learned from the earlier part of the development and available historical information into decisions at later stages. In addition, the book shares lessons learned from several select examples published in the literature since the publication of the first edition.

In particular, the book

- Shows the parallel between clinical trials and diagnostic tests and how this analogy is used to emphasize the importance of replication in drug development.
- Describes how to incorporate prior knowledge into study design and decision making at different stages of drug development.
- Explains metrics useful to address the objectives of the different stages of drug development and how to compare design options based on these metrics.
- Demonstrates why overestimation is a common problem in drug development and how adjustment should be considered to correct the overestimation.

Contents

About the Authors

Christy Chuang-Stein received a bachelor degree in mathematics from the National Taiwan University and a Ph.D. in statistics from the University of Minnesota. She retired from Pfizer as Vice President and Head of the Statistical Research and Consulting Center in July 2015, after 30 years in the pharmaceutical industry and 5 years in academia (University of Rochester). Currently, she is the owner and Principal Consultant of Chuang-Stein Consulting, LLC, and consults broadly in the areas of pharmaceutical development and evaluation.

She is a fellow of the American Statistical Association (ASA) and received the ASA's Founders' Award in 2012. She was a recipient of the Distinguished Achievement Award of the International Chinese Statistical Association in 2013 and the Distinguished Service Award from the National Institute of Statistical Sciences in 2020. She is also a repeat recipient of the Drug Information Association's Donald Francke Award for Excellence in Journal Publishing and the Thomas Teal Award for Excellence in Statistics Publishing. She is a founding editor of the journal *Pharmaceutical Statistics*.

Simon Kirby received a B.Sc. in Economics and Economic Policy from Loughborough University, an M.Sc. in Statistics from the University of Kent, a Ph.D. in Statistics from the University of Edinburgh and a BA in Mathematics from the Open University. He retired from Pfizer in 2018 after almost 20 years working as Principal Statistician, Clinical Statistics Head, Therapeutic Area Statistics Head and Consultant in the Statistical Research and Consulting Center. He is the owner of SKSTATS Limited for which he does occasional statistical consultancy.

Simon is Fellow and Chartered Statistician of the Royal Statistical Society. He previously worked as Lecturer, Senior Lecturer then Principal Lecturer in Statistics at Liverpool John Moores University and as Statistician at the UK's Institute of Food Research, Rothamsted Experimental Station and Revlon Healthcare.

Chapter 1
Clinical Testing of a New Drug

Nearly 60 percent of Americans—the highest ever—are taking prescription drugs.
—Washington Post, Nov 3 2015

1.1 Introduction

A research study reports an increase in the overall use of prescription drugs among adults (those ≥ 20 years old) between 2011 and 2012 from that between 1999 and 2000 in the United States (USA) (Kantor et al., 2015). In 1999–2000, an estimated 51% of US adults reported using any prescription drug. The estimated figure for 2011–2012 is 59%. During the same period, the prevalence of polypharmacy (use of ≥ 5 prescription drugs) increased from 8.2% to 15%. Many factors contribute to this increase, factors such as better disease prevention and management, lifestyle change, an aging population and an increase in the percentage of people who are either overweight or obese. The number of new prescription drugs developed and approved for public use every year has also greatly contributed to this increase.

Developing a new drug is a high-risk and high-reward enterprise. The high risk is reflected by the low success rate of turning a new molecular entity (NME) into an approved drug. The success rate has fluctuated over time and varied across therapeutic areas. For example, the US Food and Drug Administration published the Critical Path Initiative document in 2004 (FDA, 2004), in which FDA quoted a "current" success rate around 8% and a historical success rate of 14%.

Understandably, the success rate varies substantially across therapeutic areas (DiMasi et al., 2010, 2013). For example, the success rate of drugs for treating common bacterial infections is generally higher than that for drugs treating disorders of the central nervous system. This is in part due to the heavy use of the minimum inhibitory concentration (MIC) to help determine the appropriate dose and schedule for an NME for bacterial infections. For a microorganism studied in vitro, the MIC for an antibacterial agent is the lowest concentration of the agent which prevents detectable growth of the organism in agar or broth media under standardized conditions (Clinical and Laboratory Standards Institute, 2003). In addition to the MIC, animal models can be used to predict human response to an NME for many infections (Craig, 2003; Leggett et al., 1989). So, if an NME could deliver the desired MIC coverage without causing unacceptable side effects and if the animal model shows promising results, the NME will likely become a viable treatment option.

The success rate discussed above pertains to the clinical testing of an NME in humans. However, after an NME is synthesized, it will first be screened for biological and pharmacological activity. Preclinical testing in animals follows the biological and pharmacological screening. Preclinical testing is necessary before an NME can be tested in humans. Besides the need to understand the pharmacokinetic (PK) profile of the NME in animals, preclinical evaluation assesses the NME for its general toxicity, cardiac liability, carcinogenicity and reproductive toxicity. Some of the assessment could be done in vitro, but most is done in vivo using different animal species. The International Council for Harmonisation (ICH) has published a series of guidance documents on the technical requirements for preclinical safety evaluation of pharmaceuticals for human use. If preclinical testing suggests a reasonable PK and toxicity profile at doses likely to be used by target patients, then the NME will enter into the clinical testing stage.

Researchers have offered substantially different estimates for the success rates for the discovery and preclinical testing stages. For example, Bains (2004) estimated an approximately 30% cumulative success rate for discovery/preclinical testing combined while Hill (2008) stated a <1% success rate. Despite the difference, it is clear that the failure rate during the preclinical stage of drug development is not negligible.

In addition to the high risk, the cost of developing a new drug has increased at a faster pace than inflation. A study released by the Tuft's Center for the Study of Drug Development suggests that the average pre-tax industry cost to bring a new medicine to market was around $2.56 billion USD in 2013 money (DiMasi et al., 2016). The study included 106 investigational new drugs from ten mid- to large-sized pharmaceutical companies, and the drugs were first tested in humans during 1995–2007. Cost included clinical development up to 2013. By comparison, in 2003, the cost was about $1.04 billion in 2013 dollars. While some researchers have questioned the validity of these figures, the latest study used the same approach as that used in the previous one (DiMasi et al., 2003) in estimating the development cost. The latest study shows a substantial increase in the drug development cost over a 10-year period.

The low success rate and the high cost have motivated many pharmaceutical companies to look for better methods to make portfolio decisions. Such decisions include whether to invest in a particular NME and how to make Go/No-Go decisions concerning a particular development program. Since most development programs are likely to fail, it is important to be able to terminate a program that has a low probability to succeed as early as possible. Making efficient decisions requires designing efficient trials to acquire the needed evidence. Developing innovative designs that can enable good quantitative decisions at the earliest time has been the focus of much research in recent years.

Many books have been written about clinical trial designs to support drug development. Therefore, we will focus on methods for making quantitative decisions in this book. Because of the inseparable relationship between designs and decisions, we will also spend a good portion of this book on clinical trial designs.

In this chapter, we will offer a high-level review of clinical testing of a pharmaceutical product. We will first discuss in Sect. 1.2 the four distinct phases of clinical testing under a traditional development plan. We will discuss deviations from the traditional development plan and new regulatory approval pathways in Sect. 1.3. Section 1.4 offers some examples of recent advances in clinical trial designs. In Sect. 1.5, we briefly discuss real-world data and evidence before reflecting on the changing times in Sect. 1.6. We will conclude the chapter with a short summary in Sect. 1.7.

1.2   Clinical Development

Clinical testing of an NME to support its marketing authorization is often characterized by four phases as shown in Fig. 1.1. With some exceptions described in Sect. 1.3, three of the four phases occur before the NME is approved for marketing (pre-marketing) and the remaining one is afterward (postmarketing). The four phases are conveniently labeled as Phase 1, Phase 2, Phase 3 and Phase 4. A good description of the four phases can be found in an FDA guidance document (FDA, 1997) (Fig. 1.1).

1.2.1   Phase 1

Phase 1 trials are where an NME is first tested in human subjects. These trials are designed to investigate what the human body does to an NME in terms of absorption,

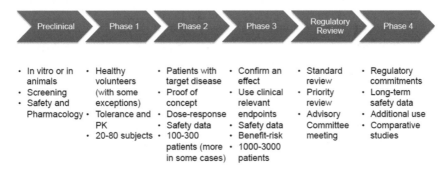

Fig. 1.1   Four phases of clinical testing

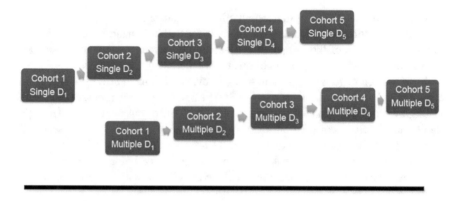

Fig. 1.2   Interwoven single- and multiple-ascending dose studies

distribution, metabolism and excretion (ADME). These are the pharmacokinetic (PK) properties of the NME. The investigation is typically conducted in healthy human volunteers, except for cytotoxic drugs. For cytotoxic drugs, Phase 1 is generally conducted in patients with very few therapeutic options due to the anticipated toxicities. When a drug is designed to target a receptor, Phase 1 trials can also include an investigation of what the NME does to the receptor.

Phase 1 trials in healthy subjects generally consist of single and multiple ascending dose cohorts. Trials studying the effect of a single dose on subjects typically precede trials studying the effect of multiple doses. Some development plans stack single-dose and multiple dose studies in such a way that there is a lag between exposing subjects to a single dose and exposing separate patients multiple times at the same dose. This strategy is shown in Fig. 1.2.

Besides collecting blood samples for PK analysis, Phase 1 trials investigate the common adverse reactions to an NME and what would be the NME's dose-limiting toxicities. We use the word "common" because the small number of subjects at this stage does not offer much opportunity to observe rare drug reactions. A typical ascending dose trial (single dose or multiple dose) randomizes subjects to a fixed dose or a control within a cohort. Observations from a cohort will be assessed to decide if another cohort should be recruited to investigate the next higher dose in a pre-specified dose range. The allowed dose range for Phase 1 testing is determined by the doses studied and adverse reactions observed in animal models.

If the NME's overall safety profile observed in Phase 1 is judged to be acceptable relative to its potential (and yet to be observed) benefit, the development will progress to the second stage (Phase 2). The number of volunteers included in Phase 1 single and multiple ascending dose studies typically ranges between 20 and 80, but could be higher if Phase 1 includes an assessment of the NME's mechanism of action or an early investigation of the NME's efficacy. The latter is a frequent feature of Phase 1 cancer trials. In these trials, a cohort of patients is often recruited at the maximum tolerated dose (MTD) to assess the NME's efficacy once the MTD is established. A good reference on designs for Phase 1 cancer trials is the book by Cheung (2011).

Other trials with a strong PK focus conducted early in the development process include bioavailability studies, drug–drug interaction studies, food effect studies and PK studies in special populations such as subjects with impaired hepatic or renal functions. Understanding an NME's PK properties in individuals with hepatic or renal function is particularly important when an NME is excreted from the body through the liver or kidneys. Understanding how the body reacts to the NME under many different, yet important, conditions is important to the planning of subsequent trials.

1.2.2 Phase 2

Phase 2 investigates what a drug does to a patient with a target disorder (i.e., the pharmacodynamics of the drug). Clinical trials at this stage are also designed to determine dose(s) whose benefit–risk profile warrants further investigation later in a confirmatory setting. Multiple doses within the dose range identified from Phase 1 are studied at this stage.

Phase 2 is typically the time when a manufacturer first learns of the beneficial effect of an NME. This stage has the highest attrition rate among the three pre-marketing phases. Therefore, if an NME is not likely to become a treatment option, it will be best to recognize this fact as soon as possible and stop further testing of the NME for the disorder already investigated. This objective plus fewer regulatory requirements at this stage offer opportunities for out-of-the-box thinking.

Testing in Phase 2 can be further divided into two stages. The first stage aims to establish the proof of concept (POC) of the NME, using a high dose (e.g., the maximum tolerated dose identified in Phase 1) to investigate the NME's efficacy. Occasionally, a sponsor may use a biomarker to verify the conjectured mechanism of the NME in a proof of mechanism (POM) study. If the study cannot establish a positive POM or POC, the development of the NME in its current formulation for the indication under investigation will stop. Because an NME is often created with the objective to treat multiple disorders, discontinuing the development for one disorder does not necessarily mean terminating the development altogether. We have seen this in the oncology area where an NME may be targeted for multiple cancer types (e.g., breast, lung and renal).

Following a positive POC, an NME will be further tested in a dose-ranging study. A dose-ranging study typically includes a control and multiple doses of the NME. A placebo is often used as the control at this stage. The new NME and the placebo could be used alone as a monotherapy or added to a patient's background therapy.

This two-step process is often referred to as Phase 2a and Phase 2b (Sheiner, 1997). To minimize the work necessary to initiate sites and obtain approvals from multiple institutional review boards, some sponsors have opted to combine the POC and the dose–response studies into one study with an unblinded interim analysis at the end of the POC stage. The sponsors will review results from the POC stage and may choose to use only data from the second stage to estimate the dose–response relationship. This strategy has the potential to increase operational efficiency by reducing the waiting period between Phase 2a and Phase 2b.

Depending on the target disorders, Phase 2 testing for a single disorder may consist of 100–300 patients. Despite strong advocacy by researchers like Sheiner (1997) to use a modeling approach to analyzing dose–response data, some sponsors continue to rely on pairwise comparisons to design and analyze dose–response studies. There have been renewed emphases from experts that the selection of dose(s) should be regarded as an estimation problem and handled by a modeling approach (EMA Dose Response Workshop, 2014). Recent research (Pinheiro et al., 2010; Thomas et al., 2014) has shown that 300 patients in a dose-ranging study may not be enough to adequately identify the optimal dose based on a preset criterion.

Ideally, Phase 2 studies should use the same endpoints to assess the benefit associated with a dose as those to be used later in Phase 3. Unfortunately, this is not always possible because the endpoint needed for Phase 3 such as survival and serious morbidity may take a longtime to obtain. In such a case, Phase 2 trials will often rely on a short-term endpoint that hopefully can predict the long-term clinical endpoint. An example is the use of progression-free survival as the endpoint in Phase 2 and overall survival in Phase 3 cancer trials.

Occasionally, a sponsor may have to conduct more than one study if the doses chosen in the initial dose–response study are not adequate to estimate the dose–response relationship. This could occur if the doses selected initially are too high (e.g., near the plateau of the dose–response curve) or not low enough. To reduce the chance of having to repeat a dose–response study, Pinheiro (2014) recommends including 4–7 doses in a wide dose range (e.g., the ratio of the maximum dose to the minimum dose ≥ 10) in the dose-finding study.

At times, different dose–response studies may need to be conducted for different diseases because a refractory disease may require a higher dose than a milder form of the same disease that has not been previously treated. Similarly, higher doses may be necessary to treat diseases considered to be harder to treat than diseases more responsive to treatment.

1.2.3 Phase 3

If the NME meets the efficacy requirement and passes the initial benefit–risk assessment, it will be further tested to confirm its efficacy. This is the final stage of clinical testing before an application is filed with regulatory agencies for marketing authorization. By this time, a commercial formulation of the NME should be available so the final testing could be conducted with the intended formulation. In the rare cases when the commercial formulation differs from the formulation used in Phase 3, a PK study will be required to show that the new formulation is bioequivalent to the previous formulation in important PK properties. For convenience, we will refer to the NME as a drug candidate (or simply a drug) from this phase on.

The US FDA generally requires two well-controlled trials to confirm a drug's effect for a target disease. This means two independent Phase 3 trials, or in some cases, a Phase 3 trial plus a well-conducted high-quality Phase 2 dose-ranging study. The primary reason for requiring two "confirmatory" trials is to ensure that a beneficial result could be replicated.

There are situations, however, when one large well-controlled Phase 3 trial is considered adequate to support marketing approval. This occurs when the first study yields highly persuasive and robust results on a clinical endpoint (e.g. mortality and serious morbidity), and it is deemed unethical by the medical community to repeat a similar study. Here, robust results mean low P-values (described in Chap. 2) for the primary (clinical) and key secondary endpoints, consistent results across multiple subgroups and few issues associated with the conduct of the studies. Interested readers should consult with the FDA guidance (FDA, 1998) on providing clinical evidence of effectiveness for human drug and biological products.

Compared with previous phases, Phase 3 enrolls a greater number of patients who are more heterogeneous in their demographic and baseline disease status. Currently, nearly all Phase 3 studies are conducted in multiple countries and in multiple geographic regions. It is at this stage that the majority of pre-marketing safety data are collected. Since a major objective of Phase 3 trials is to confirm a drug's effect, analyses focus on testing pre-specified hypotheses with adequate control for the chance of making a false positive decision. Operations at this stage require carefully protecting a trial's integrity so that trial results could be trusted. The number of patients included at this stage typically ranges between 1000 and 5000. More patients will be needed if the drug is developed for multiple disorders simultaneously. An example for multiple indications is the development of antibiotics for multiple infections.

Drugs designed to reduce the risk of a clinical endpoint may require thousands, if not tens of thousands of patients. On the other hand, drugs for orphan diseases will enroll many fewer patients. An orphan disease in the USA is defined as a condition that affects fewer than 200,000 people nationwide. Orphan diseases include well-known diseases such as cystic fibrosis and Lou Gehrig's disease (also called amyotrophic lateral sclerosis, or ALS) and less well-known rare diseases such as Duchenne muscular dystrophy (DMD). DMD affects 1 in 3600 boys.

After a drug's effect is confirmed and benefit–risk assessment supports its use in the target population, the manufacturer will file a marketing application with regulatory agencies, typically in multiple countries. Nearly, all applications are for the adult population initially. If the drug is likely to be used in the pediatric population, a manufacturer often has an ongoing pediatric development program or has a plan to initiate pediatric trials at the time of the initial marketing application. The initial marketing application may be for a single indication or for multiple indications. Once the application is approved, the drug can be made available to the public.

As explained earlier, Phase 3 is the time when the majority of safety data are collected. Safety data are crucial for sound benefit–risk assessment. The International

Council for Harmonisation describes the extent of population exposure to assess clinical safety for drugs intended for long-term treatment of non-life-threatening conditions (ICH E1). For these conditions, ICH E1 expects 1500 individuals be exposed to the drug during the clinical development program. Among the 1500 individuals, 100 patients should have been exposed to the drug for at least one year. The exposure should be at the dose levels to be marketed. So, for a new drug with a large treatment effect, the need for a reasonable safety database will likely drive the sample size decisions for confirmatory trials.

1.2.4   Phase 4

The manufacturer of a marketed drug may choose to conduct additional studies to further (1) investigate the drug in the indicated population(s) or in pediatric patients with the indicated disorder(s); (2) compare the drug head-to-head with an approved drug for the same disorder(s); (3) investigate the effect of the drug at a lower/higher dose or with different administration schedules (e.g., once a day instead of twice a day); (4) study the drug in combination with other drugs or (5) test the drug for other indications. Sometimes, a manufacturer conducts Phase 4 studies as a postmarketing commitment for regulatory approval. For example, the manufacturer may be asked to conduct additional safety studies in vulnerable populations such as elderly, pediatric, obese or pregnant patients.

Another way to characterize the four phases of drug development is by the type of studies conducted during these four phases (see ICH E8, 1997). The types of studies conducted can be described as human pharmacology studies (Phase 1), therapeutic exploratory studies (Phase 2), therapeutic confirmatory studies (Phase 3) and therapeutic use studies (Phase 4).

In addition to the aforementioned documents, the ICH has published many other documents relevant to the clinical assessment of NMEs. The ICH is always working to expand the topics on which to offer internationally harmonized guidance and to amend existing documents as science and knowledge evolve. A major recent amendment was the addition of the addendum ICH E9(R1) (2019) to ICH E9 which focuses on statistical principles for clinical trials. The addendum, on estimands and sensitivity analysis, presents a structured framework to link trial objectives to a suitable trial design and tools for estimation and hypothesis testing. The central issue is how to handle missing data in the analysis of trial data to answer the primary objectives sought by the trials.

1.3   Regulatory Review

Section 1.2 describes a traditional clinical development process. It usually takes many years for an NME to go through the first three phases. Once a marketing application is submitted, the manufacturer waits for the outcome of the regulatory review. Regulators often send queries to the manufacturer during this period for clarification or additional analyses.

In the USA, the FDA often arranges advisory committee meetings to publicly discuss submissions of NMEs or submissions that include unusual or controversial findings. Advisory committees will offer their recommendations to the agency. While these recommendations are not binding, the FDA often chooses to follow them. Before the turn of this century, the waiting period for a regulatory decision in the USA could be substantial. The review time has been significantly reduced since the beginning of the twenty-first century.

In Sects. 1.3.1 through Sect. 1.3.5, we will discuss deviations from the traditional review process that can help bring a drug with a clinically meaningful effect on serious conditions to the market faster in the USA.

In Sect. 1.3.6, we will review briefly procedures for drug approvals in the European Union.

1.3.1 Accelerated Approval

In 1992, the FDA instituted the *Accelerated Approval* regulations, allowing drugs for serious conditions that filled an unmet medical need to be approved based on a surrogate endpoint. A surrogate endpoint in this context is a measure of effect that may correlate with a real clinical endpoint but does not necessarily have a guaranteed relationship with the clinical endpoint.

Under the accelerated approval regulations, adequate and well-controlled studies that demonstrate a drug's effect on a surrogate or intermediate clinical endpoint could provide the necessary evidence for the initial marketing approval. This is the path for most cancer drug approvals in the past two decades. Even though the ultimate goal of a cancer treatment is to prolong survival, the initial approval of a cancer drug has been tumor shrinkage. The effect on tumor shrinkage is typically studied in Phase 2 trials. Some of these Phase 2 studies include only patients receiving the NME (i.e., a single arm) and rely on historical data to determine if the NME has a beneficial effect on tumor shrinkage.

With an accelerated approval, the manufacturer of a new NME for cancer still needs to conduct studies to confirm the ability of the drug to prolong survival. For this reason, accelerated approval is sometimes called *conditional* approval since there is a condition associated with the approval. A common industry practice is to start the clinical endpoint study once the effect of the NME on tumor shrinkage is confirmed. Safety data from the ongoing clinical endpoint study can be used to help augment the safety database to assist the initial regulatory review. The use of interim safety data in this fashion requires special care to protect the integrity of the clinical endpoint study.

Once a confirmatory trial verifies the clinical benefit, the FDA will generally remove the requirement. If the confirmatory trials fail to demonstrate a clinical benefit, the accelerated approval may be withdrawn. A manufacturer often has a chance to conduct multiple studies to confirm the clinical benefit before the agency takes the step to withdraw the approved indication. Even if the approval is allowed to remain for the indication, the product label will be modified to clarify that trials failed to verify clinical benefit.

1.3.2   Breakthrough Therapy

In July 2012, the US Congress signed the FDA Safety and Innovation Act. The act allows FDA to designate a drug as breakthrough therapy if (1) the drug, used alone or in combination with other drugs, is intended to treat a serious or life-threatening disease or condition; (2) preliminary clinical evidence indicates that the drug may demonstrate substantial improvement over existing therapies on at least one clinically significant endpoint. A manufacturer can submit a request to the FDA to designate a drug as breakthrough therapy. The agency has 60 days to grant or deny the request. The submission should be done prior to the meeting with the agency to review Phase 2 results.

The breakthrough therapy designation allows the manufacturer to receive intensive guidance from the agency on the drug development program. It also signals the agency's commitment to the drug program at the senior management level including an expedited review of the drug's marketing application.

Having a drug designated as a breakthrough therapy is highly desirable. In addition to a quicker agency's response to requests for feedback and a faster review timeline, a breakthrough designation increases the prestige of a drug. A requirement for a breakthrough therapy is preliminary clinical evidence of substantial improvement over existing therapies on at least one clinically meaningful endpoint. The preliminary clinical evidence could come from an early trial in a small number of subjects. Pereira et al. (2012) reported findings from an empirical investigation on how often very large treatment effects were replicated in subsequent trials of the same comparison, disease and outcome. They concluded that most large treatment effects observed in small studies became much smaller when additional trials were performed. This is a point that we will return to in later chapters of this book.

1.3.3   Priority Review

In the USA, the Prescription Drug User Act (PDUFA) came into effect in 1992. Under the Act, manufacturers of prescription drugs pay a fee when submitting an application to market the drugs. In return, the FDA agreed to improve the drug review time with specific goals. The FDA also created a two-tiered review system timeline— *standard review* and *priority review*. The act is renewable every 5 years. The 2002 amendments to PDUFA (2nd renewal) set a goal that a standard review of a new drug application be accomplished within ten months and a priority review be completed within 6 months.

A priority review designation is granted to drugs that, if approved, would contribute significantly to the treatment, diagnosis or prevention of serious conditions.

In the USA, a priority review voucher is awarded to any company that has obtained approval for a treatment for a neglected tropical disease and, in some cases, treatments with a rare pediatric disease designation (FDA, 2019a). The voucher, allowed under a provision of the Food and Drug Administration Amendments Act (H.R., 2007), is intended as an incentive to encourage companies investing in new drugs and vaccines for neglected tropical diseases or rare pediatric diseases. The voucher is transferrable.

The awarding of a priority review voucher has created an interesting phenomenon in the USA, that is, the selling of the voucher by its holder to the highest bidder in the open market. In some cases, the price paid for a voucher is hundreds of millions of US dollars. The purchaser can use the voucher toward any drug under regulatory review, hoping to get the drug to the market 6 months earlier or ahead of a rival drug that is being reviewed for the same indication contemporaneously.

1.3.4 Fast Track

Another designation that a manufacturer could seek of the FDA for their drug is *Fast Track*. A manufacturer could initiate the request at any time during the development process. The FDA will review the request and make a decision within 60 days based on whether the drug fills an unmet medical need in a serious condition.

A drug receiving the fast-track designation can expect to enjoy more frequent and timely interactions with the FDA. The manufacturer of a fast-track drug can submit sections of the new drug application for the agency review as they are being completed (rolling submission). A fast-tracked drug is eligible for accelerated approval and priority review, if other required criteria are also met (see Sect. 1.3.1 for accelerated approval and Sect. 1.3.3 for priority review). Because of more frequent communications and faster resolutions of issues, a fast-track designation often leads to earlier drug approval and access.

1.3.5 Orphan Drug

The US Congress passed the Orphan Drug Act in 1983 to provide incentives for developing treatments for orphan diseases (Kesselheim, 2010). The incentives include (1) federal funding of grants and contracts to perform clinical trials of orphan products; (2) a tax credit of 50 percent of clinical testing costs; (3) an exclusive right to market the orphan drug for 7 years from the date of marketing approval; (4) priority review by the FDA; (5) waiver of the drug application fees.

Within the class of orphan drugs, the amount of data submitted to support regulatory approval varies greatly. For example, on October 23, 2015, the FDA approved Strensiq® (asfotase alfa) as the first approved treatment for perinatal, infantile and juvenile-onset hypophosphatasia. Asfotase alfa, administered via injection three or six times a week, works by replacing the enzyme responsible for forming an essential mineral in normal bone. The latter has been shown to improve patient overall clinical outcomes.

The initial approval was based on the results from 99 patients who received asfotase alfa treatment for up to 6.5 years in four prospective, non-randomized studies. Study results showed that patients with the target condition and treated with asfotase alfa had improved overall survival compared with control patients selected from a natural history study group.

1.3.6 Drug Approval in the European Union (EU)

The first EU legislation on human medicine, triggered by the Thalidomide catastrophe and adopted in 1965, was Council Directive 65/65 on the approximation of the law relating to medicinal products. This was followed by two Council Directives in 1975. The first was on approximation of the Laws of Member States relating to analytical, pharmacotoxicological and clinical standards and protocols with respect to the testing of proprietary medicinal products. The second was on the approximation of provisions laid down by law, regulation and administrative action relating to medicinal products. The latter directive established a Committee on Proprietary Medicinal Products as an advisory committee and introduced the procedure now known as the mutual recognition procedure (Rägo & Santoso, 2008). A further directive introduced the procedure known today as the centralized procedure. In 1995, the European Medicines Agency was founded to harmonize the work of existing national medicine regulatory bodies and to protect public and animal health by assessing medicines to rigorous standards and providing partners and stakeholders with independent, science-based information on medicines (EMA: History of EMA, 2015).

There are currently two main routes for authorizing medicines in the EU (EMA: Authorization of medicines). The first is the centralized authorization procedure, whereby a manufacturer submits a single marketing authorization application to EMA. For new products, two rapporteurs are appointed from the Member States. The rapporteurs write scientific evaluation reports which are circulated to all other Committee for Medicinal products for Human Use (CHMP) members for comment. The CHMP reaches an opinion on the benefit–risk assessment by consensus or majority. If a decision is reached by a majority, then all CHMP members must accept the opinion. The second route is to make use of individual country national authorization procedures. If a manufacturer wishes to request marketing authorization in several EU Member States for a medicine that is outside the scope of the centralized procedure, it may use the mutual recognition procedure or the decentralized procedure. Currently, the great majority of new innovative medicines pass through the centralized procedure.

Similarly to the situation in the USA, there are several provisions to foster patients' early access to new medicines that address public health needs and are eligible for the centralized procedure. These include accelerated assessment which reduces the review time for medicines of major public health interest with particular regard to therapeutic innovation, conditional marketing authorization which grants authorization before complete data are available and compassionate use which allows the use of an unauthorized medicine for patients with an unmet medical need.

For additional information concerning regulatory review and approval of medicinal products in the EU, readers are encouraged to visit the EMA website (EMA: Authorisation of Medicines).

1.4 Innovative Design

In the Critical Path Initiative document mentioned earlier, the FDA identifies opportunities to help lift the perceived stagnation of drug development. The agency encourages innovations in many areas of drug discovery, development and manufacturing. In the area of clinical development, FDA encourages, among several things, more efficient clinical trial designs.

Since the 1990s, group sequential designs have been used regularly for trials involving mortality and serious morbidity, especially during Phase 3 testing. The rationale is that if there is enough evidence in an ongoing trial to demonstrate the clinical benefit of a new drug on mortality or serious morbidity, it will not be ethical to continue the trial. Similarly, if there is enough evidence to conclude that the new drug is not likely to produce a clinical benefit, there is no reason to expose patients to the drug considering the side effects inherent with all drugs.

The group sequential design is an adaptive design in that interim data are used to help decide whether some aspects of the trial should be changed (Jennison & Turnbull, 2000; Whitehead, 1997). In the late 1980s, researchers began to work on other adaptive designs beyond the traditional group sequential design.

1.4.1 Adaptive Design

Bauer et al. (2016) gave a historical overview of the history of confirmatory adaptive designs over the 25 years since 1989. The overview offers a rich literature on adaptive designs. The pace of research on adaptive designs accelerated after the publication of the FDA's Critical Path Initiative document in 2004.

Major research on adaptive features includes (1) re-estimating the sample size because of uncertainties associated with design parameters (variability, background rate, treatment effect) at the planning stage; (2) modifying the randomization ratio that dictates how patients are randomized to various treatment groups; (3) choosing among multiple treatments included in the study; (4) dropping or adding new treatments (or doses) and (5) selecting a subpopulation for future enrollment. Examples of adaptive features can be found in several recent books on adaptive designs (e.g., Chang, 2014; He et al., 2014; Menon & Zink, 2015).

Both the European Medicine Agency and the FDA have published guidance documents on adaptive designs. The EMA guidance (CHMP, 2007) focuses on adaptive designs for confirmatory trials while the FDA guidance (FDA, 2019b) covers adaptive designs for both the exploratory and confirmatory stages.

Readers who are interested in additional information on adaptive designs are encouraged to read Chap. 13.

1.4.2   Master Protocol

Another emerging trend is the use of a master protocol to screen multiple drugs simultaneously. Some refer to the resulting trial as a platform (or umbrella) trial. A platform trial could also be used to investigate a product in patients with different genotypes or phenotypes (enriched subpopulations). A more sophisticated platform trial could be conducted to study multiple treatments in multiple enriched subpopulations. Interim analyses are typically conducted in these trials to decide if a particular treatment (often with a subpopulation) could be graduated from the trial and further investigated in a confirmatory setting. Alternatively, a treatment could be dropped from the trial and a new treatment added to the trial, with the trial continuing beyond the original set of treatments. Platform trials that allow the introduction of new treatments are also called perpetual trials for this reason.

A well-known platform trial in the oncology area is the I-SPY 2 trial (Barker et al., 2009), a Phase 2 neoadjuvant trial in women with large primary cancers of the breast. Breast tumor is characterized by its response to three receptors (estrogen, progesterone and HER2), resulting in eight tumor signatures. The trial investigates multiple regimens that include investigational products from different companies. The primary endpoint is pathologic complete response at 6 months after treatment initiation. Within each tumor signature, adaptive randomization to regimens is employed. The trial may graduate or terminate a regimen according to a pre-specified rule based on an interim Bayesian prediction of Phase 3 success probability for the (regimen, signature) combination. If the regimen remains in the trial after the interim decision, assignment to that regimen will continue but be capped at a pre-specified maximum number. One major advantage of a trial like I-SPY 2 is the ability to learn during the trial on what regimen benefits which patient subpopulation and do this by borrowing information from other (regimen, signature) combinations.

While master protocols found their initial popularity in the oncology area (FDA, 2018), their usefulness is by no means restricted to oncology trials. On June 16, 2020, Oxford University announced results pertaining to the low-dose dexamethasone arm of a national trial called Randomized Evaluation of COVid-19 thERapY

(RECOVERY) conducted in the UK. RECOVERY was designed as a platform trial to test a range of potential treatments for hospitalized patients with COVID-19, an infection caused by the SARS-CoV-2 virus. It is registered as NCT04381936 in clinicaltrials.gov in the USA and EudraCT 2020-001113-21 in the EU Clinical Trials Register. Eligible and consenting patients were randomized to receive either the usual standard of care alone or the usual standard of care plus one of the multiple treatments being evaluated simultaneously with twice as many patients assigned to the standard care than any other treatment groups. Data from the trial are regularly reviewed so that any effective treatment can be identified quickly and incorporated into treatment strategies for the target patients.

One of the treatments is dexamethasone given orally or intravenously at a dose of 6 mg once daily for up to 10 days (or until hospital discharge if sooner). On June 8, recruitment to the dexamethasone arm in the study was halted since, in the view of the trial steering committee, sufficient patients had been enrolled to establish whether or not the drug had a meaningful benefit. Preliminary results were published on July 17, 2020, at NEJM.org with final results published in the New England Journal of Medicine on February 25, 2021. Following the announcement of the preliminary results, low-dose dexamethasone has been quickly incorporated into the care plan of hospitalized COVID-19 patients requiring oxygen therapy. Considering that RECOVERY was kicked off in March of 2020 with four initial treatment groups and multiple treatments were added shortly after the inception, the speed of arriving at the dexamethasone therapy was quite impressive.

Because of the increasing collaboration between public and private sectors as well as collaborations among private sector companies in screening and developing drugs, we can expect an increase in the use of platform trials in the near future.

1.4.3   Complex Innovative Trial Designs

In August 2018, the US FDA announced the plan to conduct a Complex Innovative Trial Design (CID) Pilot Meeting Program to facilitate the use of CID approaches in late-stage drug development during fiscal years 2019 to 2022. As part of the pilot program, the FDA will be allowed to publicly discuss the trial designs considered through the pilot program even though the NMEs have not yet been approved by the agency.

Sponsors who are interested in participating in the program were instructed to submit their cases to the agency. The FDA will accept two primary meeting requests and two alternates per quarter. For each meeting request granted as part of the pilot, the FDA will conduct an initial meeting and a follow-up meeting on the same CID and medical product within a span of approximately 120 days.

By design, the pilot meeting program offers sponsors whose meetings requests are granted the opportunity for increased interaction with FDA staff to discuss their proposed CID approach. Rules that govern the interactions are laid out in a draft FDA guidance for industry (FDA, 2020a).

In addition to the CID guidance, the US FDA finalized its guidance on adaptive designs in December 2019 (FDA, 2019b). The finalized guidance acknowledges the role that adaptive designs could play in drug development and signals a general openness to these designs for confirmatory trials by the agency.

1.5   Real-World Data and Evidence

In a draft guidance on submitting documents using real-world data (RWD) and real-world evidence (RWE) published in May 2019 (FDA, 2019c), the FDA described RWD as data from electronic health records, medical claims and billings, product and disease registries, patient-generated information from in-home use or other decentralized settings and other sources such as mobile devices. Using RWD to help detect new safety signals has long been a part of good pharmacovigilance practice in the industry (FDA, 2005). It is also common for manufacturers to use RWD in observational studies to satisfy parts of the postapproval safety commitments placed on their products.

The increasing availability of RWD and advances in analytic techniques has created interest, both in the public and the private sectors, to use RWD and RWE to enhance clinical research and support regulatory decision making. There is a trend to use RWD/RWE beyond safety assessment and to assist efficacy or effectiveness evaluations. Indeed, the FDA has acknowledged relevant submissions of RWD/RWE to support IND filing for randomized clinical trials, single-arm trials that use external controls, observational studies intended to help support an efficacy supplement and studies using RWE to fulfill a postmarketing requirement to further evaluate safety or effectiveness.

Despite the rising interest, there have been concerns voiced about the quality of findings from RWD. Schuemie et al. (2020) present findings from their work evaluating five commonly used statistical and epidemiological methods as applied to four large health care databases. Their results show that for most of the methods investigated by them, the operating characteristics deviate considerably from the nominal levels. The findings emphasize the need to proceed cautiously as we elevate the role of RWD/RWE beyond a secondary and supportive one.

While we focus heavily on how data from prior randomized clinical trials could help us plan future trials and make evidence-based decisions in this book, we also recognize that some of the prior data could come from RWD if such data become more complete, and we have a good handle on how to manage issues that are often associated with these data (e.g., bias resulting from treatment selection).

We include an example in Chap. 5 of using data from a natural history cohort study to judge the effect of an NME in a single-arm study for a rare disease.

1.6 Changing Times

Traditionally, pre-licensure clinical testing of a new vaccine follows the same three-phase process described in Sects. 1.2.1 to 1.2.3. Many new vaccines undergo formal large-scale Phase 4 studies to collect additional safety data. This is necessary because vaccines are typically given to a generally healthy population. It is imperative that a new vaccine has minimal side effects to support its general usage. Some manufacturers conduct additional Phase 4 studies to experiment with different number of vaccine doses or different administration schedules. It often takes between 10 and 15 years from discovering to commercializing a new vaccine.

It is understandable that the traditional development process would accelerate during disease outbreaks and pandemics. On March 23, 2014, the World Health Organization (WHO) reported cases of Ebola Virus Disease (EVD) in the forested rural region of southeastern Guinea. The identification of these early cases marked the beginning of the West Africa Ebola epidemic, the largest in history (https://www.cdc.gov/vhf/ebola/history/2014-2016-outbreak/index.html). According to Chan (2020), the outbreak prompted a huge international private–public partnership involving numerous organizations to develop a vaccine for Ebola. The Phase 1 study of Ervebo® was initiated in October 2014, and the Phase 3 dose was selected in January 2015 based on immune responses. Ervebo® was approved in December 2019. The case of Ervebo® has often been cited as a shining example of what great public–private partnership and human will could accomplish in the time of crises.

But, the development of COVID-19 vaccines shattered all previous records. The SARS-CoV-2 genome sequence was identified in January 2020. The first COVID-19 vaccine trial using the messenger RNA (mRNA) technique was initiated in March 2020. Two large-scale Phase 3 trials using this new vaccine technique were launched in July 2020 for two different vaccines. On November 9, 2020, cosponsors of one of the mRNA vaccines (Pfizer and BioNTech) announced that an interim analysis found that their vaccine was more than 90% effective in preventing the disease among trial volunteers who had no evidence of prior coronavirus infection. The announcement was followed shortly by another announcement on November 18, 2020, that the study had reached its target number of cases. (The study was designed to collect a maximum number of 164 infection cases.) Based on 170 cases of infection, the vaccine was found to be 95% effective (New York Times Health Section, November 18, 2020). No serious side effects were reported by the sponsor. On December 2, the UK authorized the Pfizer-BioNTech vaccine for emergency use and began vaccinating its population on December 8. The FDA in the USA granted its own emergency use authorization (FDA 2020b) on December 11, and the country began its vaccination program on December 14. The European Union approved the vaccine on December 21.

The other mRNA vaccine sponsor (Moderna-NIH) announced similarly promising interim results on November 16, 2020. Moderna received US emergency use authorization for its vaccine on December 18. Vaccination with the Moderna-NIH vaccine began on December 22 in the USA.

The two-dose vaccine by AstraZeneca and the University of Oxford received its first approval in the UK on December 30, 2020, and was subsequently approved by the European Union on January 29, 2021. The single-dose vaccine by Johnson and Johnson received FDA emergency use authorization on February 27, 2021. At the time of writing (March 2021), we expect to learn results from other COVID-19 vaccines in the near future. The availability of multiple highly effective vaccines has greatly enhanced our ability to fight the global pandemic.

The speed with which vaccines for COVID-19 were identified and tested is truly unprecedented. Before the pandemic, it was unimaginable to think that a new vaccine could be authorized within a year of its discovery, even if for emergency use initially. As Fu et al. (2020) pointed out, the unprecedented speed was the result of shortened discovery and preclinical timeline, streamlined clinical development, accelerated regulatory pathway and at-risk manufacturing scale-up. Compared to the traditional development pathway, every action taken to accelerate the availability of COVID-19 vaccines faced increased risks, risks that may be judged too high by manufacturers for other occasions. Nevertheless, the stories of COVID-19 vaccines have set a new precedent for what might be possible in the face of devastating global pandemics.

Besides the development of COVID-19 vaccines, the pandemic has greatly affected the investigations of many NMEs during the course of the pandemic. For much of 2020, in-person clinic visits were impeded by social distancing and lock-down requirements. Some participants may have decided to drop out from a trial altogether for fear of contracting the infection. This fear was more pronounced among seniors and trial participants who have pre-existing conditions, putting them at a higher risk for more severe consequences from the infection. Some studies were postponed, and some were placed on hold. Missing data due to missed visits and/or disrupted drug supply have created challenges for the analysis and interpretation of the data collected during the pandemic. While some general recommendations on how to handle statistical issues for clinical trials conducted during the COVID-19 pandemic have been published (e.g., see Meyer et al., 2020), the actual impact of the pandemic on trials and on the integrity of the data collected during the pandemic will need to be evaluated on a case-by-case basis in the future.

1.7   Summary

In the USA, product development has changed substantially since 1962 when the US Congress passed the Kefauver Harris (KH) Amendment to the Federal Food, Drug and Cosmetic Act of 1938 (Krantz, 1966). The amendment required drug manufacturers to prove the effectiveness and safety of their drugs in adequate and well-controlled investigations before receiving marketing approvals. This amendment set in motion the activities that led to the relatively mature state of clinical testing for new drugs today.

Still, clinical development strategies continue to change. The pursuit of personalized medicine and targeted therapies means that manufacturers will look for more nimble and adaptive pathways. Orphan diseases and rare diseases have begun to attract the attention of mid- to large-sized pharmaceutical companies. Because of the cost and risk associated with developing new drugs, we can expect to see more codevelopment between companies.

Increasingly, advocacy groups are putting pressure on pharmaceutical companies and regulators to move faster in making new drugs available, especially new drugs for previously untreatable diseases. The strong advocacy by HIV patients in the 1990s led to the rapid development and approval of many HIV drugs. More recently, parents of children with rare genetic diseases have become strong advocates for their children. They join together to form grassroots organizations to push for research on the genetic diseases inflicting their children. Some of their organizations even provide funding to support basic research. Their active participation is a new force that will undoubtedly influence the direction and outcome of drug development.

A nimble clinical development requires an infrastructure to make nimble decisions. The decisions at different stages of development need to be coordinated so that latter decisions are built upon the earlier ones for best results. This means a unified decision-making framework that is based on a core set of principles but also capable of addressing the unique needs of different stages. It is this unified decision-making framework that will be the focus of this book.

References

Bains, W. (2004). Failure rates in drug discovery and development: Will we ever get any better? *Drug Discovery World, 5*(4), 9–18.

Barker, A. D., Sigman, C. C., Kelloff, G. J., et al. (2009). I-SPY 2: An adaptive breast cancer trial design in the setting of neoadjuvant chemotherapy. *Clinical Pharmacology & Therapeutics, 86*(1), 97–100.

Bauer, P., Bretz, F., Dragalin, V., et al. (2016). 25 years of confirmatory adaptive designs: Opportunities and pitfalls. *Statistics in Medicine, 35*(3), 325–347.

Chan, I. (2020). *Opportunities and challenges in vaccine development*. Presented at a NISS-Merck workshop on vaccine development. Available at https://www.niss.org/news/nissmerck-meetup-reviews-challenges-and-potential-vaccine-development. Accessed 2 February 2021.

Chang, M. (2014). *Adaptive Design Theory and Implementation Using SAS and R* (2nd ed.). Chapman and Hall.

Cheung, Y. K. (2011). *Dose Finding by the Continual Reassessment Method*. Chapman & Hall/CRC Press.

CHMP Reflection Paper. (2007). *Methodological issues in confirmatory clinical trials planned with an adaptive design* (CHMP/EWP/2459/02).

Clinical and Laboratory Standards Institute. *Methods for dilution antimicrobial susceptibility tests for bacteria that grow aerobically*. (2003). Approved Standard Document M07 (6th ed.). CLSI, Wayne PA.

Craig, W. A. (2003). Basic pharmacodynamics of antibacterials with clinical applications to the use of β-lactams, glycopeptides, and linezolid. *Infectious Disease Clinics of North America, 17*, 479–501.

DiMasi, J. A., Hansen, R. W., & Grabowski, H. G. (2003). The price of innovation: New estimates of drug development costs. *Journal of Health Economics, 22*, 151–185.

DiMasi, J. A., Feldman, L., Seckler, A., & Wilson, A. (2010). Trends in risks associated with new drug development: Success rates for investigational drugs. *Clinical Pharmacology & Therapeutics, 87*(3), 272–277.

DiMasi, J. A., Reichert, J. M., Feldman, L., & Malins, A. (2013). Clinical approval success rates for investigational cancer drugs. *Clinical Pharmacology & Therapeutics, 94*(3), 329–335.

DiMasi, J. A., Grabowski, H. G., & Hansen, R. W. (2016). Innovation in the pharmaceutical industry: New estimates of R&D costs. *Journal of Health Economics, 47*, 20–33.

EMA: History of EMA. Available at http://www.ema.europa.eu/ema/index.jsp?curl=pages/about_us/general/general_content_000628.jsp. Accessed 2 February 2021.

EMA: Authorisation of Medicines. Available at http://www.ema.europa.eu/ema/index.jsp?curl=pages/about_us/general/general_content_000109.jsp. Accessed 2 February 2021.

EMA. (2014). European Medicines Agency/European Federation of Pharmaceutical Industries and Associations workshop on the importance of dose finding and dose selection for the successful development, licensing and lifecycle management of medicinal products. http://www.ema.europa.eu/ema/index.jsp?curl=pages/news_and_events/events/2014/06/event_detail_000993.jsp&mid=WC0b01ac058004d5c3. Accessed 2 February 2021.

FDA Guidance for Industry. (1997). *General considerations for the clinical evaluation of drugs.*

FDA Guidance for Industry. (1998). *Providing clinical evidence of effectiveness for human drug and biological products.*

FDA Innovation or Stagnation: Challenge and Opportunity on the Critical Path to New Medical Products. (2004). Available at http://wayback.archive-it.org/7993/20180125032208/https://www.fda.gov/ScienceResearch/SpecialTopics/CriticalPathInitiative/CriticalPathOpportunitiesReports/ucm077262.htm. Accessed 2 February 2021.

FDA Guidance for Industry. (2005). *Good pharmacovigilance practices and pharmacoepidemiologic assessment.*

FDA Draft Guidance to Industry. (2018). *Master protocols: Efficient clinical trial design strategies to expedite development of oncology drugs and biologics.*

FDA Draft Guidance for Industry. (2019a). *Rare pediatric disease priority review vouchers.*

FDA Guidance for Industry. (2019b). *Adaptive design clinical trials for drugs and biologics.*

FDA Draft Guidance to Industry. (2019c). *Submitting documents using real-world data and real-world evidence to FDA for drugs and biologics.*

FDA Draft Guidance for Industry. (2020a). *Interacting with the FDA on complex innovative trial designs for drugs and biological products.*

FDA Guidance for Industry. (2020b). *Emergency use authorization for vaccines to prevent COVID-19.*

Fu, B., Meng, Y., & Chen, J. (2020). *Some considerations on developing COVID-19 vaccines.* Presented at a NISS-Merck workshop on vaccine development. Available at https://www.niss.org/news/nissmerck-meetup-reviews-challenges-and-potential-vaccine-development. Accessed 18 November 2020.

He, W., Pinheiro, J., & Kuznetsova, O. M. (Eds.). (2014). *Practical considerations for adaptive trial design and implementation.* Springer.

H.R.3580 - Food and Drug Administration Amendments Act of 2007. Available at https://www.congress.gov/bill/110th-congress/house-bill/3580. Accessed 3 Feb 2021, page 150.

Hill, W. (2008). *Optimizing preclinical proof of concept, presentation as part of the MaRS Best Practices Series.* Available at http://www.slideshare.net/webgoddesscathy/optimizing-preclinical-proof-of-concept. Accessed 3 Feb 2021.

ICH E1. (1994). *The extent of population exposure to assess clinically safety for drugs intended for long-term treatment of non-life-threatening conditions.*

ICH E8. (1997). *General considerations for clinical trials.*

ICH E9(R1). (2019). *Estimands and sensitivity analysis in clinical trials.*

ICH guidances for preclinical safety evaluation of pharmaceuticals for human use.

Jennison, C., & Turnbull, B. W. (2000). *Group sequential methods with applications to clinical trials.* Chapman & Hall/CRC Press.

Kantor, E. D., Rehm, C. D., Haas, J. S., et al. (2015). Trends in prescription drug use among adults in the United States from 1999–2012. *Journal of the American Medical Association, 314*(17), 1818–1831.

Kesselheim, A. S. (2010). Innovation and the Orphan Drug Act, 1983–2009: Regulatory and clinical characteristics of approved orphan drugs. In M. J. Field, T. F. Boat (Eds.), *Rare diseases and orphan products: Accelerating research and development*. National Academies Press. Available at http://www.ncbi.nlm.nih.gov/books/NBK56187/. Accessed 3 Feb 2021.

Krantz, J. C., Jr. (1966). New drugs and the Kefauver-Harris Amendment. *Journal of New Drugs, 6*(2), 77–79.

Leggett, J. E., Fantin, B., Ebert, S., et al. (1989). Comparative antibiotic dose-effect relations at several dosing intervals in murine pneumonitis and thigh-infection models. *Journal of Infectious Diseases, 159*, 281–292.

Menon, S., & Zink, R. (2015). *Modern approaches to clinical trials using SAS®: Classical, adaptive, and Bayesian methods*. SAS Institute.

Meyer, R. D., Ratitch, B., Wolbers, M., et al. (2020). Statistical issues and recommendations for clinical trials conducted during the COVID-19 pandemic. *Statistics in Biopharmaceutical Research, 12*(4), 399–411.

New England Journal of Medicine. (2021). Dexamethasone in hospitalized patients with Covid-19. *New England Journal of Medicine, 384*(8), 693–704.

Pereira, T. V., Horwitz, R. I., & Ioannidis, J. P. A. (2012). Empirical evaluation of very large treatment effects of medical intervention. *Journal of the American Medical Association, 308*(16), 1676–1684.

Pinheiro, J., Sax, F., Antonijevic, Z., et al. (2010). Adaptive and model-based dose-ranging trials: Quantitative evaluation and recommendations. *Statistics in Biopharmaceutical Research, 2*(4), 435–454.

Pinheiro, J. (2014). *Session 2 summary—Designs & Methods. Presentation at the European Medicines Agency/European Federation of Pharmaceutical Industries and Associations workshop on the importance of dose finding and dose selection for the successful development, licensing and lifecycle management of medicinal products*. Available at http://www.ema.europa.eu/docs/en_GB/document_library/Presentation/2015/01/WC500179787.pdf. Accessed 3 Feb 2021.

Rägo, L., & Santoso, B. (2008). Drug regulation: History, present and future. In C. J. Van Boxtel, B. Santoso, I. R. Edwards (Eds.), Chapter 6 in *Drug benefits and risks: International textbook of clinical pharmacology*, (revised 2nd edn.). IOS Press and Uppsala Monitoring Centre.

Schuemie, M. J., Cepeda, M. S., Suchard, M. A., et al. (2020). How confident are we about observational findings in health care: A benchmark study. *Harvard Data Science Review, 2*.1. https://doi.org/10.1162/99608f92.147cc28e

Sheiner, L. B. (1997). Learning versus confirming in clinical drug development. *Clinical Pharmacology & Therapeutics, 61*(3), 275–291.

Thomas, N., Sweeney, K., & Somayaji, V. (2014). Meta-analysis of clinical dose–response in a large drug development portfolio. *Statistics in Biopharmaceutical Research, 6*(4), 302–317.

Whitehead, J. (1997). *The design and analysis of sequential clinical trials*. Wiley.

Chapter 2
A Frequentist Decision-Making Framework

Those who ignore Statistics are condemned to reinvent it.
—Bradley Efron

2.1 Introduction

The Frequentist approach to statistical inference involves probability via its long-run frequency interpretation. Procedures for assessing evidence and making decisions are calibrated by how they would perform were they used repeatedly. In this chapter, we consider the Frequentist approach to the testing of hypotheses and in particular to the two-action decision problem and also to the construction of confidence intervals. In the context of drug development, the two actions correspond to progressing or not progressing a drug for further development.

2.2 Statistical Hypotheses

A statistical hypothesis can be defined as "an assertion or conjecture about the distribution of one or more random variables" (Miller & Miller, 2014). Here, a random variable is a variable representing the outcome of an experiment. The possible outcomes and their probabilities are represented by a probability distribution. Statistical hypotheses can be simple, if the statistical hypothesis completely specifies the distribution, or composite if they do not.

An example of a simple hypothesis involving a drug could be if we conjecture that the number of individuals recovering from a certain illness among a population of patients treated with the drug follows a binomial distribution with a recovery proportion and that the recovery proportion is equal to 0.6.

© The Author(s), under exclusive license to Springer Nature Switzerland AG 2021
C. Chuang-Stein and S. Kirby, *Quantitative Decisions in Drug Development*, Springer Series in Pharmaceutical Statistics,
https://doi.org/10.1007/978-3-030-79731-7_2

An example of a composite hypothesis is if we conjecture that a patient's diastolic blood pressure changes when treated with a drug or a placebo can be modeled by a Normal distribution with a known and common variance and that the drug induces a greater decrease in diastolic blood pressure than the placebo.

2.3 Testing a Statistical Hypothesis

To test a statistical hypothesis, it is necessary to have another hypothesis in case the initial hypothesis is rejected. Such a hypothesis is referred to as the alternative hypothesis and is frequently denoted by H_A. The hypothesis being tested is referred to as the null hypothesis and is usually denoted by H_0. The objective is to gather enough evidence to decide whether H_0 should be rejected in favor of H_A or not to reject H_0. The latter occurs when the observed results are consistent with what could have been expected under H_0. In drug development, H_0 and H_A are usually chosen in such a way that there is a strong desire to reject H_0 and thus conclude H_A. In this sense, the hypothesis-testing paradigm is like the criminal justice system where every defendant is assumed innocent until proven guilty. The prosecutor bears the burden to collect enough evidence in order to prove beyond a reasonable doubt about the defendant's guilt.

To test a statistical hypothesis, sample data are generated from an experiment and a test statistic is calculated from the data. The test statistic is used to decide whether to accept or reject the null hypothesis. Possible values of the test statistic are divided into two sets: an acceptance region and a rejection region for H_0. The rejection region is also known as the critical region. Usually, the rejection region includes large or extreme values of the test statistic.

The above procedure can lead to two possible types of error. Rejecting the null hypothesis when it is true is called a Type I error, and the probability of this error is usually denoted by α. Accepting the null hypothesis when it is false is called a Type II error, and the probability of this is usually denoted by β. The possible outcomes of a hypothesis test, expressed in terms of correct or incorrect decisions, are illustrated in Table 2.1.

We first illustrate hypothesis testing by considering a simple null hypothesis and a simple alternative hypothesis. Consider the example about the number of individuals recovering from a particular illness after treatment with a drug. Assume that the number can be modeled by a binomial distribution with the parameter θ. Here θ represents the proportion of the population that will recover with the drug treatment. A null hypothesis can be that θ is equal to 0.6. Symbolically, we can write

Table 2.1 Possible outcomes of a hypothesis test

Decision	H_0 True	H_0 False
Accept H_0	Correct	Type II error
Reject H_0	Type I error	Correct

$$H_0: \theta = 0.6$$

We can take as our simple alternative hypothesis that the recovery proportion is equal to 0.9 and write it as

$$H_A: \theta = 0.9$$

Accepting the null hypothesis means accepting the assertion of a 60% recovery rate. Rejecting the null hypothesis means accepting the assertion of a 90% recovery rate. A Type I error corresponds to rejecting a recovery rate of 60% when this rate is true. A Type II error corresponds to accepting the 60% recovery rate when the true recovery rate is actually 90%.

Suppose that we decide to take a simple random sample of 14 subjects from the population with the illness of interest and treat them with the drug. Furthermore, suppose that we choose a testing procedure that will reject H_0 if 12 or more of the 14 subjects recover from the illness, otherwise we will accept H_0. Using binomial distributions, we can calculate the Type I error and Type II error rates associated with this testing procedure. These error probabilities are 0.04 and 0.16, respectively.

To illustrate a composite null and alternative hypothesis, we reconsider the blood pressure example. We assume that the change in diastolic blood pressure (post-treatment—baseline) for drug and placebo can both be modeled by Normal distributions, and we also assume that there is a common known variance for the two Normal distributions. A greater change (reduction) results in a more negative value for the change from baseline endpoint.

Let μ_{drug} denote the mean change in blood pressure among patients receiving the drug and $\mu_{placebo}$ the mean change in blood pressure among patients receiving the placebo. We take as our null hypothesis that the difference $\mu_{drug} - \mu_{placebo}$ is greater than or equal to zero, i.e., the drug is not more effective than the placebo in reducing the blood pressure. Symbolically, we write

$$H_0: \mu_{drug} - \mu_{placebo} \geq 0$$

For our alternative hypothesis, we speculate that the difference $\mu_{drug} - \mu_{placebo}$ is less than 0. Symbolically, we write

$$H_A: \mu_{drug} - \mu_{placebo} < 0$$

Accepting H_0 means accepting the hypothesis that the drug is not more effective in reducing the diastolic blood pressure than the placebo. Rejecting H_0 means accepting the hypothesis that the drug is more effective than the placebo in reducing the blood pressure.

To illustrate a possible testing procedure for this example, we assume that the standard deviation of the change from baseline in diastolic blood pressure over the period of interest is known to be 5 mmHg. Suppose that $2 \times n$ subjects are randomly assigned to drug or placebo so that each treatment group has n subjects. A possible test statistic is given by

$$\frac{\bar{X}_{drug} - \bar{X}_{placebo}}{\sqrt{\frac{2\sigma^2}{n}}} \tag{2.1}$$

In (2.1), $\bar{X}_{drug}$ is the sample mean change in diastolic blood pressure among patients on drug, $\bar{X}_{placebo}$ is the sample mean change in diastolic blood pressure among patients on placebo, and σ is the known standard deviation of change in diastolic blood pressure (assumed to be 5 mmHg). The test statistic is negative when the mean reduction on drug is greater than that on placebo. It becomes more negative as the reduction in diastolic blood pressure on drug becomes greater compared to placebo.

We can design a study to randomize 26 subjects in equal proportions to receive either the drug or the placebo. With $n = 13$, we can define a rejection region to consist of any value of the test statistic less than -1.645. The maximum probability of a Type I error under H_0 is 0.05, occurring when $\mu_{drug} - \mu_{placebo} = 0$. The Type II error rate depends on the value of the true difference under H_A. It can be shown that the probability of a Type II error is approximately 0.18 when $\mu_{drug} - \mu_{placebo} = -5$ mmHg.

There are many ways to construct tests. A popular test is the likelihood ratio test (Lindgren, 1993) which constructs the ratio of the maximum likelihood (the maximum probability of the observed data for a model) for values of the parameter(s) under H_0 to the maximum likelihood for any possible values of the parameter(s). Assuming that H_0 assigns values to k of r parameters, -2 times the log of the likelihood ratio constructed above has a large sample chi-square distribution with k degrees of freedom under the null hypothesis and some general regularity conditions about the distributions.

2.4   Decision Making

In drug development, accepting or rejecting a null hypothesis often leads to different actions. In the example of a simple null and alternative hypothesis involving the recovery rate from an illness, accepting the null hypothesis could mean stopping further development of a drug. Rejecting the null hypothesis could mean continuing the drug's development. A Type I error then corresponds to the decision to continue the development when the recovery rate with the drug treatment is only 60%. A Type II error corresponds to the decision to stop the development when the recovery rate is 90%.

The properties of a hypothesis test are affected by three main factors. They are sample size, Type I and II error rates. For a composite null hypothesis, we typically control the largest possible Type I error rate under the null hypothesis. For a simple alternative hypothesis, there is a single Type II error rate for a testing procedure. For a composite alternative hypothesis, as noted in the blood pressure example, the Type II error rate will vary according to the value(s) of parameter(s) permissible under the alternative hypothesis.

It is a common practice to control the Type I error rate and to evaluate the Type II error rate for different values of the sample size.

2.5 Losses and Risks

When decisions are made, it is possible to think of losses associated with each decision. Here, a loss can be positive or negative (a reward or a penalty). For the simple null and alternative hypothesis example on the recovery rate, we can denote the truth (true rate of recovery) by θ_1 for $\theta = 0.6$ or θ_2 for $\theta = 0.9$. We can also denote the decision to stop development of the drug by d_1 (decision 1) and the decision to continue by d_2 (decision 2). We can then summarize possible combinations of truth and decision as in Table 2.2 with each having an associated loss represented by $L(d_i, \theta_j)$ for $i, j = 1, 2$.

We can go one step further and define the risk associated with the decision procedure for each true state of nature. For a given true state of nature, the risk is the expected loss from the decision procedure. Under this definition, the risk for each true state of nature is given in Table 2.3.

The risk when the true recovery rate is equal to θ_1 ($\theta = 0.6$) is given by the loss when decision 1 is made (a correct decision to stop development) multiplied by the probability of this correct decision (i.e., $1 - \alpha$) plus the loss when decision 2 is made (an incorrect decision to continue development) multiplied by the probability of this incorrect decision (i.e., α).

Similarly, the risk when the true recovery rate is equal to θ_2 ($\theta = 0.9$) is given by the loss when decision 1 is made (an incorrect decision to stop) multiplied by the probability of this decision (i.e., β) plus the loss when decision 2 is made (a correct decision to continue) multiplied by the probability of this decision (i.e., $1 - \beta$).

Table 2.2 Losses for combinations of decision and true state of nature

Decision	True state of nature	
	θ_1 ($\theta = 0.6$)	θ_2 ($\theta = 0.9$)
d_1 (stop development)	$L(d_1, \theta_1)$	$L(d_1, \theta_2)$
d_2 (continue development)	$L(d_2, \theta_1)$	$L(d_2, \theta_2)$

Table 2.3 Risk for each true state of nature

True state of nature	
θ_1	θ_2
$L(d_1, \theta_1) \times (1 - \alpha) + L(d_2, \theta_1) \times \alpha$	$L(d_1, \theta_2) \times \beta + L(d_2, \theta_2) \times (1 - \beta)$

It should be noted that these risks are conditional on the true state of nature. To go further and obtain an overall risk, we would need to assign probabilities to the true state of nature as done in the Bayesian approach to inference.

While in principle a loss can be assigned to each state of nature and decision, this can be challenging in practice. This is because of the many factors involved and the uncertainties about these factors. Similarly, in the context of drug development, the reward or penalty associated with each state of nature and decision to stop or continue may be difficult to determine. By comparison, the probabilities of correct and incorrect decisions conditional on the true state of nature are easier to calculate.

2.6   The Power Function of a Test

In most situations, a drug developer is interested in a composite null hypothesis and a composite alternative hypothesis. It is, therefore, useful to define a power function that gives the probability of rejecting H_0 for various values of the parameter of interest.

Consider the blood pressure example which has a null hypothesis of

$$H_0: \mu_{drug} - \mu_{placebo} \geq 0$$

and an alternative hypothesis of

$$H_A \; \mu_{drug} - \mu_{placebo} < 0$$

Figure 2.1 shows the power function for 13 patients per group, and the decision rule of rejecting H_0 when the test statistic in (2.1) takes a value less than -1.645.

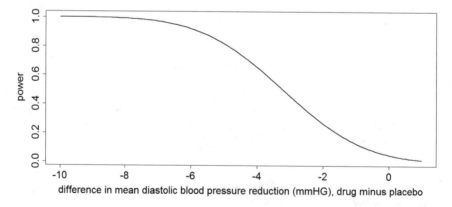

Fig. 2.1 Power function for the example described in text

It can be seen from Fig. 2.1 that the maximum Type I error rate under the null hypothesis occurs when $\mu_{drug} - \mu_{placebo} = 0$ and the power under the alternative hypothesis increases rapidly as the difference in mean change (drug–placebo) becomes more negative. As described earlier, the power when the difference in mean diastolic blood pressure decrease is equal to -5 mmHg is approximately 0.82 ($=1 - 0.18$). In general, it is desirable to conduct experiments that have high power for values of interest under the alternative hypothesis.

2.7 Determining a Sample Size for an Experiment

The power curve displayed in Fig. 2.1 is for a particular sample size, i.e., 13, for each group. Different sample sizes will give different power curves as illustrated in Fig. 2.2. As shown in Fig. 2.2, as sample size increases, the probability to reject H_0 for any $\mu_{drug} - \mu_{placebo} < 0$ increases.

The sample size used for the power curve in Fig. 2.1 was chosen by requiring a maximum Type I error rate of 5% and a Type II error rate of approximately 18% when $\mu_{drug} - \mu_{placebo} = -5$ mmHg. Such a sample size could be found by trial and error, but in many cases it is possible to write a closed-form expression for the sample size. Using the blood pressure example, we will illustrate an analytical approach that could be used to determine sample size on many occasions.

In the blood pressure example, we assume that we are interested in an experiment that will have 80% power to reject the null hypothesis when $\mu_{drug} - \mu_{placebo} = -5$. We want the Type I error rate for our decision rule to be controlled at the 5% level. The experiment will randomize the same number of patients to receive the drug and the placebo. We need to decide the sample size required for each group.

Let n denote the number of patients in each treatment group. When $\mu_{drug} - \mu_{placebo} = 0$, the difference in sample mean changes from baseline $\bar{X}_{drug} - \bar{X}_{placebo}$

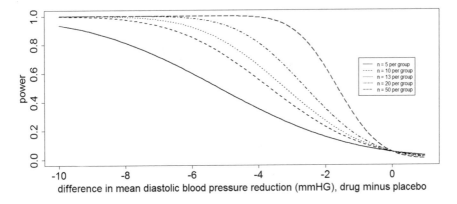

Fig. 2.2 Power curves for different sample sizes

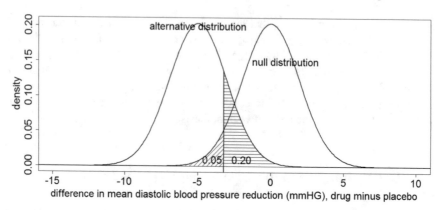

Fig. 2.3 Overlap of distributions under null and alternative hypotheses which gives desired Type I and Type II errors rates

has a Normal distribution with mean 0 and a variance equal to $\frac{2\sigma^2}{n}$. We will denote this Normal distribution by $N\left(0; \frac{2\sigma^2}{n}\right)$. This distribution is portrayed by the curve on the right in Fig. 2.3.

Under the alternative hypothesis that the true difference is equal to -5, the distribution for the difference in sample mean changes is $N\left(-5; \frac{2\sigma^2}{n}\right)$. This distribution has the same shape as $N\left(0; \frac{2\sigma^2}{n}\right)$, but is situated 5 mmHg to the left of the curve for $N\left(0; \frac{2\sigma^2}{n}\right)$. This distribution is represented by the curve on the left in Fig. 2.3.

For the Type I error rate to be 0.05, we can use the critical value of -1.645 for the test statistic. This critical value is the fifth percentile of a standard Normal distribution $N(0;1)$, because the test statistic in (2.1) has a $N(0; 1)$ distribution when $\mu_{\text{drug}} - \mu_{\text{placebo}} = 0$. This translates to the requirement in (2.2) for $\bar{X}_{\text{drug}} - \bar{X}_{\text{placebo}}$ to reject the null hypothesis. We note this requirement by the vertical line in Fig. 2.3. The area under the curve of $N\left(0; \frac{2\sigma^2}{n}\right)$ to the left of the vertical line is 0.05.

$$\bar{X}_{\text{drug}} - \bar{X}_{\text{placebo}} < -1.645 \times \sqrt{\frac{2\sigma^2}{n}} \qquad (2.2)$$

To obtain the sample size needed to give a power of 80% when $\mu_{\text{drug}} - \mu_{\text{placebo}} = -0.5$, the Normal curves should be shaped in such a way that the area to the left of the vertical line under the curve on the left (i.e., curve for $N\left(-5; \frac{2\sigma^2}{n}\right)$) is 0.80. This means that the vertical line should have an X-coordinate of $-5 + Z_{0.20} \times \sqrt{\frac{2\sigma^2}{n}}$. Here, $Z_{0.20} = 0.842$ is the upper 20th percentile of the standard Normal distribution. This new requirement plus that in (2.2) leads to the equation in (2.3).

$$-1.645 \times \sqrt{\frac{2\sigma^2}{n}} = -5 + 0.842 \times \sqrt{\frac{2\sigma^2}{n}} \tag{2.3}$$

Substituting 5 for σ in (2.3), we can solve for n, which is found to be 13 (rounding up to the nearest integer). The equation in (2.3) leads to the familiar sample size formula for a continuous endpoint for n (per group) in (2.4) with $\alpha = 0.05$, $\beta = 0.20$, $\Delta = -5$ and $\sigma = 5$ for the blood pressure example.

$$n = \frac{2\sigma^2 \times (Z_\alpha + Z_\beta)^2}{\Delta^2} \tag{2.4}$$

Kirby and Chuang-Stein (2011) apply the above approach to several other situations, along with other possible alternatives to sample sizing.

It is sometimes of interest to see for a test the treatment effect that gives a particular power for a given sample size and Type I error rate. This can be derived by, for example, solving for Δ in (2.4) as shown in (2.5).

$$\Delta = \sqrt{\frac{2\sigma^2(Z_\alpha + Z_\beta)^2}{n}} \tag{2.5}$$

2.8 The Use of a No-Decision Region

The discussion so far assumes that the acceptance of the null hypothesis is equivalent to the rejection of the alternative hypothesis and vice versa, but this is not always the case. In some situations, a no-decision region may be used such that the null hypothesis is neither accepted nor rejected when results land in this region. In drug development, the outcome of a clinical trial may not lead to a decision to stop developing the drug or continue to the next stage of development. Instead, it may lead to further data being gathered at the current stage of development. This idea is similarly used in a group sequential trial where a particular test may be carried out at each of multiple stages. Possible outcomes at each stage include the option to collect more data rather than to accept the null or alternative hypothesis (Jennison & Turnbull, 2000).

2.9 One-Sided Versus Two-Sided Tests

In the blood pressure example, we tested $H_0: \mu_{drug} - \mu_{placebo} \geq 0$ versus $H_A: \mu_{drug} - \mu_{placebo} < 0$. We considered a decision rule that called for the rejection of H_0 if the test statistic was less than -1.645. Because the rejection region consists of only those values of the test statistic that are quite negative, the test is called a one-sided test.

When the test is one sided, the allowed Type I error rate α is completely spent in one tail of the null distribution in determining the critical value for the test statistic. This is illustrated in Fig. 2.3.

There are situations when the null and alternative hypotheses are stated as H_0: $\mu_{drug} - \mu_{placebo} = 0$ and H_A: $\mu_{drug} - \mu_{placebo} \neq 0$. Under these hypotheses, very positive and very negative values of the test statistic in (2.1) would be consistent with the alternative hypothesis. So, two critical values would be needed, one for each tail of the null distribution. When the test statistic has a Normal distribution or could be approximated by a Normal distribution, a common practice is to split the allowed Type I error rate into two equal portions and assign one portion to each tail of the null distribution. For example, if the Type I error rate is set at the 5% level, each tail of the null distribution will get 2.5% probability, resulting in 1.96 and -1.96 as the critical values for the test statistic. The corresponding test is called a two-sided test.

For confirmatory trials, sponsors are typically required to formulate their tests as two-sided tests even though only one direction is of any practical interest. The real difference between a one-sided and a two-sided test is the critical values used to reject the null hypothesis. In the blood pressure example, the drug will be deemed effective if the test statistic in (2.1) is less than -1.96 under a two-sided test and less than -1.645 under a one-sided test when the allowed Type I error rate is 5%. Thus, it is harder to conclude a positive treatment effect under a two-sided test.

Despite the above, one can generally apply approaches developed for one-sided tests to two-sided tests as long as one uses the appropriate critical value. For example, we can use the sample size formula in (2.4) to determine the sample size for a two-sided test if we replace Z_α by $Z_{\alpha/2}$. The term Z_β remains the same for a two-sided test.

2.10   P-values

A P-value is one of the most fundamental concepts in hypothesis testing. A P-value is defined as the probability of obtaining a result "equal to or more extreme" than what was actually observed in support of the alternative hypothesis, assuming that the null hypothesis is true. In the blood pressure example, assume that the test statistic has a value of t_{obs}, then the P-value for the one-sided test is

$$\max_{\{\mu_{drug} - \mu_{placebo} \geq 0\}} \Pr(Z < t_{obs} | \mu_{drug} - \mu_{placebo}) \tag{2.6}$$

In (2.6), Z represents a random variable that has a standard Normal distribution $N(0; 1)$. The maximum in (2.6) occurs when $\mu_{drug} - \mu_{placebo} = 0$ and the P-value is given by $\Phi(t_{obs})$. Here $\Phi(.)$ denotes the cumulative distribution function of the standard Normal distribution.

When the test is two sided, the calculation of the P-value is a bit more involved. If $t_{obs} < 0$, then the two-sided P-value is $2 \times \Phi(t_{obs})$. If $t_{obs} > 0$, then the two-sided P-value is $2 \times \Phi(-t_{obs})$.

Since the P-value is calculated under the null hypothesis, a small P-value suggests the occurrence of an infrequent event under the conditions described by the null hypothesis. If the P-value is lower than the allowed Type I error rate, one can reject the null hypothesis since a testing procedure that calls for the rejection of the null hypothesis when the P-value is less than α will have an actual Type I error rate smaller than α. The allowed Type I error rate is also called the significance level.

The advantage of a P-value is that it is flexible and can be used to make decisions for any given Type I error rate. For this reason, a P-value is typically reported when hypotheses are tested.

2.11 Multiple Comparisons

Under the Frequentist framework, a P-value describes, for a single hypothesis test, the likelihood that one would observe a result as extreme or more extreme than the one observed in support of the alternative hypothesis, under the null hypothesis. It represents a single conditional probability.

There are many occasions when a researcher is interested in drawing inferences pertaining to multiple hypotheses in one experiment. For a clinical trial, this could mean testing for a new treatment's effect on multiple endpoints, in different patient subpopulations, at different time points of evaluation, or at different interim milestones of an ongoing study. Since a decision on each hypothesis incurs Type I and Type II errors, making decisions on multiple hypotheses could increase the probability that at least one null hypothesis is erroneously rejected. The latter is often referred to as the family-wise Type I error rate (FWER).

As an example, assume that three tests are to be conducted, each at the two-sided 5% significance level, and the test statistics for the three tests are independent of each other. Under these assumptions, the FWER is

$$\text{FWER} = 1 - (1 - 0.05)^3 = 0.143 \tag{2.7}$$

which is much higher than the 5% set for testing a single hypothesis.

While it is important to understand the level of the FWER in a trial in general, it is crucial to control the FWER for a trial designed to provide confirmatory evidence to support the registration of a pharmaceutical product. Many multiple comparison procedures (MCP) to accomplish this have been developed over the past 30 years, some of which are quite sophisticated. MCPs are also referred to as multiplicity adjustment methods.

Most MCPs require a different significance level for testing individual hypotheses than that set for the FWER. In many situations, these rules can be translated to rules that adjust the original P-values first and then compare the adjusted P-values to the pre-specified FWER. For example, the Bonferroni procedure rejects a null hypothesis H_{0j} out of K null hypotheses at an FWER of α if the P-value p_j for testing H_{0j} is less than or equal to α/K. This is equivalent to rejecting H_{0j} if the adjusted P-value, $\tilde{p}_j = K \times p_j$, is less than or equal to α.

A commonly used strategy is the hierarchical testing approach which pre-specifies the order of testing. Under this strategy, hypothesis testing will continue, and the next hypothesis in the chain of hypotheses will be tested at the FWER level α only if the current null hypothesis is rejected at the α level. This strategy is among the favorite MCPs to test for secondary endpoints after a single primary endpoint.

A good reference on traditional multiplicity adjustment methods in clinical trials is a tutorial by Dmitrienko and D'Agostino (2013).

2.12 Selective Interference

A topic closely related to multiplicity is selection. Imagine a researcher assessing the effect of a new treatment on multiple endpoints with the use of P-values and finding a P-value that is less than the customary significance level of 5%. The researcher may be tempted to publish the significant finding in a journal article without mentioning the many other tests that have been carried out. As we pointed out in Sect. 2.11, the significant finding could be a spurious finding, a case of a false positive among multiple comparisons. The selective reporting of results without making adjustment for multiplicity undoubtedly contributed to the observation that many reported positive findings could not be replicated (Ioannidis, 2005).

Selection is not limited to endpoints. It occurs with subgroups as well. Gibson (2021) illustrated the impact of selection in a case study of PRAISE-1 and PRAISE-2 trials. The PRAISE-1 trial randomized 1153 patients with severe chronic heart failure to amlodipine 10 mg or placebo in equal proportions. The randomization was stratified by ischemic or non-ischemic heart failure. The prospectively defined primary endpoint was a composite endpoint of all-cause mortality or major morbidity. The observed overall reduction in the risk for the composite endpoint was 9% (two-sided P-value $= 0.31$) with a reduction of 16% in the risk for the all-cause mortality (P-value $= 0.07$). In patients with non-ischemic heart failure, the results looked more promising with a 31% (P-value $= 0.04$) reduction in the risk for the composite endpoint and a 46% reduction (P-value < 0.001) in the risk for mortality. The impressive risk reduction in mortality observed among non-ischemic patients led to the planning of PRAISE-2.

PRAISE-2 was conducted to confirm the observed benefit of amlodipine 10 mg on all-cause mortality among non-ischemic heart failure patients. The follow-on study was designed with 90% power to detect a 25% reduction in the risk for mortality. PRAISE-2 randomized 1654 patients. The study observed a mortality rate of 33.6% in the amlodipine group and a mortality rate of 31.7% in the placebo group, showing no benefit of amlodipine in reducing the risk for mortality in this subpopulation.

Chuang-Stein and Kirby (2021) also cautioned about the selection of subgroups. They shared the case of tarenflurbil which is a selective $A\beta_{42}$-lowering agent that has been shown in vitro and in vivo to reduce $A\beta_{42}$ production. A Phase 2 trial was conducted to investigate the efficacy of two doses of tarenflurbil against placebo in a 12-month double-blind period with 12-month extension in Alzheimer's disease (AD) patients. The study enrolled 210 patients. A Phase 3 trial was initiated before all results from the Phase 2 trial were known. The Phase 3 trial initially enrolled AD patients with mild or moderate symptoms. After the analyses of the full Phase 2 data suggested that patients with mild symptoms responded better to tarenflurbil, enrollment to the Phase 3 trial was restricted to patients with mild symptoms only. Unfortunately, data on the 1684 patients with mild AD symptoms in the Phase 3 trial failed to show a significant effect of tarenflurbil in these patients.

Benjamini (2020a) put it well when he noted that selective inference is the silent killer of replicability.

2.13   Confidence Intervals

Thus far, we have focused on hypothesis tests. While their use is important, we are also usually interested in how large an effect is. It is therefore common to provide, along with a P-value, a confidence interval for the size of an effect. A confidence interval is an interval constructed such that with a certain probability, typically 0.95, the interval will contain the true unknown effect. For a probability of $(1 - \alpha)$, such an interval is known as a $100 \times (1 - \alpha)\%$ confidence interval.

One way of constructing a confidence interval is to find the set of values for the unknown true effect, Δ, that would not lead to rejection of the null hypothesis by a two-sided hypothesis test at a $100 \times \alpha\%$ significance level. Thus in the blood pressure example, we could obtain a 90% confidence interval for the true difference in means by finding the set of values for Δ which would not be rejected by a two-sided hypothesis test at the 10% significance level. Representing the observed difference in means by d, we need to find the set of values for Δ that satisfy

$$-1.645 \leq \frac{d - \Delta}{\sqrt{\frac{2*5^2}{13}}} \leq 1.645$$

By re-arranging the above, we obtain the set of values given by

$$d \pm 1.645 * \sqrt{\frac{2 * 5^2}{13}} = d \pm 3.23$$

We can construct a confidence interval for a parameter of interest after the completion of an experiment. Among intervals constructed in the above manner over repeated experiments conducted under the same conditions, approximately 90% of them will contain the true unknown difference in means. This probability is also referred to as the coverage probability of the confidence interval.

For a guide on how confidence intervals can be calculated in many different situations, we refer readers to Altman et al. (2000).

2.14   The *P*-value Controversy

As we stated earlier, the *P*-value serves the role for which it is designed. Unfortunately, undisciplined use of the *P*-value has led some to call for its elimination altogether. Some have proposed alternatives to take the place of *P*-values, and a favorite alternative put forward by the proponents of a *P*-value ban is a confidence interval for the parameter of interest. In addition to avoiding the use of the *P*-value, many consider confidence intervals to be more informative than *P*-values because confidence intervals convey two pieces of vital information instead of one.

As Chuang-Stein and Kirby (2021) point out, confidence intervals are constructed with coverage probabilities in mind. When dealing with multiple parameters originating from multiple comparisons, one needs to consider the joint coverage probability of the multiple confidence intervals when the intervals are constructed individually based on the marginal distributions of the estimates. Furthermore, Benjamini (2020b) reminds us that it is easy for our eyes to be drawn to the extreme observations and therefore focus on them. If confidence intervals are constructed in the usual manner without making any allowance for multiplicity or selection, the confidence interval based on the extreme observations will convey the wrong message as to the likely range of the corresponding parameter. This means that reporting on confidence intervals will neither solve the multiplicity nor the selective inference issues when these issues exist, unless adjustments are specifically made to address them.

We do not support the proposal to eliminate the use of *P*-values. We feel that statisticians should help the research community to better understand what a *P*-value is and what it is not. Generations of researchers have been taught, many by statisticians, *P*-values and confidence intervals in a simple, mechanical way without the required emphasis on the need to consider the context in which these summary statistics are created and should be used. There may not have been adequate discussion on how issues such as multiplicity and selection could impact the interpretation of these summary statistics. While mathematical complexity could have been used as an excuse for not doing so many years ago, the effects could easily be illustrated using simple computer simulation and graphic displays in modern times to warn of their impact. In addition, unified calls for and rigorous practice of documented transparency about the selection and number of hypotheses being tested could go a long way to enable the scientific community to evaluate the worthiness of reported results, particularly if no adjustment is made for the effect of multiplicity and/or selection.

Having said the above, we are also cognizant of the fact that some practitioners knowingly ignore the rules in their desire to publish selected positive findings to advance their own agenda. Indeed, misuse could occur despite the best statistical tutoring and well-publicized set of guiding principles. The question is—Does this fear of misuse justify the abolition of *P*-values? We think not, especially if transparency and appropriate checks are put in place as conditions of publication.

On defending the *P*-value against being regarded as the culprit for replication crisis, we share the quote from Benjamini (2021) that "it's the selection's fault – not the *P*-values,"!

2.15 Summary

Except for the Center for Devices and Radiological Health, regulatory decisions on pharmaceutical products in the USA have traditionally been made within the Frequentist framework. One major advantage of the Frequentist approach is that the validity comes from within each positive trial, and there is no need to make any assumption about data outside of the trial. The testing procedures are generally well understood, and their behaviors under various scenarios could be characterized with the help of simulations, if closed-form solutions do not exist.

The Frequentist framework can incorporate results from previous trials. In practice, a sponsor regularly uses estimates of treatment effect and variability obtained from past trials to design future trials. The estimates could come from a single trial or a meta-analysis of multiple trials. Once a trial is designed and conducted, subsequent analyses of the trial data are generally Frequentist in nature.

While the Frequentist framework has generally dominated regulatory decisions on drugs and biologics (Price & LaVange, 2014), there are some signs that this position may be changing for at least some situations. For example, the European Medicines Agency published a reflection paper on the use of extrapolation in the development of medicines for pediatric patients in 2018. When extrapolation from the adult population to the pediatric population is considered appropriate, Bayesian methods could be used to explicitly borrow information from the former to the latter. The Bayesian approach to inference is introduced in Chap. 5.

Even though we focused on significance tests and *P*-values in this chapter, it is important to remember that estimation and prediction are equally important in a Frequentist analysis. Estimation includes reporting both the point and interval estimates for the parameter of interest as discussed in Sect. 2.13. Estimation helps us judge if the observed difference is clinically meaningful. As we pointed out earlier, it is possible to have a significant *P*-value for any amount of difference as long as the sample size is large enough. Prediction allows us to draw inference based on sensible interpolation. Therefore, the interpretation of the results from an experiment should not and could not rely on significance tests or *P*-values alone.

Some researchers have recommended discounting the estimated treatment effect from past trials when using them to plan future trials. This is because of the presence of a selection bias. We will return to this topic in Chap. 12.

References

Altman, D. G., Machin, D., Bryant, T. N., & Gardner, M. J. (Eds.). (2000). *Statistics with confidence* (2nd ed.). BMJ Books.

Benjamini, Y. (2020a). Selective inference: The silent killer of replicability. *Harvard Data Science Review, 2*(4). https://doi.org/10.1162/99608f92.fc62b261

Benjamini, Y. (2020b). *Replicability problems in science: It's not the p-values' fault*, presented at a webinar hosted by the National Institute of Statistical Sciences, May 6. Accessed January 31, 2021 from https://www.niss.org/news/niss-webinar-hosts-third-webinar-use-p-values-making-decisions

Benjamini, Y. (2021). It's the selection's fault—Not the p-values': A comment on "The role of p-values in judging the strength of evidence and realistic replication expectations". *Statistics in Biopharmaceutical Research, 13*(1), 22–25.

Chuang-Stein, C., & Kirby, S. (2021). p-Values and replicability: A commentary on "The role of p-values in judging the strength of evidence and realistic replication expectations". *Statistics in Biopharmaceutical Research, 13*(1), 36–39.

Dmitrienko, A., & D'Agostino, R. D. (2013). Traditional multiplicity adjustment methods in clinical trials. *Statistics in Medicine, 32*, 5172–5218.

European Medicines Agency. (2018). *Reflection paper on the use of extrapolation in the development of medicines for paediatrics.*

Gibson, E. W. (2021). The role of p-values in judging the strength of evidence and realistic replication expectations. *Statistics in Biopharmaceutical Research, 13*(1), 6–18.

Ioannidis, J. P. A. (2005). Why most published research findings are false. *PLOS Medicine, 2*, e124.

Jennison, C., & Turnbull, B. W. (2000). *Group sequential methods with applications to clinical trials.* Chapman Hall/CRC Press.

Kirby, S., & Chuang-Stein, C. (2011). Determining sample size for classical designs (Chap 6). In A. Pong, & S. Chow (Eds.), *Handbook of adaptive designs in pharmaceutical and clinical development.* Chapman & Hall/CRC Press.

Lindgren, B. (1993). *Statistical theory* (4th ed.). Chapman & Hall/CRC Press.

Miller, I., & Miller, M. (2014). *John E. Freund's mathematical statistics* (8th ed.). Pearson.

Price, K., & LaVange, L. (2014). Bayesian methods in medical product development and regulatory reviews. *Pharmaceutical Statistics, 13*(1), 1–2.

Chapter 3
Characteristics of a Diagnostic Test

Diagnosis is foundation of therapy—and of personalized medicine.
—Janet Woodcock, CDER Director, FDA

3.1 Introduction

In medicine, a diagnostic test is often performed to diagnose a disease or to subclassify a disease regarding its severity and susceptibility to treatment. In recent years, companion diagnostics have also been developed to preselect patients for specific treatments based on their own biology. For example, when the FDA approved crizotinib for patients with ALK-positive advanced non-small cell lung cancer and vemurafenib for late-stage (metastatic) or unresectable melanoma with the BRAF V600E mutation, it stipulated that the targeted conditions be detected by FDA-approved tests.

A diagnostic test is typically based on the result from a laboratory assay. The assay measures the amount of the target entity in a sample and compares the amount to a cutoff value. The result is then expressed as a binary outcome—yes or no, present or absent, abnormal or normal, positive or negative.

When setting up an assay, a laboratory must take into account the clinical intentions of its users, optimizing the analytical procedure and selecting the operating characteristics of the assay appropriately (Oliver & Chuang-Stein, 1993). For a medical test, a key factor in deciding the above is the clinical decision points. The laboratory will set up the assay in such a way that the result is the most precise at or near the points where clinical decisions are to be made. An example is the upper and lower limits of the reference range for a safety laboratory test, when the primary consideration is to confidently identify a result as clinically abnormal or not. In this case, the precision of the assay far away from the reference range is generally less important.

In this chapter, we will first review the metrics commonly used to characterize the performance of a diagnostic test. We will discuss what it means when a diagnostic

© The Author(s), under exclusive license to Springer Nature Switzerland AG 2021
C. Chuang-Stein and S. Kirby, *Quantitative Decisions in Drug Development*, Springer Series in Pharmaceutical Statistics,
https://doi.org/10.1007/978-3-030-79731-7_3

test returns a positive or a negative result. We illustrate this by using different decision rules. We will conclude the chapter with some additional remarks.

3.2   Sensitivity and Specificity

Sackett et al. (1985) described a case of using the level of creatine kinase (CK) as a means to diagnose myocardial infarction (MI). The data came from a study conducted at the coronary care unit at the Royal Infirmary in Edinburgh in the 70s. All patients who came to the hospital and were suspected of having had an MI within the previous 48 h were admitted to the unit. There was a need to differentiate, as quickly as possible, between patients who actually had had an MI and those who had not. This would enable better patient triage and management.

The staff in the coronary care unit thought that high levels of CK might help them identify an MI sooner than measurements of enzymes (such as aspartate aminotrans-ferase) that arose later following an MI. To confirm this, they measured the CK level on admission and in the next two mornings on 360 consecutive patients who were admitted to the unit and lived long enough to have the blood samples taken.

Using ECG and autopsy, 230 patients were judged to *very probably* or *possibly* have had an MI. For simplicity, we will simply say that these patients had had an MI. The remaining 130 patients were judged to not have had an MI.

The CK values among patients who have had an MI are generally higher than those among patients who have not had an MI. However, the distributions of the two sets of values overlap. The question is what cutoff to use when using CK as the basis for diagnosing an MI. One of the possible levels is 80 IU (international unit), i.e., declaring an MI to have occurred when $CK \geq 80$ IU and not to have occurred if $CK < 80$ IU. The accuracy of this decision rule, applied to the 360 patients, is given in Table 3.1. The contents of Table 3.1 come from Sackett et al.

Among the 230 patients who have had an MI, using the decision rule will have correctly diagnosed an MI in 215 patients. This gives a correct positive rate of 93% (= 215/230). Among the 130 patients who have not had an MI, the rule will have made a correct diagnosis in 114 patients, yielding a correct negative rate of 88% (= 114/130).

Table 3.1 Results from diagnosing an MI based on $CK \geq 80$ IU

		Myocardial Infarction	
		Present	Absent
Diagnosis of an MI by CK	MI Present (CK $\geq$ 80 IU)	215 (a)	16 (b)
	MI Absent (CK < 80 IU)	15 (c)	114 (d)
	Total	230 (a + c)	130 (b + d)

Table 3.2 Results from diagnosing an MI based on CK ≥ 40 IU

		Myocardial Infarction	
		Present	Absent
Diagnosis by CK	Present (CK ≥ 40 IU)	228	43
	Absent (CK < 40 IU)	2	87
	Total	230	130

If a lower threshold, e.g., 40 IU, is used, we will get different results. The new results are given in Table 3.2. The correct positive rate is now 99% (= 228/230), and the correct negative rate is 67% (= 87/130). A lower threshold makes it easier to declare a patient to have had an MI, thus producing a higher correct positive rate among patients who have had an MI. However, the lower threshold also makes it easier to declare an MI in patients who have not had an MI, resulting in a lower correct negative rate.

Conversely, if a higher threshold than 80 IU is used, one can expect the correct positive rate to decrease while the correct negative rate to increase.

The correct positive rate of a diagnostic test is called the sensitivity of the test. The correct negative rate is called the specificity of the test. The figures we gave above are estimates of these measures based on a single sample. Using the notation in the parentheses in Table 3.1, sensitivity is given by $a/(a + c)$ and specificity given by $d/(b + d)$.

While it is desirable for a diagnostic test to have high sensitivity and high specificity, there is usually a trade-off between these two metrics as illustrated in the MI-CK example. One way to see how sensitivity and specificity trade-off with each other is to plot sensitivity on the Y-axis against (1-specificity) on the X-axis for various cutoff points. The resulting curve is called a receiver operating characteristic (ROC) curve. Because (1-specificity) represents the false positive rate (i.e., rate of an undesirable outcome), an ROC curve that ascends quickly to 100% on the Y-axis (sensitivity) while moving only slightly away from the origin on the X-axis (1-specificity) has a large area under the ROC curve and represents a highly desirable diagnostic test. In this sense, the ROC curve could be used to not only evaluate a diagnostic test but also to compare between two diagnostic tests. Readers interested in learning more about the practical aspects of analyzing ROC curves should read the book by Gonen (2007).

3.3 Positive and Negative Predictive Value

The performance of a diagnostic test is measured by its ability to give correct diagnoses among a sample of "cases" (with the condition of interest) and a sample of "controls" (without the condition). When a diagnostic test is used in practice, a critical question is how to interpret its result. Does a positive result provide definitive evidence for the presence of a condition? If the test returns a negative result, can one confidently rule out the presence of the condition?

The above questions can be answered by the positive predictive value (PPV) and the negative predictive value (NPV) of the test. In the example of using CK ≥ 80 IU to diagnose an MI, the PPV is the probability of having had an MI when CK ≥ 80 IU. The NPV is the probability of not having had an MI when CK < 80 IU. These probabilities can be derived from Bayes' Rule as shown in (3.1) and (3.2) below.

$$
\begin{aligned}
\mathrm{PPV} = \Pr(\mathrm{MI}|\mathrm{CK} \geq 80) &= \frac{\Pr(\mathrm{CK} \geq 80|\mathrm{MI}) \times \Pr(\mathrm{MI})}{\Pr(\mathrm{CK} \geq 80)} \\
&= \frac{\Pr(\mathrm{CK} \geq 80|\mathrm{MI}) \times \Pr(\mathrm{MI})}{\Pr(\mathrm{CK} \geq 80|\mathrm{MI}) \times \Pr(\mathrm{MI}) + \Pr(\mathrm{CK} \geq 80|\mathrm{No\ MI}) \times \Pr(\mathrm{No\ MI})} \\
&= \frac{\mathrm{Sensitivity} \times \Pr(\mathrm{MI})}{\mathrm{Sensitivity} \times \Pr(\mathrm{MI}) + (1 - \mathrm{Specificity}) \times (1 - \Pr(\mathrm{MI}))}
\end{aligned}
\tag{3.1}
$$

For a validated diagnostic test, we know its sensitivity and specificity. The one new term in (3.1) is the probability of having an MI, i.e., the prevalence of MI in an underlying population. The Bayes rule starts with the population prevalence and updates the population-based estimate with the test result about an individual.

In Table 3.3, we give the PPV for various combinations of (sensitivity, specificity) and MI prevalence. We include the two sets of (sensitivity, specificity) from choosing 40 IU and 80 IU as the cutoff in the top two rows. We also include additional sets of (0.80, 0.80), (0.80, 0.90), (0.90, 0.90) and (0.90, 0.95).

Table 3.3 shows some interesting trends. First, the PPV can be quite low when the prevalence is low. Second, the PPV is highly dependent on the prevalence rate. As the prevalence increases, the PPV also increases. Third, the PPV increases as sensitivity increases. Similarly, the PPV increases as specificity increases.

Similarly, one can derive the NPV through Bayes' Rule. Using the MI-CK example, the NPV is given in (3.2).

Table 3.3 PPV of a diagnostic test with various combinations of (sensitivity, specificity) and the prevalence rate

Sensitivity /specificity	Prevalence of myocardial infarction (%)					
	0.05	0.10	0.15	0.20	0.25	0.30
0.99/0.67	0.14	0.25	0.35	0.43	0.50	0.56
0.93/0.88	0.29	0.46	0.58	0.66	0.72	0.77
0.80/0.80	0.17	0.31	0.41	0.50	0.57	0.63
0.80/0.90	0.30	0.47	0.59	0.67	0.73	0.77
0.90/0.90	0.32	0.50	0.61	0.69	0.75	0.79
0.90/0.95	0.49	0.67	0.76	0.82	0.86	0.89

Table 3.4 NPV of a diagnostic test with various combinations of (sensitivity, specificity) and the prevalence rate

Sensitivity /specificity	Prevalence of myocardial infarction (%)					
	0.05	0.10	0.15	0.20	0.25	0.30
0.99/0.67	1.00	1.00	1.00	1.00	1.00	0.99
0.93/0.88	1.00	0.99	0.99	0.98	0.97	0.97
0.80/0.80	0.99	0.97	0.96	0.94	0.92	0.90
0.80/0.90	0.99	0.98	0.96	0.95	0.93	0.91
0.90/0.90	0.99	0.99	0.98	0.97	0.96	0.95
0.90/0.95	0.99	0.99	0.98	0.97	0.97	0.96

$$\text{NPV} = \frac{\text{Specificity} \times (1 - \text{Pr(MI)})}{(1 - \text{Sensitivity}) \times \text{Pr(MI)} + \text{Specificity} \times (1 - \text{Pr(MI)})} \tag{3.2}$$

We provide, in Table 3.4, the NPV for the same choices of sensitivity, specificity and prevalence as in Table 3.3. The NPV is nearly 100% for all (sensitivity, specificity) combinations considered in Table 3.4 when prevalence is 5%. Like the PPV, the NPV increases with sensitivity and specificity. Unlike the PPV, the NPV decreases as the prevalence rate increases.

3.4 Value of a Follow-On Test

Table 3.3 shows that for a condition with a 10% prevalence rate in a pertinent population, a positive diagnosis from a test with a sensitivity of 93% and a specificity of 88% will be right about 46% of the time. This means that approximately half of the time a positive result by this test in the underlying population represents a false positive diagnosis. When the false positive rate is this high, it will be logical to employ a second test, perhaps one with a higher performance quality, to confirm the positive finding before taking any important action. This logic has led health care professionals to follow up a positive skin test for tuberculosis with a chest X-ray and a suspicious mammogram with another mammogram or perhaps a biopsy.

The value of a follow-up test can be assessed quantitatively using the PPV concept. Assume that in the above example, a second test with a sensitivity of 90% and a specificity of 95% is performed following a positive result from the first test. The PPV of the second test can be calculated using the expression in (3.1) with 46% as the prevalence rate. This new prevalence rate is the PPV of the first test. The PPV of the second test can be found to be 94% as shown below. This is a much higher figure than the previous 46%.

$$\text{PPV} = \frac{0.90 \times 0.46}{0.90 \times 0.46 + (1 - 0.95) \times (1 - 0.46)} = 0.94$$

If one employs a third test with sensitivity equal to 90% and specificity equal to 95% after two consecutive positive tests, then the PPV of the third test is 99.6%. In other words, three consecutive positive results can almost assure that the positive finding is true.

In the above example with a 10% prevalence rate in the population, if the first test returns a negative result, an individual could feel 99% confident that the condition is absent. When this happens, there is generally no need to employ a second test to confirm the negative finding.

3.5 When Two Tests Are Being Done Simultaneously

In Sect. 3.4, we assume that a second test will be performed only if the first test shows a positive result. A positive diagnosis is made when both tests are positive, otherwise a negative diagnosis is made.

What can we say about the quality of the decision if we apply two tests independently, but simultaneously, and declare a positive finding only if both tests return positive results?

We will denote the two tests by T_1 and T_2. Sensitivity and specificity of the two tests are denoted by S_i and F_i, $i = 1, 2$, respectively. The decision rule of making a positive diagnosis only if the two concurrent tests return positive results has a sensitivity of $S_1 \times S_2$ and specificity of $1 - (1 - F_1) \times (1 - F_2)$. Assuming the prevalence rate is p, the PPV of this decision rule (denoted by T_1 & T_2) is

$$\mathrm{PPV}(T_1 \& T_2) = \frac{S_1 \times S_2 \times p}{S_1 \times S_2 \times p + (1 - F_1) \times (1 - F_2) \times (1 - p)} \qquad (3.3)$$

Under the sequential testing procedure in Sect. 3.4, PPV of the first test (assuming it to be T_1) is

$$\mathrm{PPV}(T_1) = \frac{S_1 \times p}{S_1 \times p + (1 - F_1) \times (1 - p)} \qquad (3.4)$$

The value of $\mathrm{PPV}(T_1)$ becomes the prevalence rate when we calculate the PPV of T_2 following a positive T_1. In other words, PPV of T_2 is now calculated to be

$$\mathrm{PPV}(T_1 \to T_2) = \frac{S_2 \times \mathrm{PPV}(T_1)}{S_2 \times \mathrm{PPV}(T_1) + (1 - F_2) \times (1 - \mathrm{PPV}(T_1))} \qquad (3.5)$$

Substituting $\mathrm{PPV}(T_1)$ in (3.5) by the expression in (3.4), we obtain the same expression for $\mathrm{PPV}(T_1 \to T_2)$ as that for $\mathrm{PPV}(T_1 \& T_2)$ in (3.3). In other words, PPV under a simultaneous testing approach is the same as that under a sequential approach.

Table 3.5 Probabilities of various outcomes from a rule that requires concordant results from two simultaneous tests to make either a positive or negative decision

		True disease state	
		Yes	No
Rule outcome	Positive	0.84	0.01
	Indecision	0.15	0.15
	Negative	0.01	0.84

An advantage of the sequential tests is the savings arising from not needing to conduct the second test if the first rest returns a negative result. However, this advantage is only meaningful if the NPV of T_1 is reasonably high and the consequence of missing a true positive is acceptable.

On the other hand, if the consequence of making a false negative diagnosis is substantial and the prevalence rate of the condition is not particularly low, a more prudent practice may be to require two consecutive negative results (out of two tests). In other words, a negative test needs to be confirmed by another negative result. Following the reasoning above, the NPV will be the same under both testing approaches.

The above observations imply that when both positive and negative finding from the first test requires confirmation, sequential testing does not have any advantage over simultaneous tests. Simultaneous testing has the advantage of getting an answer faster.

We return to the case of simultaneous testing and consider a decision rule of making a positive diagnosis if both tests return positive results and making a negative diagnosis if both tests return a negative result. This decision rule draws no conclusion when the two tests provide discordant results. When this happens, a third test is often performed to break the tie.

Using the numerical examples in Sect. 3.4, this new decision rule has a sensitivity of $0.84 (= 0.93 \times 0.90)$. The specificity is now $0.84 (= 0.88 \times 0.95)$. The performance of this new decision rule is described in Table 3.5.

Using Table 3.5, we can calculate the PPV and NPV of the modified rule under the assumption of a 10% prevalence rate.

$$\begin{aligned} \text{PPV} &= \text{Pr(Disease|Positive Outcome from Rule)} \\ &= \frac{\text{Pr(Positive|Disease)} \times 0.10}{\text{Pr(Positive|Disease)} \times 0.10 + \text{Pr(Positive|No Disease)} \times 0.90} \\ &= \frac{0.84 \times 0.10}{0.84 \times 0.10 + 0.01 \times 0.90} = 0.90 \end{aligned}$$

$$\begin{aligned} \text{NPV} &= \text{Pr(No Disease|Negative Outcome from Rule)} \\ &= \frac{\text{Pr(Negative|No Disease)} \times 0.90}{\text{Pr(Negative|Disease)} \times 0.10 + \text{Pr(Negative|No Disease)} \times 0.90} \\ &= \frac{0.84 \times 0.90}{0.01 \times 0.10 + 0.84 \times 0.90} \approx 1.00 \end{aligned}$$

Because the rule requires two negative results to give a negative conclusion, the NPV of the modified rule is higher than that of the first rule discussed in this section (i.e., requiring only one negative to make a negative diagnosis). As noted earlier, the modified rule allows the possibility of no conclusion. The probability of this outcome is approximately 15% whether the disease (condition) is present or absent.

For most of the situations covered in this book, we follow a decision rule that declares a negative finding if at least one test produces a negative result.

3.6 Summary

In this chapter, we examine the performance of a diagnostic test and the test's predictive value. A diagnosis test is essentially a decision rule that uses data to make a (generally) binary prediction. The rule can give rise to erroneous conclusions. Our ability to quantify the likelihood of these errors allows us to better formulate rules and choose among rules.

We have illustrated in this chapter how the predictive value of a diagnostic test depends on the prevalence of the condition which the test is set to diagnose. When the prevalence is extremely low (e.g., <1%), the positive predictive value of a diagnostic test is typically very low. This is why it is not recommended to conduct HIV-screening in people who are in committed monogamous relationships and who are not intravenous illicit drug users.

Although we did not discuss reproducibility in this chapter, reproducibility is an important requirement of a diagnostic test. For a diagnostic test, reproducibility means that the test will produce similar results upon rerunning the (same) sample. This requires the assay to have sufficient precision and be free from a systematic drift from the truth. For this reason, a researcher often needs to re-calibrate their assay by running control samples between separate batch runs of real samples.

We want to point out that reproducibility described above is different from taking readings from different samples of the same individual. In the latter case, the biologic variability existing among samples from the same individual could result in noticeably different results. A common example is the circulating cholesterol in plasma.

References

Gonen, M. (2007). *Analyzing receiver operating characteristic curves with SAS®* (1st ed.). SAS Press.

Oliver, L. K., Chuang-Stein, C. (1993). Laboratory data in multi-center trials: monitoring, adjustment and summarization. Chapter 6 In G. Sogliero-Gilbert (Ed.) *Drug safety assessment in clinical trials.* Marcel Dekker, New York.

Sackett, D.L., Haynes, R.B., Tugwell, P. (1985). *Clinical epidemiology. A basic science for clinical medicine.* Little, Brown and Company

Chapter 4
The Parallel Between Clinical Trials and Diagnostic Tests

Using preliminary research to approve new treatments has high costs in morbidity and healthcare dollars.
—British Medical Journal, Nov 23 2015

4.1 Introduction

During the clinical development of a new drug, a sponsor conducts a series of clinical trials to assess the safety and efficacy of the drug. We discussed the nature and objectives of these trials in Chap. 1. Although designed differently, these trials all aim to understand the new drug better.

At the end of Phase 3 testing, the sponsor needs to decide, based on the collective evidence, whether the drug meets pre-specified safety and efficacy requirements to warrant a new drug application (or a biologic license application in the case of a biologic). Once an application is filed, regulators will review and decide, based on results submitted from the sponsor, whether the drug has a favorable benefit–risk profile to be worthy of commercialization. A prerequisite for approval is a high level of confidence that the drug is beneficial, when balancing its risks against its benefits.

The end of Phase 3 is not the only time when a sponsor needs to make a decision about the likely effect of a new drug. As development progresses, a sponsor needs to decide whether to move the drug to the next phase of testing. More than that, at the end of each trial, a sponsor needs to assimilate the new information with existing knowledge to decide on the next step. This may include conducting a trial similar to the one just completed but with certain aspects of the trial modified.

Chapter 2 describes the Frequentist decision-making framework. For clinical trials, the framework is often formulated in terms of choosing between two hypotheses, the null hypothesis and the alternative hypothesis. For a superiority trial, the null hypothesis states that the new drug is not effective (i.e., the absence of an effect) and the alternative hypothesis states that the drug is effective (i.e., the presence of an effect). A trial is designed so that the ensuing test has a desired power

C. Chuang-Stein and S. Kirby, *Quantitative Decisions in Drug Development*, Springer Series in Pharmaceutical Statistics, https://doi.org/10.1007/978-3-030-79731-7_4

to reject the null hypothesis when the drug exhibits a certain level of effectiveness. Occasionally, the decision rule will result in an error in rejecting the null hypothesis, but the probability of this error is controlled at a pre-specified level. The latter is called the Type I error rate (see Sect. 2.3 in Chap. 2).

Since a major objective of all efficacy trials in drug development is to ascertain the effect of a new drug, each trial acts like a diagnostic test with a goal to detect (or diagnose) the presence of a clinically meaningful drug effect. Consider using the trial results to test the simple null hypothesis H_0: treatment effect $= 0$ versus a simple alternative hypothesis H_A: treatment effect $=$ a pre-specified clinically meaningful value. Treating the hypothesis test like a diagnostic test, the power of a hypothesis test in the Frequentist decision-making framework is the sensitivity of the diagnostic test and the Type I error rate takes the place of (1-specificity).

The above analogy between clinical trials and diagnostic tests offers us the opportunity to apply properties pertaining to diagnostic tests in Chap. 3 to clinical trials. Building on the discussion in Chap. 3, we will discuss first why replication is such a critically important concept in drug development in this chapter. We will then show why replication is not as easy as some might hope. Finally, we will reiterate the difference between statistical power and the probability of getting a positive trial. This last point becomes more important as a new drug moves through the various development stages as we will illustrate later in Chap. 9.

4.2   Why Replication Is Necessary

No isolated experiment, however significant in itself, can suffice for the experimental demonstration of any natural phenomenon; for the "one chance in a million" will undoubtedly occur, with no less and no more than its appropriate frequency, however surprised we may be that it should occur to us. —Sir R. A. Fisher.

Zuckerman et al. (2015) discussed the 21st Century Cures Act, a proposal that was eventually signed into law by the president of the USA on December 13, 2016, to jump-start the process of finding new cures for the thousands of diseases that lacked effective treatments. Zuckerman et al. questioned whether the bill, if passed and signed into law, would increase the availability of new medical products that do not necessarily work. They used Alzheimer's disease (AD) as an example. They examined data from three Alzheimer's drugs (semagacestat, bapineuzumab and latrepirdime) that failed Phase 3 testing between 2010 and 2015. They singled out AD drugs because AD is a disorder with a large unmet medical need. As of March 2021, there had been no new AD drug on the market since memantine was last approved in 2003. Besides, all the commercially available AD drugs as of March 2021 (a total of 4 of them) treat only symptoms associated with the disease and do not delay disease progression. We want to mention, though, that at the time of writing, the medical community was waiting for a decision by the US FDA on the new monoclonal antibody treatment aducanumab. Aducanumab was submitted as a potential disease-modifying agent by its developer.

The 21st Century Cures Act proposes to allow drug approval based on Phase 2 trial data for serious or life-threatening diseases. While this has become a practice for cancer drugs, the Act proposes to extend this provision to other therapeutic areas also. Citing the three consecutive late-stage failures of the AD drug candidates mentioned above, Zuckerman et al. considered this proposal problematic. All three aforementioned drugs had promising results in small Phase 2 trials but failed to replicate the results in large Phase 3 trials.

Zuckerman et al. are not alone. Kesselheim et al. (2015) examined the impact of the proposed Act on the approval of drugs intended to treat the central nervous system (CNS). They examined the failure rates of 379 CNS drugs that entered into Phase 1 trials between 1990 and 2012. They found that CNS drugs were significantly more likely than non-CNS drugs to fail at the Phase 3 stage. They concluded that the lack of efficacy of CNS drugs in general reinforced the importance of conducting Phase 3 trials when it was ethically acceptable to do so.

Other researchers have commented on the difficulty in replicating large treatment effects observed in earlier trials. Pereira et al. (2012) conducted an empirical evaluation to investigate when very large treatment effects were reported and how often they were replicated in subsequent trials of the same comparison, disease and outcome. They concluded that most large treatment effects were observed in small studies and pertaining to nonfatal outcomes, and the observed effect sizes became typically much smaller when additional trials were performed. They concluded that well-validated large effects were uncommon.

It is easy to understand the difficulty in replicating an earlier positive result using the diagnostic test analogy. Our first efficacy trial is usually a small proof-of-concept (POC) trial. This trial often has lower sensitivity or specificity or both. This is by design because of the small sample size. For illustration, we will consider a test with 80% sensitivity and 90% specificity. This corresponds to a Type I error rate of 10% and a power of 80%.

Table 3.3 in Chap. 3 shows the positive predictive value (PPV) of the test under various assumed prevalence rates of the condition to be diagnosed. In the case of a POC trial, the condition to diagnose is the presence of a clinically meaningful drug effect. The PPV of the POC trial gives the likelihood that the new drug is sufficiently effective if the POC trial yields a positive result. As we have learned in Chap. 3, the PPV is highly dependent on the "prevalence rate" of the condition to be diagnosed. In the context of drug development, we can estimate this prevalence rate by the success rate of drugs for the same disease. If the new drug is from a class of drugs with a lot of existing information on its members, we can use the success rate of drugs in the same class as an estimate for the prevalence rate.

For convenience, we use 10% as the prevalence (success) rate. According to Table 3.3, the PPV of the POC trial is 47%. In other words, the chance that the drug is effective (i.e., having a clinically meaningful effect) if the trial returns a positive result could be less than 50%. For diseases with very few prior therapeutic successes such as Alzheimer's disease, the overall success rate could be much lower than 10%.

A 5% overall success rate would result in a 30% PPV for the POC trial designed with 80% power and 10% Type I error rate.

The above results show why we need to be particularly cautious when the overall success rate among drugs intended for a specific disease is very low. This is because what we have observed in the small POC trial could have actually come from an ineffective drug. Unfortunately, developers often behave in the opposite way. When a developer observes promising results in a POC trial while rivals fail in their attempts, the developer often feels ecstatic and decides to go straight into Phase 3, convinced that they have solved the biologic secrets that have eluded their competitors.

If the positive POC trial is followed with another trial, the second trial will have a much higher PPV as shown in Chap. 3. In the current example, assume that the second trial has a sensitivity of 80% (80% power) and a specificity of 95% (5% Type I error rate). With a prevalence rate now set at 47%, the second trial will have a PPV of 93%.

This example shows the necessity of replicating an early positive finding because replication can greatly enhance our confidence that a drug is effective. A high confidence that a drug is effective is important to both the developer and the regulators.

4.3 Why Replication Is Hard

The example above did not state how likely a positive finding can be replicated. Because our ability to replicate a previous positive finding seems to be limited, researchers have been interested in estimating the probability of a successful replication. One way to phrase the question is—suppose the treatment effect was found significant at the one-sided 2.5% level and we plan to conduct an *identical* study with the same protocol (with the same sample size), what is the probability that we will again have a significant result, i.e., have a one-sided P-value < 0.025?

4.3.1 Conditional Replication Probability

For the remainder of this chapter, we assume that a drug is being compared with a placebo and the efficacy endpoint follows a Normal distribution with a known and common standard deviation in the two treatment groups. Higher values on the efficacy endpoint represent a more desirable outcome. P-value refers to one-sided P-value when the context is clear. As with other chapters in this book, we will work with a one-sided significance level in this chapter for a superiority trial. For a confirmatory trial that requires a two-sided significance level of 5%, we will work with a one-sided significance level of 2.5%.

One approach, taken by O'Neill (1997) and Hung and O'Neill (2003), is to first estimate the treatment effect size based on the P-value from the first trial. Computing the estimated treatment effect from the P-value is possible because there is a one-to-one correspondence between the two for a given sample size n per group. Let $\overline{X}_{drug}$ and $\overline{X}_{placebo}$ denotes the mean response in the drug and placebo group, $D = \overline{X}_{drug} - \overline{X}_{placebo}$, and d denotes an observed value for D. The one-sided P-value is related to the observed treatment effect size d/σ through the relationship in (4.1). In (4.1), $\Phi(.)$ is the cumulative distribution of the standard Normal distribution. In (4.1) and other equations in this chapter, P is short for the one-sided P-value from a completed study. When we need to use P for P-value (again, one-sided) from a future study, we will use the notation P(new study).

$$P = 1 - \Phi\left(\frac{d}{\sigma}\sqrt{\frac{n}{2}}\right) \tag{4.1}$$

From (4.1), one can derive the observed effect size as a function of the P-value and the sample size as in (4.2). In (4.2), $\Phi^{-1}(.)$ is the inverse function of $\Phi(.)$.

$$\frac{d}{\sigma} = \Phi^{-1}(1 - P) \times \sqrt{\frac{2}{n}} \tag{4.2}$$

O'Neill (1997) and Hung and O'Neill (2003) calculated the replication probability by assuming that the true effect size in the second trial was the same as that observed in the first study. For convenience, we will call the probability, calculated under this condition and given below, the conditional replication probability.

Conditional replication probability

$$= Pr\left(P(\text{new study}) < 0.025 | \text{ true treatment effect size} = \frac{d}{\sigma}\right)$$

One can think of the conditional replication probability as the value of the power function for testing H_0: treatment effect $= 0$ versus H_A: treatment effect > 0, evaluated at the effect size d/σ. The result is given in (4.3). In (4.3), 1.96 is the upper 97.5th percentile of the standard Normal distribution, which is the critical value that the standardized test statistic needs to exceed in order to reject the null hypothesis of no treatment effect at the one-sided significance level of 2.5%.

$$\text{Conditional replication probability} = 1 - \Phi\left(1.96 - \frac{d}{\sigma}\sqrt{\frac{n}{2}}\right)$$
$$= 1 - \Phi\left(1.96 - \Phi^{-1}(1 - P)\right) \tag{4.3}$$

Suppose that the first study has 64 patients per group in a two-arm parallel group study. This sample size has 81% power to detect an effect size of 0.5 at a one-sided 2.5% significance level. Table 4.1 gives the conditional replication probability for various one-sided P-values for this sample size. We would like to point out that while

Table 4.1 Conditional replication probability conditioning on the true effect size being the same as that observed in the first trial

One-sided P-value in the first trial	Estimated treatment effect Size (d/σ) from the first trial	Conditional replication probability
0.0001	0.657	0.961
0.0005	0.582	0.908
0.000625	0.570	0.897
0.001	0.546	0.871
0.0025	0.496	0.802
0.005	0.455	0.731
0.01	0.411	0.643
0.025	0.346	0.500

the estimated effect size d/σ is a function of the sample size in the first (completed) study, the conditional replication probability in (4.3) is not.

A striking result in Table 4.1 is the 50% conditional replication probability if the result from the first trial is just barely significant. The conditional replication probability increases as the P-value from the first trial decreases.

The probabilities in Table 4.1 were calculated assuming that the true treatment effect in the second trial was the same as the observed treatment effect in the first trial. While the observed treatment effect is generally a consistent estimate for the true treatment effect, this estimate has an inherent sampling variability. There is no guarantee that the true effect size in the second trial will be equal to the observed effect size from the first trial, especially if the sample size in the first trial is small. The need to incorporate the uncertainty in the estimate into consideration prompted the idea of an average replication probability that will be described in the next section.

4.3.2   Average Replication Probability

Chuang-Stein (2006) introduced the idea of averaging the power function over the likely values of the treatment effect, using the likelihood of these values as the weight. Consider the example in the previous section. Instead of assuming the observed treatment effect d to be the true treatment effect in the new trial, a more realistic approach is to consider a range of possible true treatment effect, based on our knowledge from the first trial. In the case of a continuous variable, one could consider a Normal distribution like the one in Fig. 4.1 to describe the range as well as the likelihood of the true treatment effect.

So, instead of calculating the probability of a significant result conditioning on the observed treatment effect being the true effect, one could first calculate the probability at any plausible value and then derive a weighted average of these probabilities

Fig. 4.1 Range of likely values for the true effect and their likelihood approximated by a Normal distribution

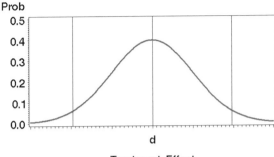

using the likelihood of the plausible values as weight. This process, formulated mathematically in (4.4), produces an average of the conditional replication probabilities. We will call this the average replication probability.

$$\text{Average replication probability} = \int \Pr\left(P(\text{new study}) < 0.025 | \frac{D}{\sigma} \right) f(D) dD$$

$$(4.4)$$

Chuang-Stein (2006) proposed to use $N\left(d; \frac{2}{n}\sigma^2\right)$, where n represents the number of subjects in each treatment group in the first trial, to describe the uncertainty in our knowledge regarding the true treatment effect. This choice is intuitive because this is the sampling distribution for the observed treatment effect.

When the difference in the mean response in the two treatment groups follows a Normal distribution, the assumption of a Normal distribution $N\left(d; \frac{2}{n}\sigma^2\right)$ to represent uncertainty about the location parameter (i.e., $\mu_{\text{drug}} - \mu_{\text{placebo}}$, difference in the population mean response) results in a closed-form expression for (4.4). The closed-form expression is derived from the fact that the unconditional distribution of $\overline{X}_{\text{drug}} - \overline{X}_{\text{placebo}}$ is $N\left(d; \frac{4}{n}\sigma^2\right)$. The inclusion of the uncertainty in the treatment effect doubles the variance of the distribution of $\overline{X}_{\text{drug}} - \overline{X}_{\text{placebo}}$. Using this distribution, one can calculate the unconditional probability $\Pr\left(\overline{X}_{\text{drug}} - \overline{X}_{\text{placebo}} > 1.96 \times \sqrt{\frac{2}{n}}\sigma\right)$ in the second trial, yielding the result in (4.5).

$$\text{Average replication probability} = 1 - \Phi\left(\frac{1}{\sqrt{2}}\left(1.96 - \frac{d}{\sigma}\sqrt{\frac{n}{2}} \right) \right)$$

$$= 1 - \Phi\left(\frac{1}{\sqrt{2}}(1.96 - \Phi^{-1}(1 - P)) \right) \quad (4.5)$$

The difference between (4.3) and (4.5) is the extra term $1/\sqrt{2}$ inside the function $\Phi(.)$ in (4.5). When the first trial produces a significant treatment effect, the term inside the cumulative function $\Phi(.)$ is negative. The term $1/\sqrt{2}$ shrinks the absolute value of the term, leading to a larger value for $\Phi(.)$ and a smaller average replication

Table 4.2 Average replication probability for various one-sided P-values

One-sided P-value in the first trial	Conditional replication probability	Average replication probability
0.0001	0.961	0.893
0.0005	0.908	0.827
0.000625	0.897	0.815
0.001	0.871	0.788
0.0025	0.802	0.725
0.005	0.731	0.668
0.01	0.643	0.602
0.025	0.500	0.500

probability compared to the conditional replication probability. Like the conditional replication probability, the average replication probability does not depend on n. This is because all the information about the first trial is conveyed through the P-value when σ is assumed known.

For our example, the average replication probabilities are given in Table 4.2. For comparison purpose, we include the conditional replication probabilities in Table 4.2 also.

4.3.3 When the Second Trial Has a Different Sample Size

The calculations in Sects. 4.3.1 and 4.3.2 assume that the second trial has the same sample size as the first one. But, this does not need to be the case. In drug development, a sponsor may want to replicate an earlier positive efficacy result with a larger study (e.g., using the same protocol and same investigators, but a different sample size). This is similar to employing a diagnostic test with a higher quality to confirm an earlier positive finding. In addition, a larger trial may offer a better chance to observe adverse drug reactions.

Suppose that the first study has m patients per group and the second study plans to enroll n patients per group. The unconditional distribution of $\overline{X}_{\text{drug}} - \overline{X}_{\text{placebo}}$ is now $N\left(d; \left(\frac{2}{n} + \frac{2}{m}\right)\sigma^2\right)$. Under this distribution, the probability $\Pr\left(\overline{X}_{\text{drug}} - \overline{X}_{\text{placebo}} > 1.96 \times \sqrt{\frac{2}{n}}\sigma\right)$ is given by the right-hand side of (4.6).

$$\text{Average replication probability} = 1 - \Phi\left(\sqrt{\frac{n}{m+n}}\left(1.96 \times \sqrt{\frac{m}{n}} - \Phi^{-1}(1-P)\right)\right)$$

$$(4.6)$$

Returning to our earlier example, suppose a team is choosing between 100 or 200 patients per group in the second trial to replicate a previous positive finding based

Table 4.3 Average probability of replicating an earlier positive finding in a new trial with two possible choices of sample size per group	One-sided P-value in the first trial	Average replication Probability, $n = 100$	Average replication probability, $n = 200$
	0.0001	0.953	0.988
	0.0005	0.911	0.971
	0.000625	0.902	0.967
	0.001	0.883	0.958
	0.0025	0.833	0.930
	0.005	0.784	0.899
	0.01	0.723	0.855
	0.025	0.620	0.771

on 64 patients per group. The team wonders what the average replication probability would be. The team could substitute 64 for m and 100 (200) for n in (4.6) and arrive at the results in Table 4.3.

The average replication probability increases as the sample size for the new trial increases. This is easy to understand since the power of a hypothesis test increases with sample size and the average replication probability is just a weighted average of the statistical power at possible values of the treatment effect.

We would like to remind our readers that we work on the P-value scale in this chapter. For an observed treatment effect in a smaller study to produce the same P-value as that in a larger study, the observed treatment effect in the smaller study has to be numerically larger (assuming that larger values are more desirable). This can be seen from (4.1) or (4.2). This is different from the situation when we work on the treatment effect scale and hope to replicate the treatment effect observed in an earlier trial.

4.4 Differentiate Between Statistical Power and the Probability of a Successful Trial

Assuming that the success of a trial is defined by having a P-value smaller than the pre-specified significance level, the average replication probability can be regarded as the probability of getting a successful trial. This probability takes into account our knowledge about the effect of a new treatment and the uncertainty in our knowledge. While the calculation of the average replication probability builds on the concept of statistical power, it differs from statistical power because the average replication probability does not condition on a specific treatment effect.

As the development program progresses, we will have more information about a new drug. The information could be integrated to convey our cumulative knowledge about the drug. This integrated knowledge could take the place of the distribution $f(.)$ in (4.4).

Another difference between statistical power and the success probability is that we can make the statistical power close to 100% by simply increasing the sample size. By comparison, if evidence about a new drug is scanty or prior evidence suggests a very small treatment effect, then the success probability will be low even if the next trial has a very large sample size. In this regard, the success probability offers useful information beyond statistical power, especially when the development has moved to the late stage. We will revisit this point in Chap. 9 and particularly in Sect. 9.3.

4.5 Replicability

Benjamini (2020) defined replicability of results as "replicating the entire study, from enlisting subjects through collecting data, and analyzing the results, in a similar but not necessarily identical way, yet get essentially the same results." He argued that independent replication of results with P-value < 0.05 by 2 investigators is scientifically stronger than a single P-value < 0.005. Benjamini (2020) noted that replicating others' work is a way of life in the scientific world.

It is important to differentiate between replicability and reproducibility. Reproducibility is the ability to get the same results (e.g., tables and figures) as reported by others from the original data through separate and independent analysis. Replicability, on the other hand, refers to the generation of new data in additional experiments to validate previously reported results.

In this chapter, we treat the terms *replicability* and *replication* interchangeably. In the context of drug development, both refer to our ability to observe a positive treatment effect in a subsequent trial after a positive finding initially. The average replication probability we introduced in this chapter is an effort to quantify this probability.

There has been an increasing interest in the root cause for the disappointingly low replication probability in scientific research (Gibson, 2020). This has led to numerous debates on the basis upon which we draw inferences. We discussed some factors that have contributed to the replication crisis in Chap. 2 (see Sects. 2.10–2.13). Among these factors, selective inference is a major contributor.

There are other forms of selection that can inflate our expectation of a positive treatment effect. By design, a drug developer only moves forward candidates that have demonstrated positive results in earlier trials. This selection, while logical, creates a selection bias in estimating treatment effects in these selected trials. We will return to this topic in Chap. 12.

4.6 Summary

Replication is a cornerstone for establishing credible scientific evidence. This is part of the reason why the US Food and Drug Administration usually requires at least two adequate and well-controlled studies, each convincing on its own, to establish the effectiveness of a new pharmaceutical product.

In this chapter, we examine replication from different perspectives. From our experience, we have found the analogy between clinical trials at the various stages of a product development and diagnostic tests with different precision very useful. It is easy to communicate to non-statistician colleagues the critical role of replication by using this analogy. This analogy is not new. It was used in a paper by Lee and Zelen (2000) at the turn of the century. Despite its early use, the analogy does not appear to have been broadly picked up by statisticians or drug developers.

Chuang-Stein and Kirby (2014) encouraged statisticians to remain cool-headed in the presence of overwhelming positive but isolated trial results. They also encouraged statisticians to help dispel the myth surrounding the shrinking or disappearing treatment effect to non-statistician colleagues. The latter is the focus of Chap. 12.

For simplicity, we dichotomized a drug to have a clinically meaningful treatment effect or not. This simplification reflects the binary outcome of the drug approval process. At times, the threshold for a meaningful treatment effect may be determined by an effect necessary to make the drug commercially competitive. Despite the implicit assumption of a threshold for the dichotomization, we did not incorporate any requirement on the size of the estimated treatment effect in any replication probability calculation in this chapter. We will discuss the inclusion of this additional requirement as part of the definition of a successful trial in Sect. 9.3 in Chap. 9.

References

Benjamini, Y. (2020). *Replicability problems in science: It's not the p-values' fault*, presented at a webinar hosted by the National Institute of Statistical Sciences, May 6. Available at https://www.niss.org/news/niss-webinar-hosts-third-webinar-use-p-values-making-decisions. Accessed 12 February 2021.

Chuang-Stein, C. (2006). Sample size and the probability of a successful trial. *Pharmaceutical Statistics, 5*(4), 305–309.

Chuang-Stein, C., & Kirby, S. (2014). The shrinking or disappearing observed treatment effect. *Pharmaceutical Statistics, 13*(5), 277–280.

Gibson, E. W. (2020). The role of p-values in judging the strength of evidence and realistic replication expectations. *Statistics in Biopharmaceutical Research*. https://doi.org/10.1080/19466315.2020.1724560

Hung, H. M. J., & O'Neill, R. T. (2003). Utilities of the P-value distribution associated with effect size in clinical trials. *Biometrical Journal, 45*(6), 659–669.

Kesselheim, A. S., Hwang, T. J., & Franklin, J. M. (2015). Two decades of new drug development for central nervous system disorders. *Nature Reviews Drug Discovery, 14*(12), 815–816.

Lee, S. J., & Zelen, M. (2000). Clinical trials and sample size considerations: Another perspective. *Statistical Science, 15*(2), 95–110.

O'Neill, R. T. (1997). Secondary endpoints cannot be validly analyzed if the primary endpoint does not demonstrate clear statistical significance. *Controlled Clinical Trials, 18*(6), 550–556.

Pereira, T. V., Horwitz, R. I., & Ioannidis, J. P. A. (2012). Empirical evaluation of very large treatment effects of medical intervention. *Journal of the American Medical Association, 308*(16), 1676–1684.

Zuckerman, D. M., Jury, N. J., & Sicox, C. E. (2015). 21st century cures act and similar policy efforts: at what cost? *British Medical Journal, 351*, h6122.

Chapter 5
Incorporating Information from Completed Trials and Other Sources in Future Trial Planning

Data! Data! Data! I can't make bricks without clay.
—Sir Arthur Conan Doyle

5.1 Introduction

In Chap. 4, we looked at calculating the average replication probability by averaging the conditional replication probability for a given treatment effect using a weight which reflects the likelihood of the given treatment effect. In this chapter, we consider the Bayesian approach to inference which allows distributions for unknown parameters such as a parameter representing a treatment effect. In this framework, the average replication probability with likelihood replaced by a prior distribution for the treatment effect becomes a probability known as an assurance probability (O'Hagan et al., 2005). We consider how a prior distribution may be obtained from the results of a previous trial and used to calculate an assurance probability for a new trial.

We proceed to look at various closed-form expressions for assurance probabilities where the probability of interest is the probability of a statistically significant result at some pre-specified significance level. When a closed-form expression for an assurance calculation is not available, we illustrate how a simulation approach can be used to carry out the calculation. We also consider assurance calculations where, in addition to requiring that a null hypothesis is rejected, a second requirement is placed on the observed treatment effect.

We assume that for a treatment to be successful, the true treatment effect needs to be greater than some minimum value. We go on to consider the PPV and NPV of a new trial using a prior distribution for the treatment effect. These quantities give summaries of the worth of a positive or negative result from a planned trial with respect to correctly identifying whether the true treatment effect is at least as big as desired.

C. Chuang-Stein and S. Kirby, *Quantitative Decisions in Drug Development*, Springer Series in Pharmaceutical Statistics, https://doi.org/10.1007/978-3-030-79731-7_5

It may be the case that there are a number of previous clinical trials which can be considered similar to a planned trial. If this is the case, then a Bayesian hierarchical model can be used to derive a prior. We briefly outline this approach.

There are times when it may not be possible or appropriate to use the results from previous trials of the same drug to derive a prior distribution for an unknown treatment effect. In such cases, we need to consider alternative approaches. For example, for a Phase 2 proof-of-concept study of an unprecedented compound, one alternative is to consider using a prior distribution representing the treatment effect sizes observed in previous Phase 2 proof-of-concept studies for other unprecedented compounds. Another alternative is to elicit a prior distribution from experts.

For Phase 2b and Phase 3 trials, other alternative approaches include using PK/PD modeling and/or model-based meta-analysis (MBMA) to obtain a plausible prior distribution for the treatment effect expected in Phase 2b or Phase 3 trials. We include two examples of an MBMA using a PK/PD model in this chapter.

In the final part of the chapter, we consider the important topic of the use of historical control data. There may be compelling ethical, logistical and financial reasons for using historical control data. We share an example where historical control data were used in the evaluation and ultimate approval of Brineura® (cerliponase alfa) by the US FDA in 2017 for slowing the loss of ambulation in symptomatic pediatric patients 3 years or older with late infantile neuronal ceroid lipofuscinosis type 2.

5.2 The Bayesian Approach to Inference

The Bayesian approach to inference enables relevant information to be included in an analysis. This is done by using a prior distribution $p(\theta)$ which represents our understanding or beliefs for unknown parameters θ (Hobbs & Carlin, 2008). Inference is conducted on the posterior distribution for θ given the data using Bayes rule. Using y to denote a vector of data, the Bayes rule generates the posterior distribution of θ given y, i.e., $p(\theta|y)$ as shown in (5.1)

$$p(\theta|y) = \frac{p(\theta, y)}{p(y)} = \frac{p(y|\theta)p(\theta)}{\int p(y|\theta)p(\theta)d\theta} \tag{5.1}$$

The posterior distribution $p(\theta|y)$ is equal to the likelihood of the data, $p(y|\theta)$, multiplied by the prior distribution $p(\theta)$ and divided by the probability of the data. Thus, prior information about the parameters is combined with data to produce an updated distribution for the parameters. This posterior distribution may then be used as a prior distribution with future data. The posterior distribution can also be used to calculate values and probabilities of interest for the parameters.

The integral in (5.1) and further required integrals may be difficult to solve directly but can be evaluated numerically using modern Markov chain Monte Carlo methods (Lunn et al., 2013) as programmed in Statistics packages such as WinBUGS

(WinBUGS) and OpenBUGS (OpenBUGS) and in the SAS procedure PROC MCMC
(SAS, 2020).

5.3 Bayesian Average Power and Assurance

O'Hagan et al. (2005) defined assurance as

$$\int P(R|\boldsymbol{\theta})p(\boldsymbol{\theta})d\boldsymbol{\theta} \tag{5.2}$$

where R is an event of interest such as rejecting the null hypothesis, $p(R|\boldsymbol{\theta})$ is the
probability of R given $\boldsymbol{\theta}$ and $p(\boldsymbol{\theta})$ is the prior probability distribution for $\boldsymbol{\theta}$. If we let R
represent rejection of a null hypothesis, then the assurance probability is the expected
(or average) power where the averaging is with respect to the prior distribution. The
average replication probability described in Chapter 4 is a special case of assurance
where average is with respect to the sampling distribution of an estimator for $\boldsymbol{\theta}$,
obtained from the previous trial.

Thus, if we have a prior distribution we can use (5.2) to calculate the expected
power for a new trial with a particular trial design. The advantage of calculating the
expected power, as summarized in Chap. 4, is that given a relevant prior the assurance
probability takes account of uncertainty in the treatment effect to give a more realistic
assessment of the probability of rejecting the null hypothesis.

Suppose there is a previous trial with data that can be considered exchangeable
with the data to be produced from a planned trial, then we can use the results from
the previous trial to generate a prior distribution for the treatment effect for the
planned trial. Informally, exchangeable here means that the data to be obtained in
the planned trial are expected to be similar to that obtained in the previous trial. One
way to generate a prior distribution using data from a previous trial is to start with
a so-called vague, objective or reference prior and to combine this prior with the
data from the trial using Bayes rule as described above. Such a prior is only weakly
informative about the treatment effect so that the posterior distribution obtained is
dominated by the data from the trial. The posterior distribution then becomes the
prior distribution for the next trial and can be used in a calculation of an assurance
probability.

As an example, we consider the mean of a Normal distribution with known variance. If we initially start with a Normal prior distribution with mean μ_0 and variance
τ_0^2 and combine this with the likelihood for n independent observations $y_1, \ldots y_n$ from
a Normal distribution with mean θ and known variance σ^2, the posterior distribution
is Normal with mean

$$\mu_n = \frac{\frac{1}{\tau_0^2}\mu_0 + \frac{n}{\sigma^2}\bar{y}}{\frac{1}{\tau_0^2} + \frac{n}{\sigma^2}} \tag{5.3}$$

and variance τ_n^2 where

$$\frac{1}{\tau_n^2} = \frac{1}{\tau_0^2} + \frac{n}{\sigma^2} \tag{5.4}$$

and $\bar{y}$ is the mean of $\{y_i, i = 1,\ldots,n\}$. Letting the prior precision $\frac{1}{\tau_0^2}$ become small (or τ_0^2 to become very large) corresponds to the use of a vague prior distribution and the posterior distribution then tends to a Normal distribution with mean $\bar{y}$ and variance $\frac{\sigma^2}{n}$. This distribution is the same as the sampling distribution of the mean from a Normal distribution with a known variance.

Trying to define a vague prior is an old problem in Statistics, and some care needs to be taken to ensure that the prior used is not more informative than desired. For many common situations, suitable vague priors are readily available (Lunn et al., 2013). When there are a number of previous trials which can be considered to be similar to the planned trial, we can alternatively consider the use of a Bayesian hierarchical model to generate a suitable prior distribution. We will return to this topic later in this chapter.

5.4 Closed-Form Expressions for Assurance and the Simulation Approach

One closed-form expression for the assurance probability for rejecting the null hypothesis

$$H_0 : \mu_{\text{drug}} - \mu_{\text{placebo}} \leq 0$$

versus the one-sided alternative

$$H_A : \mu_{\text{drug}} - \mu_{\text{placebo}} > 0$$

using a critical value for a one-sided test has already been given in Chap. 4 for the case where the difference in sample mean responses in two treatment groups follows a Normal distribution and a Normal "prior" $N\left(d; \frac{2\sigma^2}{n}\right)$ is used. Assuming a one-sided significance level of α, the assurance probability can be written slightly more generally as in (5.5). For a confirmatory trial, α typically takes the value of 0.025.

$$P\left(\bar{X}_{\text{drug}} - \bar{X}_{\text{placebo}} > \sqrt{\tau}Z_\alpha\right) = 1 - \Phi\left(\frac{\sqrt{\tau}Z_\alpha - d}{\sqrt{\tau + \frac{2}{n}\sigma^2}}\right) \tag{5.5}$$

In (5.5), $\tau = \frac{\sigma^2}{n_{\mathrm{drug}}} + \frac{\sigma^2}{n_{\mathrm{placebo}}}$ is the variance for the difference in sample means for the planned trial when n_{drug} and n_{placebo} subjects receive drug and placebo, respectively. The assurance probability in (5.5) is equivalent to the average replication probability when the sample size for the two studies is allowed to differ as discussed in Sect. 4.3.3.

One can compare the expression in (5.5) to the power function for declaring a significant treatment effect when the true effect is given by d in (5.6).

$$\text{Power(treatment effect is } d) = 1 - \Phi\left(\frac{\sqrt{\tau}Z_\alpha - d}{\sqrt{\tau}}\right) \tag{5.6}$$

When $\sqrt{\tau}Z_\alpha = d$. (the numerator of the expression inside $\Phi(.)$ in (5.5) and (5.6) are equal to 0), both the assurance and the power are 50%. When $\sqrt{\tau}Z_\alpha > d$, both the assurance and the power are less than 50%, but the assurance will be greater than the power. When $\sqrt{\tau}Z_\alpha < d$, both the assurance and the power are greater than 50% with power greater than the assurance.

For a non-inferiority trial with n patients in each treatment group, assume that the null hypothesis is formulated as $\Delta \leq -\Delta*$ where Δ is the true difference in treatment means and $\Delta* (>0)$ is a clinically meaningful difference. For a difference in means which is Normally distributed and the same prior as used above for testing for superiority, it can be shown that the assurance probability can be calculated as

$$P\left(\overline{X}_{\mathrm{drug}} - \overline{X}_{\mathrm{placebo}} > -\Delta* + \sqrt{\tau}Z_\alpha\right) = 1 - \Phi\left(\frac{\sqrt{\tau}Z_\alpha - d - \Delta*}{\sqrt{\tau + \frac{2}{n}\sigma^2}}\right) \tag{5.7}$$

Similar to the expression in (5.5), α is typically set at 0.025 for confirmatory non-inferiority trials.

Further examples of closed-form expressions for assurance calculations are given in O'Hagan et al. (2005).

In general, closed-form expressions for the assurance probability may not be available. When this is the case, we can use simulation to estimate an assurance probability to the desired degree of precision. To illustrate this, we consider the case of a one-sided test for superiority as above but now assume that the common variance is unknown with a prior distribution. In this case, we can simulate an assurance probability using the following steps:

1. Select the total number of iterations N. Set the counter for iteration number I to 1 and initiate the number of significant results P to zero.
2. Sample Δ and σ^2 from their joint prior distribution (if the priors are assumed independent then the joint distribution is the product of the priors).
3. Simulate a difference in sample means $(\overline{x}_{\mathrm{drug}} - \overline{x}_{\mathrm{placebo}})$ and a sample variance $\hat{\sigma}^2$ using the sampled Δ and σ^2.
4. Increment P if the test statistic $t = \frac{\overline{x}_{\mathrm{drug}} - \overline{x}_{\mathrm{placebo}}}{\sqrt{\frac{\hat{\sigma}^2}{n_{\mathrm{drug}}} + \frac{\hat{\sigma}^2}{n_{\mathrm{placebo}}}}} \geq t_{\alpha, n_{\mathrm{drug}} + n_{\mathrm{placebo}} - 2}$.
5. Increment I. If $I < N$ then go to Step 2.

6.   Estimate the assurance probability by dividing P by N.

The above steps produce an estimate for the assurance probability which in this case is defined as the probability of rejecting a null hypothesis. One can also use the above steps to calculate the probability that the treatment effect is statistically significant, and the true treatment effect is at least equal to some value Δ_{min}. This joint probability can be obtained by adding the requirement $\Delta > \Delta_{min}$ at Step 4.

Instead of defining a trial success by a statistically significant treatment effect, one could require additionally that the observed (or estimated) treatment effect be greater than Δ_0. In this case, we need to add the requirement $\bar{x}_{drug} - \bar{x}_{placebo} > \Delta_0$ at Step 4 when calculating the assurance probability.

Throughout the rest of the book, we use the simulation approach to calculating assurance and related probabilities. We take this approach for consistency and ease of generalization because closed-form expressions for assurance probabilities only exist for simple situations. In practice, the precision of simulation results can be made sufficiently high by employing a large number of simulation runs. In addition, we feel that describing the simulation steps can help readers better understand the definition of an expression and the impact of the various components making up the expression.

5.5   PPV and NPV for a Planned Trial

The positive predictive value (PPV) and negative predictive value (NPV), introduced in Chap. 3, can be written for an additional required minimum true treatment effect, Δ_{min}, in a trial as

$$PPV = P(\Delta \geq \Delta_{min}|Pos) = \frac{P(Pos \text{ and } \Delta \geq \Delta_{min})}{P(Pos)}$$

and

$$NPV = P(\Delta < \Delta_{min}|Neg) = \frac{P(Neg \text{ and } \Delta < \Delta_{min})}{P(Neg)}$$

where *Pos* represents rejection of the null hypothesis and *Neg* represents failure to reject the null hypothesis. Both the numerator and denominator in each case can be derived from assurance calculations given a prior probability distribution for the treatment effect.

To illustrate, we take a modified example from the literature (Kowalski et al., 2008a, 2008b). The example relates to a compound SC-75416 which was a selective COX-2 inhibitor being developed for the treatment of acute and chronic pain. The endpoint of interest in a planned dental pain study was TOTPAR6, the total pain relief over the first 6 h post tooth extraction. TOTPAR6 is a time-weighted sum of

Table 5.1 Classification of decisions for combinations of decision and truth

		Truth		Total
		$\Delta < 3$	$\Delta \geq 3$	
Decision	Do not reject H_0	Correct No-Go	Incorrect No-Go	P(No-Go)
	Reject H_0	Incorrect Go	Correct Go	P(Go)
	Total	$P(\Delta < 3)$	$P(\Delta \geq 3)$	1.00

the pain relief (PR) scores over the 6-h period (see (5.9) in Sect. 5.9). The PR score at each hourly time point is measured on a 5-point Likert scale (0–4, PR $= 0$, no relief; PR $= 4$, complete relief). Therefore, TOTPAR6 can take a value between 0 and 24 with higher values corresponding to more pain relief.

The prior distribution for the treatment effect was derived from a PK/PD model, a topic we return to later in this chapter but for now we simply note that the modeling gave a Normal prior distribution for the treatment effect (over 400 mg ibuprofen) with mean 3.27 and standard deviation 0.60. We assume that the difference in mean TOTPAR6 for a new study is Normally distributed and that the common standard deviation of TOTPAR6 is 7. The new study is planned to be a parallel group study with 100 patients in each of the two groups (SC-75416 and ibuprofen).

Suppose that a successful trial is defined by rejecting the one-sided null hypothesis

$$\mu_{\text{drug}} - \mu_{\text{placebo}} \leq 0$$

at the 2.5% significance level. We require the true treatment effect to be at least 3 points in favor of the drug treatment (over 400 mg ibuprofen) for the new drug to be of interest. We can use the simulation steps similar to those described in Sect. 5.4 to calculate the probabilities in Table 5.1 with the prior described above (i.e., $N(3.27;(0.6)^2)$). As the common standard deviation is assumed known and is not estimated, a Z-test is used for the difference in means. The results obtained below differ little from those that would be obtained if the standard deviation were estimated and a t-test used. In general, there will be little difference between the use of a Z-test and a t-test for the sample sizes usually used in clinical trials. We assume that failure to reject the null hypothesis results in a No-Go decision and rejection of the null hypothesis leads to a Go decision.

Based on 10,000 simulation samples using the Statistics package R (R Core Team, 2020), we obtained the estimated probabilities in Table 5.2.

We can see that the probability for rejecting the null hypothesis is 0.88, but we can also see that this includes a probability of 0.25 of rejecting the null hypothesis when the true treatment effect is not as big as the desired 3-point difference.

We can work out the estimated PPV and NPV using the estimated probabilities in Table 5.2. Doing this, we obtain

$$\text{PPV} = \frac{0.63}{0.88} = 0.72$$

Table 5.2 Estimated probabilities for combinations of decision and truth for 10,000 simulated trials

		Truth		Total
		$\Delta < 3$	$\Delta \geq 3$	
Decision	Do not reject H$_0$	0.08	0.04	0.12
	Reject H$_0$	0.25	0.63	0.88
	Total	0.33	0.67	1.00

and

$$\text{NPV} = \frac{0.08}{0.12} = 0.67$$

Thus, a positive result gives a probability of 0.72 that the true treatment effect is greater than or equal to the required 3 points. We can compare this with the probability of getting a difference of at least 3 points before the trial, which was 0.67. Thus, a positive result would increase our confidence that the true treatment difference is at least 3 points from 67 to 72%. Similarly, a negative result increases the probability of a treatment difference less than 3 from 33 to 67%.

5.6 Forming a Prior Distribution from a Number of Similar Previous Trials

It may be the case that the results from a number of previous trials are available when a new trial is being planned. If the parameters representing the treatment effects can be viewed as exchangeable, then we can consider using a Bayesian hierarchical model to combine information from these past trials. As described previously, exchangeable is informally taken to mean similar.

A Bayesian hierarchical model (Spiegelhalter et al., 2004) assumes that parameters of interest are drawn from some common prior distribution. The Normal hierarchical model assumes that the parameters representing the treatment effect in the different trials, say $\theta_1, \ldots, \theta_K$, have a Normal distribution so

$$\theta_k \sim N(\mu; \tau^2), \ k = 1, \ldots, K$$

The parameters μ and τ are in turn assigned prior distributions, usually vague and estimated from the data.

A prior for a new trial can be formed by using the posterior distribution for θ obtained from combining the data for the previous trials with the hierarchical prior distribution.

Bayesian hierarchical modeling can also be used to derive a predictive distribution for a response for a marketed biological drug when a manufacturer desires to develop a biosimilar. In this case, the trial results for the marketed drug are used to derive the predictive distribution for the response which is expected to be similar to that for the biosimilar. In this setting, a nonparametric model for the responses in different trials may be more appropriate than the assumption of a Normal distribution (Lunn et al., 2013).

5.7   Standard Prior Distributions

It may be the case that there are no previous data for a compound that can satisfactorily be relied upon to form a prior distribution for a treatment effect. For example, this may arise for a Phase 2 proof-of-concept study when no previous efficacy data exist. In these circumstances, it may be possible to obtain a relevant standard prior distribution using data from other compounds.

For the particular case of a Phase 2 proof-of-concept study, we can consider using a mixture distribution (Cornfield, 1969) which represents efficacy results for previous similar compounds. To illustrate, we conjecture that for a particular pain compound we can find previous dental pain study results for other relevant compounds that lead to using the following mixture prior for the endpoint TOTPAR6. We place a lump of 20% of the prior at the value 0 to represent the proportion of similar compounds found to have no effect. We then take the remaining 80% to be a Normal distribution centered at the assumed historical average among compounds with some effect which we take to be 2.5 with a standard deviation of 0.8. The standard deviation is also assumed to come from the same historical results. This mixture prior distribution is shown in Fig. 5.1 with the lump centered at 0 and given a width of 0.1. The use of 0.1 as the width makes the point mass visible as a bar in Fig. 5.1.

To show the effect of this prior, we use it with the same planned dental pain study as considered above, but consider the study now as a proof-of-concept study without any previous efficacy data for the compound and use a Z-test with a one-sided 5%

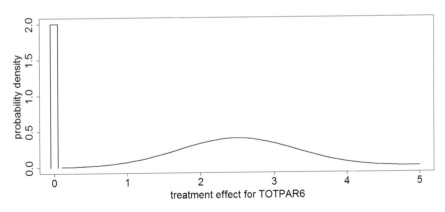

Fig. 5.1 Mixture prior distribution for the dental pain example

Table 5.3 Estimated probabilities for combinations of decision and truth for 10,000 simulated trials

		Truth		Total
		$\Delta < 3$	$\Delta \geq 3$	
Decision	Do not reject H_0	0.38	0.01	0.39
	Reject H_0	0.41	0.20	0.61
	Total	0.79	0.21	1.00

significance level. Estimated probabilities from the simulation approach for 10,000 samples for a given random number seed are given in Table 5.3.

We can see that the PPV is $0.20/0.61 = 0.33$ so that there is a one-third chance that the true treatment effect is at least 3 points on the TOTPAR6 scale after a positive outcome from the POC trial.

5.8 Elicitation of a Prior Distribution from Experts

Another option when no previous data for a compound that can satisfactorily be relied on to form a prior distribution exists is to elicit a prior distribution from experts.

Kinnersley and Day (2013) give an overview of methods of elicitation. After noting that an expert can be defined in a number of ways, they go on to consider frameworks for conducting an elicitation session. They list six steps described in Choy et al. (2009) which are present in a number of frameworks. These six steps are:

- determining the purpose and motivation for using prior information
- specifying the relevant expert knowledge available
- formulating the statistical model
- designing effective and efficient numerical encoding
- managing uncertainty
- designing a practical elicitation protocol.

Kinnersley and Day (2013) note that none of the frameworks for elicitation they describe uses the more prescriptive questioning advocated by Kynn (2008). The prescriptive questioning advocated by Kynn is based on her assessment of recent advances in the psychology and cognitive models literature.

Kinnersley and Day include in their paper a protocol developed for an elicitation session for a hypothetical clinical trial using the SHELF (O'Hagan et al., 2006) system. The protocol contains sections on endpoint definition, evidence, plausible treatment effect range and a description of the chips in bins elicitation method (Gore, 1987), probability distribution fitting for each expert, group elicitation, probability distribution fitting for the group with feedback and chosen distribution with discussion.

Walley et al. (2015) describe elicitation of prior distributions for the placebo response and treatment effect for a case study in chronic kidney disease. The prior distribution for the placebo response was equivalent to approximately 113 subjects in a parallel study design and was used both to assess the study design and in the analysis. In contrast, the prior distribution for the treatment effect was used only to assess the study design.

Kinnersley and Day conclude in their paper that further empirical research on the feasibility of conducting elicitation is required as well as more research to establish the measurement science properties of the available elicitation instruments in the clinical trial domain.

5.9 Prior Distributions from PK/PD Modeling and Model-Based Meta-Analysis

It may be the case, particularly for Phase 2b and Phase 3 trials, that there is not a previous trial for the same endpoint and same population as intended for a Phase 3 trial. This can come about because of the practice of using shorter term endpoints in early Phase 2 trials and/or the tendency for the patient population to become more heterogeneous as development moves to Phase 3. In these cases, it may be considered inappropriate to directly extrapolate a Phase 2 result to a different endpoint and/or to a markedly different population.

PK/PD modeling is the modeling of a pharmacodynamic (PD) response (what the drug does to the body for a certain response) using pharmacokinetic (PK) (what the body does to the drug) data. The most common PK data used in PK/PD modeling are drug concentrations. PK/PD modeling may be able to address the issues of using a different endpoint or enrolling a different population by applying a plausible model for the PK/PD relationship for the endpoint of interest in different types of individuals. Such a model may be assumed from known clinical pharmacology theory or modeling strength borrowed from other compounds expected to have a similar PK/PD relationship. If the model is fitted using a Bayesian approach, then the posterior distribution for the treatment effect can be obtained from the model.

Model-based meta-analysis (MBMA) is the meta-analysis of data using a model (Lalonde et al., 2007). While it can be argued that most meta-analyses assume a parametric model, the terminology is taken here to mean a model based on clinical pharmacology theory. Thus, a PK/PD analysis as described above could be a meta-analysis combining data from different sources using an appropriate PK/PD model. Alternatively, a model-based meta-analysis might be a meta-analysis of dose–response relationships using a dose–response model. The idea is to borrow strength about unknown relationships from other compounds that can be considered similar to the compound of interest. If the fitting is carried out using Bayesian methods, then a posterior distribution for the treatment effect of interest can be obtained.

An example of an MBMA involving the use of a PK/PD model is given by the COX-2 inhibitor compound development program referred to in Sect. 5.5 (Kowalski et al., 2008a). For this compound, a logistic-Normal PK/PD model was developed to model the pain relief (PR) scores at time t_j described in Sect. 5.5. The model was

$$logit\left(Pr\left(PR_{ij} \geq m|\eta_i\right)\right) = f_p\left(t_j, m\right) + f_d\left(c_{ij}\right) + \left(t_j\right)^{\chi}\eta_i \qquad (5.8)$$

where PR_{ij} denotes pain relief for the ith subject at time t_j on the 5-point scale (0–4) represented by m, η_i is a random effect for the ith subject, $f_p(t_j, m)$ is a function describing the placebo-time effect, $f_d(c_{ij})$ is a function describing the drug effect as a function of the observed plasma concentration c_{ij}, and χ (the exponent of t_j) is a variance scale parameter to allow for interpatient variability to depend on time. Kowalski et al. (2008a) proposed submodels for f_p and f_d. It was assumed that all non-steroidal anti-inflammatory drugs (NSAIDs, which include COX-2 inhibitors) can achieve the same maximum drug effect and they differ only in potency.

Kowalski et al. estimated the logit model in (5.8) for $m = 1,\dots, 4$ using data from SC-75416, rofecoxib and valdecoxib postoral surgery pain studies. Three of the valdecoxib studies contained 400 mg ibuprofen as an active control. They used the estimated logit model together with a dropout model to simulate PR scores and dropout time for each of 50,000 hypothetical patients at each of the doses of the drugs included in the studies. The simulated PR scores at the simulated dropout times were set to missing and replaced by the last "observed" simulated PR score before dropout. We want to remind our readers that the work by Kowalski et al. was done at a time when "last observation carried forward" approach was a common approach for handling missing data. More principled approaches to manage missing data have emerged in the past decade.

The PR score-time profile for each hypothetical patient (indexed by i) was used to calculate the TOTPAR6 for the patient using the equation in (5.9). In (5.9), t_0 is set to 0. The mean of the 50,000 TOTPAR6s is an estimate for the population mean at a specific dose of a drug. These estimates were compared to their observed counterparts from studies to check for the goodness of fit of the models. The means were then used to simulate data to evaluate study designs.

$$TOTPAR6_i = \sum_{j=1}^{6} PR_{ij} \times \left(t_j - t_{j-1}\right) \qquad (5.9)$$

Milligan et al. (2013) gave an example of using PK/PD modeling to estimate the clinical benefit and risk of a new anticoagulant when planning a Phase 2 dose-ranging study of the drug in patients following total hip and knee replacement surgery. Benefit of the new anticoagulant was to be measured in terms of venous thromboembolism (VTE) prevention, and risk was to be measured in terms of major bleeding (MB) incidence. At the time the Phase 2 study was planned, there were no data on the drug's effect on VTE prevention and MB risk. But, there were data on the drug's effect in inhibiting thrombin generation through an in vitro PD assay. The development team built a PK/PD model, linking results from the in vitro PD assay to clinical outcomes of VTE and MB. Data used in the estimation of the model came from 21 other anticoagulant compounds. The model is a logistic regression model that specifies the same shape of the dose–response relationship but different potencies across different compounds.

The fitted model was used to predict the effect of the new anticoagulant on VTE and MB at various doses, based on the drug's effect in inhibiting thrombin generation. This information was used to determine the dose range for the Phase 2 dose-ranging study. The PK/PD modeling together with a design that allowed doses to be dropped or added led to a successful Phase 2 trial. We describe in details how the modeling work led to the choice of the dose range and how the uncertainty surrounding this choice led the developer of the new anticoagulant to conduct an adaptive dose-ranging study in Chap. 13 (see Sect. 13.5).

The development of PK/PD models to synthesize prior data requires collaboration among multiple disciplines. The process demands good clinical, pharmacological and statistical principles. Close collaboration will have the best chance to produce the most interpretable models that take into consideration sources of variability and are transparent in their assumptions.

5.10 The Use of Historical Control Data

So far, we have focused on prior information that may shed light on the effect of a new treatment. In this section, we will focus on prior information pertaining to a control that could be used in an upcoming trial.

As noted by Galwey (2016), there are compelling ethical, logistical and financial reasons for supplementing the evidence from a new trial with historical control data. Many methods have been proposed in the literature and these have been summarized recently by, for example, the Drug Information Association Adaptive Design Scientific Working Group (Ghadessi et al., 2020). We review some of these methods here. An example of an evaluation of a design for a particular method of using historical control data is described in Chap. 7.

Before we review some of the methods for using historical control data, we briefly consider potential sources and some criteria for the selection of appropriate control data.

Historical control data can come from a number of different sources (Ghadessi et al., 2020). The best source is prior trials of the same investigational product or of other treatments intended for the same target population. Other sources include an individual patient's medical history and patient registries. Patient registries are organized systems that use observational methods to collect specified outcomes in a population of interest. A further source is natural history trials that track the natural course of a disease. These differ from registries in that they can be designed to collect very comprehensive data to describe the disease. As noted by Ghadessi et al., care must be taken about the possibility of patient selection bias when patients selected from these sources do not match those planned for the new trial.

There may be many biases in using historical controls. Ghadessi et al. suggest minimizing them by starting with choosing high quality historical control data and designing the new study in patients with characteristics well-represented in historical controls. Adapting criteria suggested by Pocock (1976), they propose choosing historical controls with the same inclusion/exclusion criteria, type of study design, well-known prognostic factors, study quality and treatment for the control group. They also propose including concurrent controls or adjusting for time dependent shifts.

We now consider some quantitative methods for using appropriately chosen historical control data.

5.10.1 Methods When There Are No Concurrent Controls

Ideally, at least some current controls will be included in a clinical trial, but there may be cases where this is not possible or there is a high degree of confidence that historical control data adequately represent the responses that would be observed in the current trial. In this situation, methods that have been suggested for use include "threshold crossing" (Eichler et al., 2016) and propensity score methods (Rosenbaum & Rubin, 1985).

Threshold crossing seeks to define thresholds for success and futility for a single-arm study from data on historical controls. The method proceeds as follows. First, agree on an appropriate definition of an estimand. Next, agree on rules for estimation of the counterfactual, the average outcome on control corresponding to a group of patients who received a new experimental treatment. Third, select a historical control cohort and estimate the counterfactual. Finally, set an efficacy and possibly a futility threshold. The threshold will be the benchmark for the primary analysis. After the single-arm study is conducted and the primary analysis is performed, additional steps include carrying out sensitivity analyses and transitioning to subsequent steps determined by the outcome and the action plan.

A propensity score is the probability of treatment assignment conditional on observed baseline covariates (Rosenbaum & Rubin, 1983). A propensity score is commonly estimated using logistic regression as in (5.10),

$$\text{logit}(Z_i) = X_i \boldsymbol{\beta} \qquad (5.10)$$

where Z is an indicator variable denoting the treatment received ($Z = 0$ for control treatment and $Z = 1$ for active treatment), X_i is the vector of measured baseline variables for the i-th individual and $\boldsymbol{\beta}$ is a vector of regression coefficients.

Austin (2011) noted that the propensity score is a balancing score that summarizes the information in the available (measured) prognostic variables. Because of this, conditional on the propensity score, the distribution of measured baseline covariates is similar between the treated and untreated subjects. As a result, propensity scores can be used to estimate a treatment effect for a single-arm clinical trial provided appropriate historical control data are available.

Propensity scores have been used in several methods to remove/reduce the effects of confounding variables when estimating treatment effects. These methods include matching patients using the propensity score, stratifying patients using the propensity score, weighing response to a treatment by the inverse of the propensity score for that treatment, and including a propensity score as a covariate in a multivariable model.

Matching is probably the most widely used method. The method forms matched sets of treated and control patients who share similar propensity scores to allow for comparability. The matching of patients can be done in different ways. A common approach is to match treated and untreated subjects who are closest to one another as measured by difference in the logit of the propensity scores subject to some maximum allowed difference. It has been suggested by Austin (Austin, 2011) that this maximum allowed difference or caliper should be 0.2 of the standard deviation of the propensity score. Once a matched sample has been formed, the treatment effect can be estimated by comparing outcomes in the matched sample.

In the extreme case, matching may be done using measured baseline covariates directly. In 2017, the Food and Drug Administration (FDA) in the USA approved Brineura® (cerliponase alga) for slowing the loss of ambulation in symptomatic pediatric patients 3 years or older with late infantile neuronal ceroid lipofuscinosis type 2 (CLN2). CLN2 is a rare, devastating neurological degenerative disease of early childhood with a relatively predictable clinical course. Prior to the Brineura approval, there was no available therapy for CLN2. Most of the materials for the remaining of this section come from the Statistical Review Report for Brineura (2017) by the FDA.

The submission package includes the following studies:

- Study 901: a natural history cohort study containing registry data. Out of 69 patients in the cohort, 42 patients were judged to be evaluable based on patient characteristics and available assessments pertinent to the submission.
- Study 201: a single-arm, 1st-in-human, dose-escalation study (24 patients enrolled, 23 completed)
- Study 202: extension of Study 201

The CLN2 rating scale was used to assess a patient's CLN2 condition in Study 201/202 and Study 901. The full-length version of the scale includes four domains (Motor, Language, Visual and Seizure). Each domain has four categories (scores 0–3) with higher categories representing a more desirable health state. A two-item short-form version, consisting of Motor and Language, was used in all of the studies. The sponsor initially proposed to use the Motor–Language total score, or rather the mean rate of decline in the total score, as the primary endpoint. The sponsor proposed to apply a one sample t-test using data in Study 201/202 with information from Study 901 as a reference.

FDA reviewers examined the administrations of the abbreviated CLN2 rating scale and found substantial differences in how they were administered in Study 201/202 and Study 901. Not only were different rater instructions were used, other different methods such as prospective and retrospective assessment were also used in Study 901 based on parental interviews with long recall periods and post hoc medical record reviews (i.e., not done by clinicians in real time). Comparing available video clips, FDA reviewers found a tendency for the Study 201/202 clinicians to offer higher Language ratings. In their opinions, the inconsistent Language domain ratings impede the interpretation and direct comparison in the proposed primary endpoint between Study 201/202 and Study 901.

By comparison, the majority of rating discrepancies observed in the Motor domain were 1-category differences. After much discussion, the FDA advised the sponsor to change the primary efficacy analysis to a responder analysis in the matched population with a responder defined as an absence of "0 or an unreversed 2-category (raw)" decline in Motor score. An unreversed 2-category decline means any decline of 2-categories or more that had not reverted to a 1-category decline (or better) as of the last recorded observation. An unreversed score of zero is a decline to 0 that had not reverted to a higher category (i.e., 1, 2 or 3) at the last recorded observation.

Matching between patients in Study 201/202 and those in Study 901 was done using 3 criteria. They are baseline Motor score, age ±3 months, and genotype defined as 0, 1 or 2 key mutations. If there was a 1 to multiple or multiple to 1 match, further matching variables were considered in the following order: detailed genotype, gender, and age of first symptom (seizure; if no seizure, look at other symptoms). The matching resulted in 17 matched pairs of patients with data at 48, 72 and 96 weeks.

Extensive discussions took place between the sponsor and the agency. In addition to endpoint selection and the analysis population, there were questions on the primary time point of evaluation, which analytical method to use and what additional analysis to conduct beyond the matched population analyses. Ultimately, the 96-week responder data in the matched populations demonstrated some sign of efficacy based on the McNemar's Exact test. This observation was supported by additional analyses of other endpoints and analyses that used all available data.

So, while data from a natural history study played an important role in the evaluation of Brineura, the evaluation was challenged by the many issues brought on by the completely historical nature of the control data in this submission. This was evidenced by the numerous correspondences between the sponsor and the US FDA and the multiple changes to the Statistical Analysis Plan.

5.10.2   Methods for Augmenting Concurrent Control Data

A key distinction for methods that augment the concurrent controls in a clinical trial with historical control data is between static and dynamic borrowing of the historical control data (Ghadessi et al., 2020). Static borrowing sets a fixed level of borrowing irrespective of evidence about consistency between the past and current data. Dynamic borrowing, in contrast, controls the level of borrowing based on the consistency of the historical control and concurrent control data.

Among some static borrowing methods, a very basic assumption is to consider that the historical control data can be pooled with the concurrent control data. This assumes that any difference is purely due to sampling variation and consequently reflects a strong assumption about the data.

A popular static borrowing method is the use of a power prior which has emerged as a useful class of informative priors when historical data are available. Ibrahim et al. (2015) describe the basic formulation of the power prior in (5.11)

$$\pi(\theta|D_0, a_0) \propto L(\theta|D_0)^{a_0}\pi_0(\theta) \tag{5.11}$$

where $0 \leq a_0 \leq 1$ is a scalar parameter, $\pi_0(\theta)$ is the initial prior for θ (the parameter of interest) before the historical data D_0 were observed, and $L(\theta|D_0)$ is the likelihood function for the historical data D_0. In many applications, $\pi_0(\theta)$ is taken to be an improper prior. Since the scalar parameter a_0 in (5.11) is between 0 and 1, the power prior in (5.11) could downweight the contribution of the historical control data.

Another static borrowing method is given by Pocock's method (Pocock, 1976; Rosmalen et al, 2018) where the historical data are assumed to be a potentially biased representation of the data in the current trial and the between-trial variance (heterogeneity) has to be specified. For a single historical control trial, the between-trial difference is defined as

$$\delta = \theta_{C_D} - \theta_{C_H}$$

where θ_{C_D} represents the response of the current controls and θ_{C_H} the response of the historical controls. Pocock's method assumes the difference is distributed as

$$\delta \sim N\left(0, \sigma_b^2\right)$$

Pocock proposed pre-specifying the between-trial variance σ_b^2 because it is likely to be poorly estimated. The above specification can be extended to include historical control data from multiple trials.

A number of dynamic borrowing methods have also been suggested. We will briefly describe five of them: test then pool, power priors without a fixed power, commensurate priors, meta-analytic predictive (MAP) priors and robust MAP priors.

The test then pool approach applies the simple idea of comparing the historical control data with the concurrent control data for consistency using a hypothesis test. If the hypothesis test is not rejected, then it is considered acceptable to pool the historical control data with concurrent control data; otherwise, the historical control data cannot be used.

We have already briefly described the power prior approach with a fixed value for the power a_0. The method can be extended to allow for a variable power decided from the data (Neuenschwander et al., 2009).

The commensurate prior approach assumes that the historic response for the controls is a non-systematically biased version of the current response (Hobbs et al., 2012; Lim et al., 2018). This approach is equivalent to Pocock's approach for control data from a single historical trial except that the between-trial variance σ_b^2 is estimated and not set in advance (van Rosmalen et al., 2018).

The meta-analytic predictive (MAP) approach assumes that, for an endpoint following a Normal distribution, the model parameters for all trials are exchangeable and drawn from the same Normal distribution (Neuenschwander et al., 2010). Consequently, we have

$$\theta_{C_{H_k}} = \mu_\theta + \eta_k, \ k = 1, \ldots, K \text{ and } \theta_{C_D} = \mu_\theta + \eta_{K+1}$$

where $\theta_{C_{H_k}}$ is the response for the kth historical control arm and θ_{C_D} is the response for the concurrent control arm, μ_θ is the population mean for these parameters and $\eta_k(k = 1, \ldots, K + 1)$ is distributed as

$$\eta_k \sim N\left(0, \sigma_\eta^2\right)$$

It is important to note that the MAP approach differs from conventional meta-analysis in that it aims to predict θ_{C_D} (the response) and not the overall mean μ_θ.

Schmidli et al. (2014) proposed a robust version of the MAP approach. Under their approach, the MAP prior is first estimated using only historical data. (it should be noted that applying this MAP prior as a prior for the control in the current trial yields the same posterior distribution for the control as performing a meta-analysis of all control data, under the above model, at the end of the trial). A less informative component is then added to the MAP prior to give a mixture prior

$$w \times \pi_{\text{MAP}} + (1 - w) \times \pi_{\text{robust}}$$

where w is a weight between 0 and 1, π_{MAP} is the MAP prior and π_{robust} is a less informative component. The weight w is given an initial value which, once data are observed, is adapted to produce a prior that provides the best prediction for the observed data (Lunn et al., 2013). The greater the consistency between the historical control data and the concurrent control data is, the larger the updated value of w will be.

Viele et al. (2014) compared a number of the methods for borrowing information from historical controls and concluded that the methods are most useful when historic and concurrent controls have similar responses. We will illustrate the use of a robustified MAP prior in a proof-of-concept trial in Chap. 7 (see Sect. 7.10.2).

5.11   Discussion

The focus of this chapter is on how to incorporate information from completed trials to help plan future trials of a new drug. Here, completed trials could mean trials involving the new drug under investigation or any trials that may provide pertinent information on the new drug. The examples of a new Cox-2 inhibitor and a new anticoagulant show how studies of other drugs could be used to help predict the effect of a new drug.

The Bayesian approach begins with a prior distribution that represents our knowledge or belief about the parameter (or parameters) of interest. The prior is joined by the likelihood function of trial data to form the posterior distribution. This posterior distribution can then be used as a prior distribution for planning the next trial and calculating assurance and/or other probabilities.

We also discuss how to select the prior. We review several options in this chapter. If an informative prior cannot be obtained, then diffuse or non-informative priors can be used.

The process to identify a prior raises the question of whether the sampling distribution of an estimate for the parameter (or parameters) could play the role of a prior distribution. After all, the majority of the commonly used approaches produce unbiased and consistent estimates when selective inference is not an issue. The standard deviation of the sampling distribution describes our uncertainty about using the estimate(s) as an approximation to the parameter(s) of interest. So, for the purpose of describing our uncertainty about the parameter(s), the sampling distribution could be a reasonable choice for this objective. We will discuss in Chap. 12 how the location parameter (typically the mean) of a sampling distribution could be adjusted to reduce the bias resulting from selection so that the adjusted sampling distribution would be a more appropriate prior for the treatment effect than the original sampling distribution.

In Chaps. 3 and 4, we used the sampling distributions to calculate the average replication probability and the average power. The calculation of these quantities is the same as that of assurance except that sampling distributions were used instead of a posterior distribution arising from an expert-provided prior or a non-informative prior. While the origins of the prior distributions differ under these two approaches, we believe both approaches are valuable in incorporating our uncertainty about the parameters when planning a future trial or assessing the operating characteristics of a study design in conjunction with a decision rule.

The use of historical control data has been an emerging topic over the last two decades because of the demand for analyses which rely on historical control data and the growing availability of historical control data. We described some methods for using historical control data in Sect. 5.10. We covered a regulatory case where approval was based on comparing a single-arm study to data from a natural history study. In addition, we refer readers to an example of an evaluation of a design using the robust MAP prior approach in Chap. 7 (See Sect. 7.10.2).

References

Austin, P. C. (2011). An introduction to propensity score methods for reducing the effects of confounding in observational studies. *Multivariate Behavioral Research, 46*(3), 399–424.

Choy, S. L., O'Leary, R., & Mengersen, K. (2009). Elicitation by design in ecology: Using expert opinion to inform priors for Bayesian statistical models. *Ecology, 90*(1), 265–277.

Cornfield, J. (1969). The Bayesian outlook and its application. *Biometrics, 25*(4), 617–657.

Eichler, H.-G., Bloechl-Daum, B., Bauer, P., et al. (2016). "Threshold-crossing": A useful way to establish the counterfactual in clinical trials? *Clinical Pharmacology and Therapeutics, 100*(6), 699–712.

FDA Statistical Reviews of Brineura. (2017). Available at https://www.accessdata.fda.gov/drugsa tfda_docs/nda/2017/761052Orig1s000TOC.cfm. Accessed 8 February 2021.

Galwey, N. W. (2016). Supplementation of a clinical trial by historical control data: Is the prospect of dynamic borrowing an illusion? *Statistics in Medicine, 36*(6), 899–916.

Ghadessi, M., Tang, R., Zhou, J., et al. (2020). A roadmap to using historical controls in clinical trials—by Drug Information Association Adaptive Design Scientific Working Group (DIA-ADSWG). *Orphanet Journal of Rare Diseases.* https://doi.org/10.1186/s13023-020-1332-x

Gore, S. M. (1987). Biostatistics and the medical research council. *Medical Research Council News, 35*, 19–21.

Hobbs, B. P., & Carlin, B. P. (2008). Practical Bayesian design and analysis for drug and device clinical trials. *Journal of Biopharmaceutical Statistics, 18*(1), 54–80.

Hobbs, B. P., Sargent, D. J., & Carlin, B. P. (2012). Commensurate priors for incorporating historical information in clinical trials using general and generalized linear models. *Bayesian Analysis, 7*(3), 639–674.

Ibrahim, J. G., Chen, M.-H., Gwon, Y., & Chen, F. (2015). The power prior: Theory and applications. *Statistics in Medicine, 34*(28), 3724–3749.

Kinnersley, N., & Day, S. (2013). Structured approach to the elicitation of expert beliefs for a Bayesian-designed clinical trial: a case study. *Pharmaceutical Statistics, 12*, 104–113.

Kowalski, K. G., Olson, S., Remmers, A. E., & Hutmacher, M. M. (2008a). Modeling and simulation to support dose selection and clinical development of SC-75416, a selective COX-2 inhibitor for the treatment of acute and chronic pain. *Clinical Pharmacology & Therapeutics, 83*(6), 857–866.

Kowalski, K. G., French, J. L., Smith, M. K., & Hutmacher, M. M. (2008b). A model-based framework for quantitative decision-making in drug development. *Presented at the American Conference on Pharmacometrics*, Tucson AZ, March 12. Abstract available at https://www.go-acop.org/assets/Legacy_ACOPs/2008ACOP/Main_Program_Presentations/abstract_kowalski.pdf. Accessed Feb 9 2021.

Kynn, M. (2008). The 'heuristics and biases' bias in expert elicitation. *Journal of the Royal Statistical Society, Series A, 171*(1), 239–264.

Lalonde, R. L., Kowalski, K. G., & Hutmacher, M. M., et al. (2007). Model-based drug development. *Clinical Pharmacology & Therapeutics, 82*(1), 21–32.

Lim, J., Walley, R., Yuan, J., et al. (2018). Minimizing patient burden through the use of historical subject-level data in innovative confirmatory trials: Review of methods and opportunities. *Therapeutic Innovation & Regulatory Science, 52*(5), 546–559.

Lunn, D., Jackson, C., Best, N., et al. (2013). *The BUGS book: A practical introduction to Bayesian analysis.* Chapman Hall/CRC Press.

Milligan, P. A., Brown, M. J., Marchant, B., et al. (2013). Model-based drug development: A rational approach to efficiently accelerate drug development. *Clinical Pharmacology & Therapeutics, 93*(6), 502–514.

Neuenschwander, B., Branson, M., & Spiegelhalter, D. (2009). A note on the power prior. *Statistics in Medicine, 28*, 3562–3566.

Neuenschwander, B., Capkun-Niggli, G., Branson, M., & Spiegelhalter, D. J. (2010). Summarizing information on controls in clinical trials. *Clinical Trials, 7*, 5–18.

O'Hagan, A., Buck, C.E., Daneshkhah, A. et al. (2006). *Uncertain judgements: Eliciting experts' probabilities.* Wiley.

O'Hagan, A., Stevens, J. W., & Campbell, M. J. (2005). Assurance in clinical trial design. *Pharmaceutical Statistics, 4*(3), 187–201.

OpenBUGS. Available at http://www.openbugs.net/w/FrontPage.

Pocock, S. J. (1976). The combination of randomized and historical controls in clinical trials. *Journal of Chronic Diseases, 29*(3), 175–188.

R Core Team. (2020). R: A language and environment for statistical computing. R Foundation for Statistical Computing, Vienna, Austria. ISBN 3-900051-07-0. http://www.R-project.org/.

Rosenbaum, P. R., & Rubin, D. B. (1983). The central role of the propensity score in observational studies for causal effects. *Biometrika, 70*(1), 41–55.

Rosenbaum, P. R., & Rubin, D. B. (1985). Constructing a control group using multivariate matched sampling methods that incorporate the propensity score. *The American Statistician, 39*(1), 33–38.

van Rosmalen, J., Dejardin, D., van Norden, Y., et al. (2018). Including historical data in the analysis of clinical trials: Is it worth the effort? *Statistical Methods in Medical Research, 27*(10), 3167–3182.

SAS (2020) SAS/Stat® User's Guide, Version 15.2. SAS Institute Inc., Cary NC.

Schmidli, H., Gsteiger, S., Roychoudhury, S., et al. (2014). Robust meta-analytic-predictive priors in clinical trials with historical control information. *Biometrics, 70*(4), 1023–1032.

Spiegelhalter, D. J., Abrams, K. R., & Myles, J. P. (2004). *Bayesian approaches to clinical trials and health-care evaluation.* Wiley.

Viele, K., Berry, S., Neuenschwander, B., et al. (2014). Use of historical control data for assessing treatment effects in clinical trials. *Pharmaceutical Statistics, 13*(1), 41–54.

Walley, R. J., Smith, C. L., Gale, J. D., & Woodward, P. (2015). Advantages of a wholly Bayesian approach to assessing efficacy in early drug development: A case study. *Pharmaceutical Statistics, 14*, 205–215.

WinBUGS. Available at http://www.mrc-bsu.cam.ac.uk/software/bugs/the-bugs-project-winbugs/.

Chapter 6
Choosing Metrics Appropriate for Different Stages of Drug Development

Without a standard there is no logical basis for making a decision or taking action.
—Joseph M. Juran

6.1 Introduction

There are many ways to design a study and set up a decision rule. Some decision rules, while appearing different, actually have very similar properties. It is, therefore, helpful to have metrics that can summarize important properties of a study design and decision rule so that designs and decision rules can be compared.

In the Frequentist framework, Type I and Type II error rates can be viewed as the default metrics. In the diagnostic world, sensitivity and specificity are well-accepted metrics. As we illustrated in Chap. 5, the ability to incorporate prior information into the design and decision process makes it possible to develop metrics that also incorporate prior information.

Chapter 1 discusses the objectives of the various stages of clinical development. As studies and decision rules are designed to address diverse objectives, it is natural to expect metrics chosen for different development stages to reflect these diverse objectives. Consequently, while some metrics may be relevant to all stages, others may be more appropriate for one stage than for others.

In this chapter, we will focus on metrics for determining if a new drug is efficacious. The focus on efficacy is due to the generally well-defined endpoints to decide the beneficial effect of a new drug. Nevertheless, the approach is equally applicable to safety endpoints if there are specific safety endpoints that can be used to anchor design considerations and decision rules.

In Sect. 6.2, we will focus on metrics for a proof-of-concept study. We will focus on dose-ranging studies and confirmatory trials in Sects. 6.3 and 6.4, respectively. In Sect. 6.5, we discuss two additional success metrics, the probability of program success (POPS) and the probability of compound success (POCS). We will discuss

© The Author(s), under exclusive license to Springer Nature Switzerland AG 2021
C. Chuang-Stein and S. Kirby, *Quantitative Decisions in Drug Development*, Springer Series in Pharmaceutical Statistics,
https://doi.org/10.1007/978-3-030-79731-7_6

briefly the use of the expected net present value as another metric in Sect. 6.6, but leave the detailed illustration of its calculation to Chap. 11 (see Sect. 11.3). In Sect. 6.6, we will also offer our readers several points to consider when selecting distributions to describe our knowledge about the effect of a new drug.

6.2 Metrics for Proof-of-Concept Studies

In Table 2.1, we described the two types of error associated with testing a simple null hypothesis H_0 against a simple alternative hypothesis H_A. The probabilities of these two types of error as well as those of correct decisions under H_0 and H_A are given in parentheses in Table 6.1.

The probabilities in Table 6.1 are conditional probabilities, conditioning on H_0 or H_A being true. The marginal probabilities are 100% in each column. A common choice for the Type I error rate α in a POC study is 10%, and a common choice for the Type II error rate β is 20%. While β is twice the value of α in this case, the ratio of the actual likelihood of a false negative to a false positive error depends on how often H_0 (or H_A) is true.

For example, if past experience in developing drugs for a particular disorder suggests a 10% success rate (i.e., H_0 of no drug effect is correct 90% of the time), this probability could be used in conjunction with the conditional probabilities in Table 6.1 to construct the unconditional probabilities in Table 6.2.

The probability of correct decisions is $0.90 \times (1 - \alpha) + 0.10 \times (1 - \beta)$. The probability of incorrect decisions is $0.90 \times \alpha + 0.10 \times \beta$. For $\alpha = 0.10$ and $\beta = 0.20$, these probabilities are 89% and 11%. Under the same assumptions, the probability of a false positive (9%) is 4.5 times that of a false negative (2%).

Since POC is usually the first time a sponsor investigates the efficacy of a drug, any speculation on the likelihood that the drug possesses a sufficient effect is likely

Table 6.1 Type I and Type II errors and their rates in testing H_0 versus H_A

	H_0 True	H_0 False
Accept H_0	Correct decision $(1 - \alpha)$	Type II error (β)
Reject H_0	Type I error (α)	Correct decision $(1 - \beta)$
Total probability	1.00	1.00

Table 6.2 Unconditional probabilities of various actions in testing H_0 versus H_A

	H_0 True	H_0 False
Accept H_0	$0.90 \times (1 - \alpha)$	$0.10 \times \beta$
Reject H_0	$0.90 \times \alpha$	$0.10 \times (1 - \beta)$
Total probability	0.90	0.10

to come from external sources. Occasionally, a sponsor may be able to construct a portfolio prior from other drugs for the same indication or drugs with the same mode of action. This is possible in a well-understood disease area with many treatment options. When a portfolio prior is possible and considered reasonable, one could consider a decision rule based on the posterior probability that the drug effect exceeds a pre-specified threshold. One can evaluate the properties of such a Bayesian decision rule as one does a Frequentist one.

More often, an informative prior is not possible or not considered reliable. In such cases, it will be better to focus on the operating characteristics of a Frequentist decision framework laid out in Table 6.1. Nevertheless, it is useful to bear in mind that because of the generally low success rate in drug development, a sponsor is more likely to commit a false positive error than a false negative error at this stage.

6.3 Metrics for Dose-Ranging Studies

According to Ruberg (1995a, 1995b), the primary objectives of a dose-ranging study are to detect a dose–response relationship, to identify clinical relevance of the response, to select a target dose and to estimate the dose–response relationship. Since some of these objectives can be addressed together, the characteristics of a design and a chosen analytical strategy to address these objectives can be assessed by the following three metrics.

Metric #1   Probability to correctly detect a positive dose–response relationship.
Metric #2   Probability to correctly identify a target dose, given that a positive dose–response relationship has been concluded. A target dose could be a dose with a minimum treatment effect or a dose that has a desired effect from the commercial perspective.
Metric #3   Relative average prediction error obtained by averaging the absolute differences between the estimated and the true dose–response values at each of the doses included in the study, and dividing the average by the absolute target effect.

The above three metrics were used by Pinheiro et al. (2010) in assessing different design options and analytical strategies in dose-ranging studies. The second metric measures the accuracy of dose selection, while the third metric assesses the average adequacy of the estimated effect at the doses included in the study.

Calculating the above metrics requires (1) estimating a dose–response relationship; (2) using the estimated dose–response relationship or a testing strategy to identify a target dose; (3) testing for a positive dose–response relationship. The required activities do not need to follow this order because one can test a positive dose–response relationship without first fitting a dose–response model as we show in Sect. 6.3.2.

6.3.1 Estimating a Dose–response Relationship

Estimating a dose–response relationship is fundamental in the analysis of a dose-ranging study. This is implied in the ICH E4 guidance document, which states that dose–response study designs should emphasize the "elucidation of the dose–response function". In this section, we will review some common dose–response models used to explore the dose–response relationship.

Let $E(Y_i)$ denote the mean response at the dose d_i. For convenience, we assume that large values of Y_i are more desirable.

6.3.1.1 E_{max} Model

Even though the Emax model originally came from describing the concentration–effect relationship based on pharmacological considerations, an Emax model has also been found to be very useful in describing dose–response relationships. Thomas et al. (2014a) reported that the sigmoid Emax model described the dose–response data well for the 33 small molecules in Pfizer's portfolio that completed Phase 2 studies between 1998 and 2009 and met the inclusion criteria for their investigation. The only exception is a single compound that had a non-monotone dose–response. Thomas et al. (2014b) reported additional work examining dose–response data for small molecules approved by the US FDA between 2009 and 2014. They found that most dose–response relationships looked like hyperbolic Emax curves.

The adequacy of the Emax model to describe dose–response relationship for biologics has been assessed by Wu et al. (2018) who examined 71 distinct biologics in 91 placebo-controlled dose–response studies published between 1995 and 2014. They found that 82% of the biologics they investigated conform to a consistent dose–response relationship that could be described by the Emax model.

The Emax model relates $E(Y_i)$ to d_i in (6.1). In (6.1), E_0 represents the mean response of the placebo group and E_{max} the maximum mean increase in the experimental group over the placebo group. ED_{50} represents the dose that gives a mean response of $E_{max}/2$ over the placebo. The parameter λ (> 0) determines the shape of the curve and is often called the "Hill" parameter. For the same E_0 and E_{max}, the larger λ is away from 1, the more sharply and quickly the dose–response curve of $E(Y_i)$ versus d_i rises to its maximum of $E_0 + E_{max}$. On the other hand, the smaller λ is away from 1, the slower the dose–response curve rises to its maximum. This relationship is shown in Fig. 6.1 for select λ values. The model in (6.1) is called a 4-parameter E_{max} model because it contains four unknown parameters.

$$E(Y_i|d_i) = E_0 + E_{max} \times \frac{d_i^{\lambda}}{\left(ED_{50}^{\lambda} + d_i^{\lambda}\right)} \tag{6.1}$$

The model reduces to a 3-parameter Emax model if λ is set to 1. When $\lambda = 1$, ED_{90} (the dose that produces 90% of the Emax response over the placebo) is 9 times

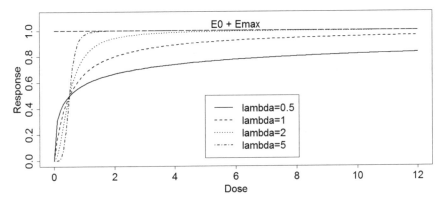

Fig. 6.1 Dose–response curves under a 4-parameter E_{max} model for different choices of the Hill parameter λ

the ED_{50}. By comparison, when $\lambda = 2$, ED_{90} is only 3 times the ED_{50}. When $\lambda = 0.5$, ED_{90} is 81 times the ED_{50}. These results reflect a faster or a slower rise of the dose–response curve when $\lambda = 2$ or 0.5, compared to when $\lambda = 1$.

The 4-parameter Emax model in (6.1) is sometimes written as in (6.2) for ease of computation. In (6.2), $b = -E_{max}, a = E_0 - b, c = 1/ED_{50}$.

$$E(Y_i|d_i) = a + \frac{b}{1 + (c \times d_i)^{\lambda}} \tag{6.2}$$

The sigmoid E_{max} model can approximate most common monotone dose–response curves (Thomas, 2006). The maximum likelihood method can be used to estimate the parameters in (6.1) when the endpoint follows a Normal distribution. When the endpoint is binary, an E_{max} model can still be used, but constraints need to be placed on the parameters to limit the probabilities between 0 and 1 (see Sect. 8.2). The optimization can be carried out using the Gauss Newton or the partial linear (Seber & Wild, 2003) optimization algorithms. One can use the historical control effect, the largest imaginable treatment effect relative to the control, the middle of the dose range and $1.91/\log_{10}$(dose range) as initial values for E_0, E_{max}, ED_{50} and λ, respectively (MacDougall, 2006). Unfortunately, convergence is not guaranteed. This can happen when data do not contain sufficient information to allow unique estimation of the parameters. An example is when the maximum possible response is not well defined by the available data.

When convergence fails under a 4-parameter Emax model, one could try a simpler model such as the 3-parameter Emax model, a linear log-dose or linear model (see Sect. 6.3.1.2). Another option is to apply a Bayesian approach. Under the Bayesian approach, priors are assigned to the 4 parameters and posterior probabilities are computed. For convenience, this approach typically assumes independence among the 4 priors. Thomas (2006) found that even relatively diffuse priors could improve maximum likelihood estimation in situations when the design provides little information about some parameters in the model. Examples include when all doses are on the plateau of the dose–response curve or when the signal-to-noise ratio is low. In these situations, maximum likelihood estimation tends to be unstable and Bayesian estimation could be useful for dose selection instead.

In many cases, historical information is available to allow the construction of a reasonable prior for E_0. Otherwise, a diffuse prior could be used for E_0. When information from a POC study and data on other drugs in the same class are available, one can use such information to build a prior for E_{max}, although the POC study may not be able to go up toward E_{max}. When the dose-ranging study is the first study to collect efficacy information about a new drug (i.e., a POC trial was not conducted), it will be better to use a conservative prior that has a high probability of suggesting no drug effect for E_{max}.

Thomas et al. (2014) found that among the set of small molecules they examined, the Hill parameter λ was concentrated near 1.0 and it was uncommon for λ to be greater than 1.5. They also found that the ratio of ED_{50} to the projected ED_{50} based on pharmacometric projection fell within the (1/10, 10) range with more than 90% of the cases with the highest concentration between (0.5, 4). These findings could be used to form prior distributions for λ and ED_{50}. Examples of Bayesian Emax dose–response modeling can be found in Jones et al. (2011), Tan et al. (2011) and Banerjee and Christensen (2015). We will return to this subject in more detail in Chap. 8, including the selection of priors for the parameters in a 4-parameter Emax model (Sect. 8.6.1).

Another approach to get around the convergence problem is to place a "box" around allowed parameter estimates and use Profile Likelihood to make inferences about estimands of interest (Brain et al., 2014). This can be done because although the estimates for the parameters in the usual parameterization given by (6.1) may not converge despite it being the true model, parameters for mean responses at the doses included or parameters for the doses required to produce given possible effects will usually converge when (6.1) is the correct model. To obtain an estimate for a mean responses or the dose required to give an effect of interest and corresponding confidence intervals, model (6.1) is re-parameterized as

$$E(Y_i|d_i) = E_0 + \frac{\Delta \times d_i^\lambda}{ED_\Delta^\lambda + \left(d_i^\lambda - ED_\Delta^\lambda\right)\left(\frac{\exp(\alpha)}{1+\exp(\alpha)}\right)} \tag{6.3}$$

where Δ is the expected difference from placebo at a given dose ED_Δ and $\frac{\Delta}{E_{max}} = \frac{\exp(\alpha)}{1+\exp(\alpha)}$.

The profile likelihood for Δ can be obtained by taking in turn each of a discretized range of possible values for Δ for a given ED_Δ and maximizing the likelihood for the remaining parameters. This gives the so-called profile likelihood for Δ. The profile likelihood for ED_Δ for a given Δ may be obtained in a similar way. The profile likelihood can then be used to obtain an approximate 95% confidence interval by finding values for the parameter of interest where the F test for the ratio of the residual sum of squares to the minimum residual sum of squares is not significant at the 5% level. The limits for each parameter should be set large enough so that the likelihood surface outside of the limits is approximately flat as the parameter goes beyond the limits.

6.3.1.2 Other Dose–response Models

Bretz et al. (2005) proposed a testing procedure that allowed multiple dose–response curves to be included in a proposed multiple comparison procedure involving dose–response models. In addition to the Emax model, they considered the following dose–response models.

Linear log-dose: $E_0 + \theta \times \log(d_i + 1)$.

Linear: $E_0 + \delta \times d_i$
Scaled exponential: $E_0 + E_1 \times \exp(d_i/\delta)$.
Quadratic (umbrella): $E_0 + \beta_1 \times d_i + \beta_2 \times d_i^2$
Logistic: $E_0 + E_{max}/\{1 + \exp[(ED_{50} - d_i)/\delta]\}$.

These are among the most commonly employed dose–response curves in analyzing dose-ranging studies or in conducting research on dose-ranging design options (Bornkamp et al., 2007; Patel et al., 2012; Pinheiro et al., 2010). We show them in Fig. 6.2 with the maximum effect fixed at 0.8 and the maximum dose scaled to be 1 for all dose–response curves.

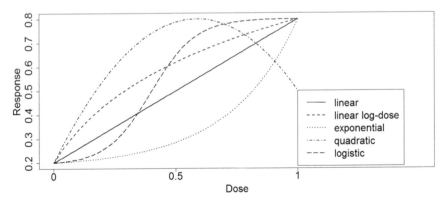

Fig. 6.2 Five commonly used dose–response curves besides E_{max}

6.3.2 Testing for a Positive Dose–response Relationship

Assuming a monotone increasing dose–response relationship with D different doses $\{d_i, i = 1,\ldots, D\}$ and a placebo $d_0 = 0$, the simplest test for a positive dose–response relationship is a trend test. Under a trend test, a linear contrast $\sum_{i=0}^{D} c_i \times E(Y_i) = 0$ with $\sum_{i=0}^{D} c_i = 0$ is tested against $\sum_{i=0}^{D} c_i \times E(Y_i) > 0$. For example, if $D = 4$, a choice for $\{c_i, i = 0,\ldots,4\}$ could be $\{-2, -1, 0, 1, 2\}$. Alternatively, one can also employ tests for $H_0\colon E(Y_0) = E(Y_1) = \ldots = E(Y_D)$ against a monotone alternative $H_A\colon E(Y_0) \leq E(Y_1) \leq \ldots \leq E(Y_D)$ with at least one of the inequalities being a strict inequality (Robertson et al., 1988). Another frequently used strategy that takes advantage of an assumed monotone dose–response relationship is a sequential test starting with the highest dose.

Under the same monotonicity assumption, one could fit a linear log-dose or linear dose–response model and test if θ (linear log-dose) or δ (linear) is positive (see Sect. 6.3.1.2 for what θ and δ represent).

Other commonly used tests include Dunnett's test comparing each dose against the control (Dunnett, 1955), pairwise comparisons or a global test. When the dose–response relationship is indeed monotone, these tests tend to have less power to detect the positive dose–response relationship than those mentioned above because they do not take advantage of the monotonicity assumption.

Bretz et al. (2005) proposed a procedure (MCP-Mod) that applied the idea of a multiple comparison procedure to dose–response models. The procedure, including both testing and estimating a dose–response relationship, can be briefly described in the following steps:

1. Specify a set of candidate models (e.g., Emax, linear log, linear, quadratic, exponential and logistic);
2. Convert each model to a simple linear regression model in its parameters by supplying guesses for the non-linear parameters (e.g., supplying guesses for λ and ED_{50} in an Emax model, supplying a guess for δ in a scaled exponential model);
3. Fit the linearized models obtained in Step 2 and compute the t-statistics for testing the slope parameters. Obtain the maximum t-statistic (recall that we assume higher values to be more desirable).
4. Use the multivariate t-distribution under the null hypothesis of no dose–response relationship to find the critical value for the maximum t-statistic. If the maximum t-statistic is greater than the critical value, the null hypothesis of no dose–response relationship is rejected. This multiple comparison procedure controls the family-wide Type I error rate for the set of null hypotheses that the regression coefficient for each of the identified set of candidate curves is zero.
5. Choose a linearized dose–response model (e.g., the one producing the maximum t-statistic). Estimate the parameters in the model as they originally appear (i.e., no linearization).
6. Use the estimated model in Step 5 to estimate the response at each dose and the dose that produces a pre-specified value on effect.

A detailed description of the R package MCP-Mod for implementing the MCP-Mod methodology can be found in Bornkamp, Pinheiro and Bretz (2009).

6.3.3 Calculating the Metrics

For a design and an analytical approach, the metric of correctly detecting a positive dose–response relationship (Metric #1) under several likely dose–response models can be regarded as the power to detect a positive dose–response relationship. The power can be calculated using simulation. In the simulation, for each dose–response model, we will first use the model to generate the dose–response data according to the design specifications. The generated data will be analyzed by the chosen analytical approach. This process will be repeated for, say 10,000 times. The proportion of times when the analytical approach concludes a positive dose–response relationship will be used as an estimate for the power. The metric will be calculated for each of the likely dose–response models and a flat dose–response model. When the dose–response relationship is flat, the metric provides the Type I error rate for erroneously concluding a positive dose–response relationship when it does not exist.

As for the metric of correctly identifying a target dose (Metric #2), we can evaluate the dose-selection accuracy by counting the percentage of times that a selected dose falls within a target dose interval among the simulation runs that result in an identification of a positive dose–response relationship. In other words, Metric #2 is conditional on the identification of a positive dose–response relationship first. This concept was used in Bornkamp et al. (2007) and Pinheiro et al. (2010). A target dose interval can be defined as an interval of doses that have an effect within a certain neighborhood of the target effect. An example of this neighborhood could be $\pm 10\%$ of the target effect.

For a true dose–response model, one could identify the target dose interval by using the target effect and the rule about a neighborhood. If the maximum effect under the dose–response model is very low, a target dose interval may not exist. In the simulation, one can use the simulated data to identify the lowest dose that is predicted to have the target effect. The identification could be done through a fitted dose–response curve or a pre-specified testing procedure. The choice of the lowest dose reflects the general preference for using the lowest dose among all doses with the desired effect in order to minimize adverse drug reactions. If the identified dose falls within the target dose interval, this counts toward the number of times when a target dose is correctly identified.

Instead of calculating Metric #1 and Metric #2 separately, one can calculate a combined metric for the probability of declaring a positive dose–response relationship and correctly identifying a target dose. Alternatively, one could simply examine the probability of correctly identifying a target dose if the sample size is too low to allow a reasonable power to detect a positive dose–response relationship. Under these two choices, the probability of correctly identifying a target dose is no longer a conditional probability, conditioning on declaring a positive dose–response relationship first.

Metric #3 measures the goodness of fit of the dose–response model. This metric requires the fitting of a dose–response model. The fitted model is compared to the true dose–response model in each simulation run to get an estimate for the prediction error. The average of the estimates over repeated runs and divided by the target effect will yield a value for Metric #3 for the particular combination of dose–response model, study design and the analytical approach.

6.4 Metrics for Confirmatory Studies

In Chap. 5, we discussed various strategies to incorporate prior information into decision making. By the time a drug development moves into the confirmatory stage, there is usually a fair amount of information about the drug. Such information, together with relevant information from other drugs from the same class or perhaps even drugs for the same indication, could be used to help a developer make internal decisions at this stage.

Since a primary objective of a confirmatory trial is to confirm the efficacy of a new drug through hypothesis tests, a developer needs to think beyond statistical power. As we discussed before, power is a conditional probability of getting a successful outcome, conditioning on the drug having a certain clinical effect. In addition to this conditional probability, a developer should also ask questions about the unconditional probability of a successful outcome. A successful outcome in this context could mean a significant P-value on the primary efficacy endpoint in the primary analysis population, or a significant P-value with an added requirement that the estimated treatment effect be at least of a certain magnitude.

In addition to asking about the probability of study success (POSS), it is important to estimate the positive and negative predictive value of the new study. Furthermore, we need to know the probability of making correct decisions at this stage. Consequently, we recommend the following metrics in addition to the traditional power consideration for confirmatory studies:

Metric #1: Probability of study success (POSS).

Metric #2: Positive and negative predictive value of the study.

Metric #3: Probability of making a correct decision.

Let us return to the example of chronic pain in Chap. 5. Suppose that the prior data on the effect of a new pain drug over a marketed product ibuprofen, measured by the total pain relief over 6 h (TOTPAR6) on the visual analog scale and denoted by Δ, suggests that the effect of the new drug over ibuprofen could be described by a Normal distribution $N(3.27;(0.6)^2)$. Considering the number of pain medicines available on the market and the safety profile of drugs in the same class, the developer is interested in developing the new drug only if the true effect of the drug relative

Table 6.3 Joint probabilities of (truth, action) under an assumed prior for the truth, based on 10,000 repetitions in simulation

Decision	Truth		Total
	$\Delta < 3$	$\Delta \geq 3$	
Accept $\Delta < 3$	0.23	0.15	0.38
Accept $\Delta \geq 3$	0.10	0.52	0.62
Total	0.33	0.67	1.00

to ibuprofen is at least 3 units. But of course, the developer does not know the true effect of the drug.

Using $N(3.27;(0.6)^2)$ for Δ, the probability that $\Delta \geq 3$, i.e., $\Pr(\Delta \geq 3.0 | \text{prior data})$, is 67% as shown in Table 5.2.

Based on past experience, the standard deviation of TOTPAR6 is 7 units. Suppose that the sponsor is considering a study that will randomize patients to the new drug or ibuprofen in equal proportions so that each group will have 225 patients. Furthermore, suppose that the developer will accept the hypothesis that the drug has the desired effect ($\Delta \geq 3$) if the comparison between the two groups yields a one-sided P-value significant at the 2.5% level <u>and</u> the observed mean responses between the two groups differ by at least 3 units. If one of these two criteria is not met, the developer will not proceed with the development.

Using simulation with 10,000 repetitions, we obtained the results in Table 6.3.

Table 6.3 suggests that the probability of a successful study (i.e., accepting $\Delta \geq 3$, Metric #1) is 62%. This figure includes a 10% chance of accepting $\Delta \geq 3$ when $\Delta < 3$, an erroneous decision. The positive predictive value of the study together with the associated decision rule is 84% (=0.52/0.62, Metric #2). The negative predictive value is 61% (=0.23/0.38, Metric #2). The probability of making a correct decision is 75% (=0.23 + 0.52, Metric #3).

6.5 Other Types of Success Probabilities

In Sect. 6.4, we focused on the probability of a successful trial. The discussion pertains to a single trial. In this section, we describe two additional success metrics.

6.5.1 Probability of Program Success (POPS)

When the development of a drug moves into the confirmatory stage, a developer may also want to examine the probability that the confirmatory program will be successful. A successful confirmatory program typically requires two successful trials (out of the two trials conducted). For disorders where a successful outcome is not guaranteed even with approved products (such as anti-depressants), a developer may need to conduct three or four Phase 3 trials with success defined by having at least 2 positive trials among those conducted.

For convenience, we will denote the program-level success probability by POPS (probability of program success). This terminology was used in Wang et al. (2015) who considered POPS for clinical programs with multiple trials and binary outcomes. Wang, Liu and Schindler calculated POPS by incorporating prior and interim data from all ongoing Phase 3 trials to decide whether a clinical program would be successful. They suggested that a developer might want to consider abandoning a program early if the estimated POPS is very low.

Assume that a confirmatory program includes two Phase 3 trials and both trials need to be successful for the confirmatory program to be successful. Furthermore, assume that the parameter of interest is denoted by θ and the available information about θ can be described by the distribution $p(\theta)$. Then POPS can be estimated by

$$\int \text{Prob(Both trials are successful}|\theta)p(\theta)d\theta$$
$$= \int \text{Prob(Trial 1 is successful}|\theta) \times$$
$$\text{Prob(Trial 2 is successful}|\theta)p(\theta)d(\theta) \qquad (6.4)$$

To calculate POPS through simulation, one can take the follow steps:

1. Sample θ from $p(\theta)$;
2. Conditioning on θ, calculate the probabilities that the first and the second trial will be successful individually;
3. Multiply the two success probabilities together;
4. Repeat the above process, say, 10,000 times and add the product of the two success probabilities from each simulation run together;
5. Divide the sum in Step 4 by 10,000 to obtain an approximation to POPS.

In the pain medicine example, suppose the developer plans to run two trials of the same design (same protocol with 225 patients per group) and the definition of a successful trial is the same as before (significant P-value and an observed treatment effect of 3 units or more). Using $N(3.27;(0.6)^2)$ as a distribution for the treatment effect, we obtained an estimate for the POPS of 45% based on 10,000 simulation runs. This is lower than the POSS of an individual trial (i.e., 62%), but is higher than multiplying 0.62 by 0.62.

When a successful program is defined by having at least two positive trials out of 3 trials, the calculation can proceed similarly. In this case, the simulation steps can be described as follows:

1. Sample θ from $p(\theta)$;
2. Conditioning on θ, calculate the success probability of each trial;
3. Use the probabilities obtained in Step 2 to calculate the probability that all trials are unsuccessful and the probability that exactly one trial is successful. Subtract

the sum of these two probabilities from 1 to obtain the probability that at least 2 trials are successful;
4. Repeat the above process, say, 10,000 times and add the probability of at least two successful trials from each run together;
5. Divide the sum in Step 4 by 10,000 to obtain an approximation to POPS.

The fourth step above can be modified to handle other definitions of a successful program.

6.5.2 Probability of Compound Success

At any time during the development of a drug, a developer could ask about the likelihood that the new drug has the target commercial profile. While the estimated likelihood could be highly unreliable at the beginning of the development due to the paucity of drug-specific data, the estimate will get more reliable as data pertaining to the drug begin to accumulate. In the example of the pain medicine, PK/PD modeling together with available data suggests a distribution $N(3.27;(0.6)^2)$ for the treatment effect at some point in the development process. If the target profile mandates a treatment effect to be at least 3 units on TOTPAR6, then the probability that the drug will meet this profile is 67%.

We will call the above probability the probability of compound success, or POCS. This probability is continuously updated as more data become available. A starting point for the POCS of a new drug could be the historical success rate.

Unlike POSS and POPS, POCS is completely derived from past data and does not depend on any future study or program under planning. However, POCS is an integral part of the POSS and POPS estimation since POCS typically appears as a marginal probability as shown in Table 6.3.

When Bayesian analysis is used to fit an Emax model, the resulting posterior distributions can be used to answer questions such as the probability that the new drug will produce a target effect or the probability that a higher dose produces an effect higher than a lower dose by a certain amount. In other words, the calculation of POCS-like metrics is a part of the analysis itself, enabled by the Bayesian framework.

6.6 Discussion

The metrics discussed in this chapter may depend on factors such as disease state, gender, geographic region and medical practice because the effect of the new drug is a function of these factors. When this is the case, it is important to build these covariates into the treatment effect model and incorporate them when calculating the metrics. For example, if the effect of a new drug is suspected to be twice as large in patients with a severe form of a disease than patients with a mild/moderate manifestation, POSS will depend on the percentage of severe patients relative to mild/moderate patients in the study. All things being equal, a study that enrolls a higher percentage of severe patients will have a higher POSS than a study enrolling a smaller percentage of severe patients. Because of this, a developer could enrich a study by enrolling a higher percentage of severe patients than is usually represented in the disease population. Similarly, the calculation of POCS should reflect the success probability in the most likely target population. If one is not sure what the ultimate indicated population will be, POCS could be calculated for a broad and for an enriched population. Therefore, it is critical to always state clearly the distributions and the assumptions that go into the calculation of any metric.

In some situations, different data sources and assumptions will result in different distributions for a treatment effect. For example, when borrowing information from other drugs to build a model relating a biomarker to a clinical endpoint, a developer may include all drugs for the same indication or include only drugs with the same mechanism. Rather than trying to integrate the data sources and reconcile the assumptions in these situations, it may be better to calculate the metrics under different distributions and obtain a range of values for the metric. One may calculate the average or the median of these values. In general, we recommend reporting the range to convey the degree of uncertainty about the metric.

For some disorders, Phase 3 trials may employ endpoints different from those in Phase 2 trials. For example, a long-term Phase 3 trial investigating a lipid-reducing regimen typically uses a major adverse cardiovascular event as the primary endpoint while Phase 2 trials focus on the regimen's effect on lipid reduction. In this case, translating an observed efficacy on lipid to that on the clinical endpoint requires the development of a model relating these two endpoints to each other. Fortunately, this is possible (and has been done) in the case of lipid-reducing agents because there is a rich literature on these agents. However, when the disease is rare such as the Duchenne muscular dystrophy (DMD), relating a drug's effect on levels of the protein dystrophin to that on a patient's ability to perform basic tasks such as rising from the floor and walking for six minutes is difficult when no drug has yet shown an effect on the 6-min walk endpoint. This was the situation with DMD treatments even after four drugs have been approved for DMD as of March 2021. Among the four drugs approved, three were approved through the accelerated approval pathway and are still being investigated for their clinical benefit. One drug, EMFLAZA ® has received a regular approval by demonstrating a benefit in increasing the average muscle strength and showing some numerical benefit in prolonging the average time to loss of ambulation among individuals suffering from DMD.

One needs to be vigilant about the choice of data sources when developing the distribution for the treatment effect. Take tarenflurbil as an example. Tarenflurbil was investigated as a treatment for Alzheimer's disease (AD). A Phase 2 trial was conducted between November 3, 2003 and April 24, 2006, in Canada and UK. The study, including a 12-month double-blind treatment period and a 12-month extension, enrolled 210 patients (Wilcock et al., 2008). A Phase 3 study began in February 2005 in the USA. The Phase 3 study initially enrolled both mild and moderate AD patients. The enrollment was subsequently restricted to only mild patients when results from the Phase 2 study showed that patients with mild AD had a better response to tarenflurbil. The Phase 3 study enrolled 1,684 mild AD patients and showed no treatment benefit with tarenflurbil (Green et al., 2009).

Is the above a case of subgroup analysis gone wild? When evidence comes from subgroup analyses, especially an unplanned one, one needs to be wary of the source and cognizant of the impact of selection bias. We have used this example to illustrate the impact of selective inference in Sect. 2.12 of Chap. 2. We will return to the general topic of selection bias in Chap. 12.

The peril of using potentially inappropriate distributions for the effect of a new treatment is by no means limited to subgroups. Increasingly, developers are conducting global confirmatory trials in multiple geographic regions to enable simultaneous product registrations in multiple markets. Because of the diversity of patients in Phase 3 trials, it is critical to know how translatable results from Phase 2 trials with limited investigator sites are to Phase 3 trials with sites all over the world. Launching a confirmatory multi-regional trial when there is little knowledge on how patients in most regions are likely to respond is risky. There are examples of failed global confirmatory trials when the single Phase 2 trial was conducted in a population unrepresentative of the general population planned for Phase 3 trials. For example, the number one (out of the top 10) Phase 3 failure in 2010 compiled by the Biotech Industry's Daily Monitor FierceBiotech was Dimebon (FierceBiotech Report, 2010). Dimebon was a new drug intended to treat Alzheimer's disease. Dimebon's global Phase 3 program was based on a single positive Phase 2 trial conducted in Russia.

The examples above illustrate the need to understand the data source and how results from the data source will be used. One measure that can help reduce the influence of an overly optimistic data source is to replicate prior findings in a closely related setting before launching a full-blown Phase 3 program. In the case of tarenflurbil, this could mean to replicate the effect in mild AD patients first. In the case of Dimebon, this could mean conducting a second Phase 2 study in western European countries and the USA.

All the metrics discussed in this chapter so far are based on scientific data even though the decision on the target value may have been influenced by commercial consideration. Nevertheless, the speed to market is always on the mind of a developer. This is because a longer remaining patent life at the point of product launch typically means a higher net revenue for the product. The need to take speed into consideration has motivated some researchers to propose using the expected net present value (NPV) as a metric in considering different strategies for a Phase 2 program (Patel et al., 2012) or in a decision-analytical approach (Burman et al., 2007). We will discuss the calculation of the expected NPV in detail in Chap. 11 (see Sect. 11.3). Despite the published and ongoing work, our experience suggests that up until now NPV has been used more in portfolio decision analysis than decisions pertaining to clinical development strategies.

In Chaps. 7–10, we will discuss designs options and how to use the metrics discussed in this chapter to help compare and select designs for the various stages of drug development.

Similarly to what we stated in Sect. 5.4, we use simulation to estimate the value of a metric in this and subsequent chapters of this book. We adopt this approach for consistency and ease of generalization because closed-form expressions for metrics only exist for simple situations. Since the precision of simulation results can be made sufficiently high by employing a large number of simulation runs, using simulation to estimate the value of a metric should not affect the quality of the estimation even when a closed-form expression exists for the metric. In addition, describing the simulation steps makes it easier to understand the definition of a metric and the impact of the various components making up the metric.

References

Banerjee, A., & Christensen, J. (2015). Bayesian dose response. In S. M. Menon & R. C. Zink (Eds.), *Modern Approaches to clinical trials using SAS®: classical, adaptive, and Bayesian methods* (pp. 225–246). SAS Press.

Bornkamp, B., Bretz, F., Dmitrienko, A., et al. (2007). Innovative approaches for designing and analyzing adaptive dose-ranging trials. *Journal of Biopharmaceutical Statistics, 17*(6), 965–995.

Bornkamp, B., Pinheiro, J., & Bretz, F. (2009). MCPMod: An R package for the design and analysis of dose-finding studies. *Journal of Statistical Software, 29*(7), published in February.

Brain, P., Kirby, S., & Larionov, R. (2014). Fitting Emax models to clinical trial dose-response data when the high dose asymptote is ill defined. *Pharmaceutical Statistics, 13*(6), 364–370.

Bretz, F., Pinheiro, J., & Branson, M. (2005). Combining multiple comparisons and modeling techniques in dose-response studies. *Biometrics, 61*(3), 738–748.

Burman, C. F., Grieve, A. P., & Senn, S. (2007). Decision analysis in drug development. In A. Dmitrienko, C. Chuang-Stein, & R. D'Agostino (Eds.), *Pharmaceutical statistics using SAS®: A practical guide* (pp. 385–428). Cary NC, SAS Institute.

Dunnett, C. W. (1955). A multiple comparison procedure for comparing several treatments with a control. *Journal of the American Statistical Association, 50*(272), 1096–1121.

FierceBiotech Report. The top 10 phase III failures of 2010. Available at http://www.fiercebiotech.com/special-reports/top-10-phase-iii-failures-2010#ixzz13Nwfm52q. Accessed 15 February 2021.

Green, R. C., Schneider, L. S., Amato, D. A., et al. (2009). Effect of tarenflurbil on cognitive decline and activities of daily living in patients with mild Alzheimer disease: A randomized controlled trial. *Journal of the American Medical Association, 302*(23), 2557–2564.

Jones, B., Layton, G., Richardson, H., & Thomas, N. (2011). Model-based Bayesian adaptive dose finding designs for a phase II trial. *Statistics in Biopharmaceutical Research, 3*(2), 276–287.

MacDougall, J. (2006). Analysis of Dose–response studies-Emax model. In N Ting (Ed.), *Dose–finding in drug development*. Springer.

Patel, N., Bolognese, J., Chuang-Stein, C., et al. (2012). Designing phase 2 trials based on program-level considerations: A case study for neuropathic pain. *Drug Information Journal, 46*(4), 439–454.

Pinheiro, J., Sax, F., Antonijevic, Z., et al. (2010). Adaptive and model-based dose-ranging trials: Quantitative evaluation and recommendations. *Statistics in Biopharmaceutical Research, 2*(4), 435–454.

Robertson, T., Wright, F. T., & Dykstra, R. L. (1988). *Order restricted statistical inference*. Wiley.

Ruberg, S. J. (1995). Dose-response studies I: Some design considerations. *Journal of Biopharmaceutical Statistics, 5*(1), 1–14.

Ruberg, S. J. (1995). Dose-response studies II: Analysis and interpretation. *Journal of Biopharmaceutical Statistics, 5*(1), 15–42.

Seber, G. A. F., & Wild, C. J. (2003). *Nonlinear regression*. Wiley.

Tan, H., Gruben, D., French, J., & Thomas, N. (2011). A case study of model-based Bayesian dose response estimation. *Statistics in Medicine, 30*(21), 2622–2633.

Thomas, N. (2006). Hypothesis testing and Bayesian estimation using a sigmoid Emax model applied to sparse dose-response designs. *Journal of Biopharmaceutical Statistics, 16*(5), 657–677.

Thomas, N., Sweeney, K., & Somayaji, V. (2014). Meta-analysis of clinical dose–response in a large drug development portfolio. *Statistics in Biopharmaceutical Research, 6*(4), 302–317.

Thomas, N., Roy, D., Somayaji, V., & Sweeney, K. (2014b). *Meta-analyses of clinical dose response*. Presentation at the European Medicines Agency/European Federation of Pharmaceutical Industries and Associations workshop on the importance of dose finding and dose selection for the successful development, licensing and lifecycle management of medicinal products. Available at http://www.ema.europa.eu/docs/en_GB/document_library/Presentation/2015/01/WC500179795.pdf. Accessed 15 February 2021.

Wang, M., Liu, G. F., & Schindler, J. (2015). Evaluation of program success for programs with multiple trials in binary outcomes. *Pharmaceutical Statistics, 14*(3), 172–179.

Wilcock, G. K., Black, S. E., Hendrix, S. B. et al. Tarenflurbil Phase II Study Investigators. (2008). Efficacy and safety of tarenflurbil in mild to moderate Alzheimer's disease: A randomized phase II trial. *Lancet Neurology, 7*(6), 483–493.

Wu, J., Banerjee, A., Jin, B., et al. (2018). Clinical dose-response for a broad set of biological products: A model-based meta-analysis. *Statistical Methods in Medical Research, 27*(9), 2694–2721.

Chapter 7
Designing Proof-of-Concept Trials with Desired Characteristics

Prove all things; hold fast that which is good.
— *King James Bible*

7.1 Introduction

A proof-of-concept (POC) study is a key stage in drug development when the developer finds out if a compound has any effect on the endpoint of interest and if so, whether the size of the effect warrants investment in further development. A large observed effect can lead to a greatly accelerated development program although, as we have discussed in Chap. 4, there can be dangers in using an unreplicated result to make a major acceleration decision.

Good decisions dictate that good compounds have a large probability of being progressed, and poor compounds have a large probability of being stopped.

When designing a trial, we need to consider how results from the trial will be used to make decisions. If the information from the trial is inadequate, the decisions will not enjoy the kind of quality we have come to expect of good decisions. Therefore, the design together with the decision rule should dictate how many subjects are needed for a particular design type. In this chapter, we will first discuss how this can be done using a Frequentist approach for a parallel group design when the responses for an endpoint are assumed to be Normally and independently distributed with a known constant variance. We then consider the case of binary data and the use of a Bayesian approach.

A number of approaches have been used for making a decision for a POC study. In this chapter, we review five of these approaches. The approaches are the traditional hypothesis-testing approach, the Early Signal of Efficacy (ESoE) approach, the approach implemented in the Learn Phase Development Assessment Tool (LPDAT) and two approaches that can be considered as special cases of the LPDAT approach.

C. Chuang-Stein and S. Kirby, *Quantitative Decisions in Drug Development*, Springer Series in Pharmaceutical Statistics,
https://doi.org/10.1007/978-3-030-79731-7_7

We then review the metrics that can be used to evaluate POC trial designs, as briefly described in Chap. 6 (see Sect. 6.2).

As described in Chap. 5, if a prior distribution for the treatment effect is to be used to evaluate a trial design, a key consideration is how this prior distribution is obtained. One possibility, which we will focus on, is to use a standard prior derived from relevant historical results. Such a prior could be the mixture of essentially a probability of no effect and a distribution where there is some treatment effect. This prior allows for the possibility that a compound has no effect. On the other hand, if there is a high degree of confidence that a compound will have an effect then a prior which allows only nonzero treatment effects may be more appropriate. Another possibility at this stage of development is to use a prior distribution which is elicited from expert opinion (O'Hagan et al., 2006). We briefly consider using a prior distribution elicited from expert opinion in Sect. 7.5.

For simplicity, we use the word "designs" to mean the designs and the companion decision rules. We consider numerical examples for trial designs derived from the five approaches to show how the designs can be evaluated and compared.

7.2 Five Approaches to Decision Making

In this chapter, we assume that large values on the endpoint are more desirable and we measure the effect of a new drug by calculating the difference in the mean response between the new drug and a comparator (i.e., new drug - comparator). A more positive difference means a greater drug effect. We denote the true effect of the new drug relative to the comparator by Δ. We focus on a continuous endpoint in Sect. 7.2 through Sect. 7.6 and extend the discussions to a binary endpoint in Sect. 7.8.

7.2.1 The Traditional Hypothesis-Testing Approach

The traditional approach to decision making for a POC trial follows the hypothesis-testing framework set out in Chap. 2. The null hypothesis of no treatment effect against a comparator

$$H_0 : \Delta \leq 0$$

is tested against the following alternative hypothesis of a positive treatment effect

$$H_A : \Delta > 0$$

If the null hypothesis is rejected using a one-sided test at a pre-specified $100\alpha\%$ significance level, then the trial result is considered positive and the decision is made to continue with development. Otherwise, the development of the compound is stopped.

7.2.2 The ESoE Approach

The ESoE approach requires that two critical values C_1 and C_2 ($C_1 < C_2$) be pre-specified for a test statistic like that in (7.1). In (7.1), $\overline{X}_{drug}$ denotes the mean response of patients receiving the new drug, $\overline{X}_{control}$ denotes the mean response of patients in the control group, n denotes the number of patients in each group, and σ is the common standard deviation for the endpoint. We assume that σ is known.

$$Z = \frac{\overline{X}_{drug} - \overline{X}_{control}}{\sqrt{\frac{2\sigma^2}{n}}} \tag{7.1}$$

If the test statistic is less than C_1, then a Kill decision is made. If the value of the test statistic is above C_2, then an Accelerate decision is made. Values between C_1 and C_2 lead to a Pause decision and staged development of a compound. The critical values C_1 and C_2 are determined by the probabilities one is willing to accept for accelerating an ineffective drug and an effective drug (or to Kill an ineffective and an effective drug). We will return to the subject of C_1 and C_2 in Sect. 7.3.2.

The ESoE approach strictly speaking does not lead to a POC study, but since one of its outcomes may lead to POC being declared we include it in the category of POC study designs. The study leads to one of three possible decision outcomes. They are Kill (or Stop), Pause and Accelerate. Clinical trial designs with three possible decision outcomes have also previously been considered by Hong and Wang (2007), Shuster (2002), Sargent et al. (2001), Thall et al. (1995), Storer (1992), Emerson and Tritchler (1987) and Fleming (1982). The idea of the ESoE approach is to have a small screening design which quickly leads to a decision.

The rationale for the ESoE approach is actually a portfolio level one (Brown et al., 2012). The portfolio rationale is to swiftly identify compounds with no effect or likely to have the target effect of interest and to separate these compounds from compounds which require more staged investment to see if they have the required target treatment effect.

7.2.3 The LPDAT Approach

The LPDAT approach proceeds by constructing two one-sided confidence intervals for the treatment effect which are joined together and then making Go/No-Go/Pause decisions according to where the constructed interval lies with respect to two values, the minimum acceptable value (MAV) and a target value (TV).

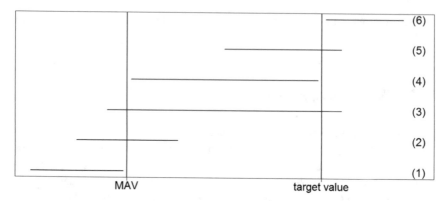

Fig. 7.1 Six possible configurations for LPDAT confidence interval relative to MAV and target value

More specifically, under the LPDAT approach, a lower $100(1 - \alpha_1)\%$ confidence interval (L_{α_1}, ∞) and an upper $100(1 - \alpha_2)\%$ confidence interval $(-\infty, U_{\alpha_2})$ are constructed for the true treatment effect. These two intervals are then combined into a two-sided confidence interval $(L_{\alpha_1}, U_{\alpha_2})$. The position of the constructed interval relative to the MAV and TV results in six possible outcomes (from the bottom to the top in Fig. 7.1):

(1)   Both L_{α_1} and U_{α_2} are below MAV;
(2) L_{α_1} is below MAV, and U_{α_2} is between MAV and TV;
(3) L_{α_1} is below MAV and U_{α_2} is above TV;
(4)   Both L_{α_1} and U_{α_2} are between MAV and TV;
(5) L_{α_1} is between MAV and TV, and U_{α_2} is above TV;
(6)   Both L_{α_1} and U_{α_2} are above TV.

Each of the six possible outcomes can be associated with a Go decision, a Stop decision or a decision to Pause. Usually, outcomes (1) and (2) are associated with a Stop decision because there is evidence against the treatment effect being as big as the desired TV effect and there is evidence that the treatment effect could be less than the MAV. Outcomes (5) and (6) are typically associated with Go decisions because there is evidence that the treatment effect is greater than the MAV and could be greater than TV. Outcomes (3) and (4) are in between and tend to lead to No-Go or Pause decisions.

A slightly modified version of the LPDAT approach is to refer to a lower reference value (LRV), instead of an MAV. The LRV can be 0, implying that any advantage over a comparator is considered minimally acceptable.

The rationale for the LPDAT approach, as usually implemented, is that when making a Go decision we need to have some confidence that the true treatment effect is greater than TV while at the same time being reassured that it is unlikely to be less than the MAV.

If the decision rule stipulates Go for outcomes (5) and (6), Pause for outcomes (3) and (4), Stop for outcomes (1) and (2), then the probability of a Go decision when

$\Delta = $ MAV is at most α_1 and the probability of a Stop decision when $\Delta = $ TV is at most α_2.

We note that although LPDAT was derived using a Frequentist framework it is possible to consider a parallel Bayesian approach which is based on posterior credible intervals. We consider this and Bayesian alternatives to the other decision-making procedures in Sect. 7.9.

7.2.4 The TV Approach

An approach that has received some attention recently is to require that for a positive result the observed treatment effect $\hat{\Delta}$ exceed some target value TV, i.e.,

$$\hat{\Delta} > TV$$

and to also require that the null hypothesis of no difference from a comparator be rejected using a one-sided test against the appropriate alternative at a pre-specified $100\alpha\%$ significance level.

The rationale for a Go decision under this approach is to have at least 50% confidence that the true treatment effect is greater than TV, while at the same time an unbiased and symmetrically distributed estimator $\hat{\Delta}$ has sufficient precision for us to be confident that the true treatment effect is greater than 0.

It should be noted that the TV approach can be regarded as a special case of the LPDAT one with $\alpha_2 = 0.50$, $\alpha_1 = \alpha$, and LRV $= 0$.

7.2.5 The TV$_{MCID}$ Approach

The TV approach described above can be modified to still require that the observed effect $\hat{\Delta}$ be greater than TV, but also require that the null hypothesis H_0: $\Delta \leq$ MCID is rejected in favor of H_A: $\Delta >$ MCID at a pre-specified $100\alpha\%$ significance level using a one-sided test. Here MCID represents a minimum clinically important difference for the effect of a new drug relative to a comparator.

The rationale for a Go decision under this approach is to have at least 50% confidence that the true treatment effect is greater than TV, while at the same time an unbiased and symmetrically distributed estimator $\hat{\Delta}$ has sufficient precision for us to be confident that the true treatment effect is greater than MCID.

The TV$_{MCID}$ approach can be regarded as a special case of the LPDAT approach with $\alpha_2 = 0.50$, $\alpha_1 = \alpha$, and MAV $= $ MCID.

7.2.6 A Comparison of the Five Approaches

The differences between the five approaches mainly reflect their different objectives. The traditional hypothesis-testing approach is concerned with detecting compounds that achieve the MCID level of efficacy. By comparison, the other four approaches focus on a target level of efficacy which is greater than the MCID. An ESoE design is a small screening design whose main purpose is to clearly separate compounds worth accelerating or needing to be killed from the remaining compounds. The LPDAT approach has the same facility as the ESoE for a Pause decision but is concerned with achieving evidence of exceeding a minimum acceptable value and a target value. Finally, TV and TV$_{\text{MCID}}$ are special cases of the LPDAT approach which require the observed effect to exceed the target value.

   Given the different objectives of the five approaches, it is possible to describe their strengths and weaknesses. For example, the traditional hypothesis-testing approach will have a low probability of missing a compound with the MCID level of efficacy but can also have high probabilities of continuing development for effects smaller than the MCID. The ESoE design can pick out clear winners and losers but may result in a Pause decision for a large percentage of compounds due to its small size. The LPDAT design can give high confidence that a treatment effect is greater than the MAV with some confidence of being greater than the target value but the sample size required may be large. Finally, TV and TV$_{\text{MCID}}$ designs give simple rules in terms of the value the observed effect needs to exceed but may have low precision and Kill a bigger percentage of compounds with the target level of efficacy than desired.

   We describe an example scenario in Sect. 7.6 in which some of the points made above are illustrated.

7.3 Criteria for Determining Sample Size

In this section, we consider how to determine the sample size for trials whose data will be used to support decision making under the five approaches described in Sect. 7.2. We consider the two-group parallel design and the case when the responses for the primary endpoint are Normally and independently distributed with known constant variance. Extensions to other common settings are straightforward.

   In what follows we denote values for the primary efficacy endpoint by X_{ij} for $i = 1, 2$ and $j = 1$ to n where $i = 1$ represents the treatment of interest (e.g., the new drug), $i = 2$ represents a comparator and there are n subjects allocated to each treatment. We assume that the X_{ij}'s are Normally and independently distributed with known common variance σ^2 and mean μ_i.

   We let $\overline{X}_i$ denote the mean of X_{ij}, $j = 1, ..., n$, $\Delta = \mu_1 - \mu_2$ and Z_γ the upper 100γth percentile of the standard Normal distribution N(0;1). For simplicity, we assume that $\overline{X}_1 - \overline{X}_2$ is used as an estimator for Δ. Furthermore, we use Lγ to denote the lower limit of a lower $100(1 - \gamma)\%$ confidence interval $(L\gamma, \infty)$ and $U\gamma$ to denote the upper limit of an upper $100(1 - \gamma)\%$ confidence interval $(-\infty, U\gamma)$.

7.3.1 The Traditional Hypothesis-Testing Approach

To derive a sample size for the traditional hypothesis-testing approach, we need to specify the significance level for the test and a power requirement, e.g., $100(1 - \beta)\%$ when the true treatment effect is equal to the MCID. The required sample size per group (n) can be found from the well-known formula (Matthews, 2000) provided in Chap. 2.

$$n = \frac{(Z_\alpha + Z_\beta)^2 2\sigma^2}{(\Delta_{MCID})^2}$$

where Δ_{MCID} is the treatment effect equal to the MCID.

7.3.2 The Early Signal of Efficacy Approach

To determine a sample size, we rely on the following Accelerate and Kill functions

$$A(t) = P(Z > C_2 | \delta = t)$$

$$K(t) = P(Z < C_1 | \delta = t)$$

where Z is defined in (7.1). Under the assumptions of a Normal distribution and known variance, Z has a standard Normal distribution.

A sample size can be determined by specifying $A(0)$ and $A(\Delta_{ESoE})$ or alternatively by specifying $K(0)$ and $K(\Delta_{ESoE})$ where Δ_{ESoE} represents a target level of efficacy needed to bring the new drug to a patient population. The corresponding expressions for the sample size in each group are

$$n_A = \frac{2\sigma^2 \left(Z_{A(0)} + Z_{1-A(\Delta_{ESoE})} \right)^2}{(\Delta_{ESoE})^2}$$

and

$$n_K = \frac{2\sigma^2 \left(Z_{K(0)} + Z_{1-K(\Delta_{ESoE})} \right)^2}{(\Delta_{ESoE})^2}$$

For a sample size determined by, for example, $A(0)$ and $A(\Delta_{ESoE})$, one can determine $K(\Delta_{ESoE})$ for a desirable level of $K(0)$. The sample size that satisfies both sets of requirements on $A(t)$ and $K(t)$ at $t = 0$ and $t = \Delta_{ESoE}$ can be determined by $\max(n_A, n_K)$.

7.3.3   The LPDAT Approach

The required sample size for the LPDAT approach depends on the classification of the six possible outcomes described in Sect. 7.2.3 as Stop, Pause and Go and on the desired operating characteristics. To enable a comparison with the other approaches, we consider the following decisions: outcomes (1), (2) and (4) in Fig. 7.1 lead to a Stop decision; outcomes (5) and (6) lead to a Go (the reader should note that in Sect. 7.2.3 outcome (4) was classified as a Pause). A decision to Pause is thus only made when $L_{\alpha 1}$ is below MAV and $U_{\alpha 2}$ is above TV (i.e., outcome (3) in Sect. 7.2.3). The rationale for a Pause decision in this case is the lack of precision in the treatment effect estimate (as reflected by a wide confidence interval) that suggests the need for additional information to make a Go or Stop decision.

To calculate the sample size, we consider the desired probabilities of Stop and Go decisions when Δ (the true difference in means) is equal to MAV or to the target value TV. By construction the probability of stopping when Δ equals to TV is α_2. The probability of a Go when Δ equals to MAV is α_1 provided that the requirement of $L_{\alpha 1} > $ MAV dominates the requirement of $U_{\alpha 2} > $ TV when $\Delta = $ MAV. This leaves the probability of Go when $\Delta = $ TV and the probability of Stop when $\Delta = $ MAV to be determined. In this chapter, we assume that the second of these is set equal to 0.5 representing a level of efficacy for which the sponsor is indifferent if the decision is to Stop or otherwise. The probability of a Go when $\Delta = $ TV can then be obtained by calculation for a given sample size.

In general, if we only specify α_1 and α_2, we can vary the sample size and find the Stop probability at $\Delta = $ MAV for a given sample size. The sample size that gives us an acceptable level for this Stop probability can be selected as the sample size for the study. The tool LPDAT was developed to enable this selection by computing the Go/Stop/Pause probabilities for a set of sample sizes and rules specified by the users.

7.3.4   The TV and TV_{MCID} Approaches

The sample size for these two approaches can be obtained by the requirement on precision. One way to implement this is to require that the value of the following test statistic

$$\frac{\overline{X}_1 - \overline{X}_2 - d}{\sqrt{\frac{2\sigma^2}{n}}} \tag{7.2}$$

be equal to the critical value Z_α when $\overline{x}_1 - \overline{x}_2$ is equal to the target value. In (7.2), d is zero for the TV approach and MCID for the TV$_{MCID}$ approach.

7.4 Metrics for a Proof-of-Concept Study

The metric of most interest at the POC stage is likely to be the probability of a correct decision. A correct decision could be correctly distinguishing between no effect and some effect or, more stringently, correctly distinguishing between an effect less than the targeted effect and an effect at least equal to the target effect.

A correct decision is comprised of two components, a correct negative decision and a correct positive decision. At the POC stage given the relative infrequency of effective drugs, it is likely to be more important to have a high probability of a correct negative decision than a correct positive decision. That being said, we want to acknowledge situations when a serious unmet medical need may justify the acceptance of a higher false positive rate. In the following sections, we will see for a given scenario, how the different trial designs trade off correct negative and correct positive decisions.

As described in Chap. 6 (see Sect. 6.2) the two types of error can be evaluated conditional on the truth or unconditionally if the probability of the truth can be reasonably specified. For the former, we can look at the Frequentist operating characteristics for a particular trial design. For the latter we can make use of a prior distribution for the treatment effect, as previously described. In the next section, we discuss possible ways of obtaining a prior distribution for the treatment effect at the POC study stage.

7.5 Prior Distributions for the Treatment Effect

As described in Chap. 5, we can use a prior distribution for the treatment effect to evaluate a design. At the POC study stage, it is unlikely that there will be much previous information about the effect of the new drug for the relevant endpoint and population of interest. Consequently, the main approaches to obtaining a prior are likely to be the use of historical results for other similar compounds and elicitation of expert opinion.

We described in Chap. 5 (see Sect. 5.7) the use of a mixture distribution as a prior when a new compound might not have any effect. Alternatively, if the compound is precedented or it is felt that the compound has a very convincing mode of mechanism, a prior with a distribution of nonzero treatment effects may be used.

For situations, where it is felt that there is no relevant prior information from previous trials it is possible to try to derive a prior from expert opinion as discussed in Sect. 5.8 (Kinnersley & Day, 2013; Walley et al., 2015).

Whether eliciting a prior distribution is likely to be useful depends strongly on the experts having relevant information and if they do, whether this information can be appropriately summarized as a distribution for the treatment effect. We want to caution against the tendency to be overly optimistic when conjecturing treatment effect. There are many examples in drug development where expert opinion was that a compound should work but trial results proved otherwise. Thus, a good deal of caution is needed if this approach is to be used. If it is established that the expert opinion is really based on previous trial results, then it might be better to use these results directly to obtain a prior distribution.

7.6 An Example of Evaluating POC Trial Designs for Desired Characteristics

We consider a particular scenario to show how proof-of-concept trial designs can be evaluated to see if they possess the desired characteristics.

Following the notation in Sect. 7.3, we assume that the MCID defined in the traditional hypothesis-testing approach is equal to MAV in the LPDAT approach and that the difference of interest, Δ_{ESoE}, for the ESoE approach is the same as the target value in the LPDAT approach and the target values for the TV approaches. With these assumptions, we refer just to MCID when meaning MCID or MAV and just to TV when meaning the same target value for ESoE, LPDAT and the two TV approaches. We return to these assumptions later.

We use the idea of an effect size (Cohen, 1988) defined as Δ/σ. We consider the scenario where the MCID is an effect size of 0.3 and the target value is an effect size of 0.5.

To sample size the trial using each of the five approaches, we make some additional assumptions:

1. We assume a one-sided 2.5% significance test and a required power of 80% for the traditional hypothesis-testing approach (Trad).
2. For ESoE, we set $K(TV) = 0.05$, $K(0) = 0.80$, $A(0) = 0.05$ and $A(TV) = 0.80$. The choice of $A(TV) = 0.80$ can be viewed as analogous to the use of 80% power in the traditional approach. For the scenario considered, the sample size obtained for ESoE is less than half of that for the traditional approach. Recall that the ESoE design aims for a significant saving compared with the traditional approach by focusing on treatments with a substantial benefit. For situations where the ESoE sample size is greater than half of that for the traditional approach, we recommend that a sponsor considers capping the sample size at half that of the traditional approach. This may result in the

Table 7.1 Sample sizes per group for five different approaches

Approach	Sample size
Trad	$n = 175$
ESoE	$n = 50$
LPDAT (MAV = MCID)	$n = 135$
TV	$n = 22$
TV_{MCID}	$n = 136$

possibility that the trial is underpowered so this recommendation needs to be considered carefully to see if it is suitable for a particular situation.

3. For LPDAT, we use a lower one-sided 80% confidence interval (i.e., $\alpha_1 = 0.20$) and an upper one-sided 95% confidence interval (i.e., $\alpha_2 = 0.05$). We set the probability of Stop when $\Delta = MAV$ at 0.5. These confidence levels are similar to those that have been used by the originators of the LPDAT method in their examples.

4. For the TV approaches (TV and TV_{MCID}), we use a lower one-sided 95% confidence interval to assess the requirement on precision (i.e., $\alpha_1 = 0.05$).

Using the methods of sample sizing described in Sect. 7.3, we obtained the sample sizes per group for the studies to support the five approaches in Table 7.1. The differences in the sample size reflect differences in objectives and demands of the new treatment. As a result, the designs will have different operating characteristics.

In what follows we refer to a Go decision as meaning Go or Accelerate and a Stop decision as meaning Stop or Kill a compound. A Pause decision means that further data are needed before a Go or Stop decision can be made.

7.6.1 Conditional Evaluation of the Trial Designs

To examine the conditional properties of each trial design, we look at its operating characteristics. We do this by graphing the probability of Stop and Go and where relevant, the probability of a Pause decision for a range of the true treatment effect of interest.

The graphs for Go, Stop and Pause probabilities we obtained for the five designs are shown in order in Figs. 7.2, 7.3 and 7.4. All probabilities are calculated exactly using Normal distributions with σ assumed known and equal to 1. The use of t-distributions would lead to very similar probabilities. The biggest differences would be for the TV approach because of its smaller sample size but even for this approach the differences would be small and the qualitative conclusions remain the same.

First, we consider the case when a correct Go decision can only occur when the true treatment effect size is greater than the MCID of 0.3. From Fig. 7.2, one can see that the probability of a correct Go decision is highest initially for effect sizes just greater than 0.3 for the traditional and ESoE designs. As the effect size becomes

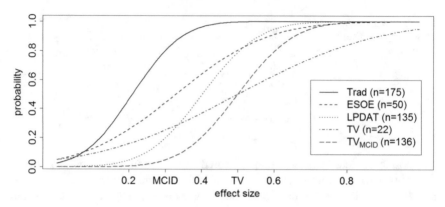

Fig. 7.2 Probability of a Go decision for five different approaches

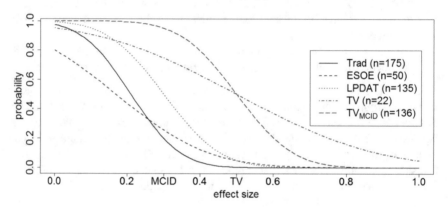

Fig. 7.3 Probability of a Stop decision for five different approaches

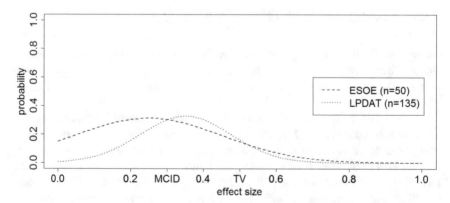

Fig. 7.4 Probability of a Pause decision for two different approaches

larger, the probability for the ESoE and LPDAT designs becomes close but are above the probabilities for the TV and TV$_{MCID}$ designs. For bigger effect sizes (e.g., $\geq$ 0.8) the probability for traditional, ESoE, LPDAT and TV$_{MCID}$ designs converge above that for the TV design before the probability for the TV design catches up for extremely large effect sizes.

In the above situations, the probability of a correct Stop decision shown in Fig. 7.3 is the greatest for the TV$_{MCID}$ design. The probability of stopping for the LPDAT, Trad and TV designs is also initially big for small values of the true treatment effect. The probabilities of stopping for the LPDAT and Trad designs then fall away rapidly as the true treatment effect approaches the MCID.

If a correct positive decision can occur only when the true treatment effect is at least 0.5, then the probability of a correct positive decision is virtually 1.0 under the traditional approach. The next biggest probabilities of a correct positive decision when the treatment effect size is 0.5 or above are for the LPDAT and ESoE designs. The two designs continue to generate the next biggest probabilities of a correct positive decision until the treatment effect size reaches around 0.8 when the TV$_{MCID}$ design has a similar probability. Even at an effect size of 1.0, historically a very large effect size, the probability of a correct positive decision for the TV design is less than that for the other four designs.

The probability of a correct negative decision when the treatment effect size is less than 0.5 is very high for the TV and TV$_{MCID}$ designs. The ordering of the probabilities for the remaining designs, from biggest to smallest is, similar to the case when MCID is set at 0.3, LPDAT then traditional then ESoE until Δ is greater than 0.25 when the ordering of the probabilities for the traditional and ESoE designs swap over.

We also note that the probability of a Pause decision for the ESoE design is generally greater than that for the LPDAT design and that the highest Pause probability under these two designs is around 0.3. A developer needs to decide if this level of a Pause probability is acceptable.

The choice of design will depend on the desirability of the different operating characteristics, the definition of correct positive and correct negative decisions and the resources needed for a particular design. If a positive decision is regarded as a correct decision when the treatment effect size is greater than or equal to the MCID, then the traditional or ESoE designs might be preferred. If a positive decision is regarded, however, as a correct decision when the treatment effect is greater than or equal to the target effect then one of the designs other than the traditional design may be preferred.

We want to remind our readers that the above comparisons are for the purpose of illustration only. Differences in sample sizes and the rationales behind the designs will result in different operating characteristics. In practice, if we want a new treatment to have an (true) effect size greater than 0.5 to consider the new treatment worthy of development, it will not be appropriate to size the study to detect an effect size of 0.3 as in the traditional approach. Sizing a study this way will not only require more resources than necessary, but will also incur a high probability of an incorrect Go decision.

7.6.2 Unconditional Evaluation of the Trial Designs

In this section, we illustrate how one may evaluate the trial designs unconditionally using a prior that reflects the sort of effect size seen for all compounds in the pharmaceutical industry in the recent past. One way to represent the collective experience on the effect size is a mixture prior with 80% of the mixture having a point mass at zero and the remaining 20% having a Normal distribution centered at 0.5 with standard deviation of 0.17. One could also consider a more Pessimistic prior that is a 90%-10% mixture distribution. Under the first distribution, 10% of compounds have an effect size greater than or equal to 0.5. This 10% success rate agrees approximately with that which can be derived from the data in Hay et al. (2014) for all indications—see Fig. 1 in this publication.

We assume first that our criterion for a correct Go decision requires that the true treatment effect is equal to or greater than the MCID (defined to be an effect size of 0.3 in this chapter).

With these assumptions, we include in Tables 7.2, 7.3, 7.4, 7.5 and 7.6 the estimated probabilities for correct and incorrect decisions. The estimated probabilities are obtained using simulation with the same 10,000 samples for the treatment effect for each approach but different independent samples generated as the data for each design given the simulated treatment effect. Given a simulated value for the treatment effect from the prior distribution, as in Sect. 7.6.1, Normal distributions with σ set equal to 1 are used to calculate probabilities. The use of t distributions would give very similar final estimated probabilities to those reported below.

From the above tables, we can draw up Table 7.7 of PPV and NPV values, defined as $\Pr(\Delta \geq MCID \mid Go\ decision)$ and $\Pr(\Delta < MCID \mid Stop\ decision)$.

Table 7.2 Estimated unconditional probabilities for traditional trial design from 10,000 simulated trials

		Truth		
		$\Delta < MCID$	$\Delta \geq MCID$	
Decision	Stop	0.79	0.00	0.79
	Go	0.03	0.18	0.21
		0.82	0.18	

Table 7.3 Estimated unconditional probabilities for ESoE trial design from 10,000 simulated trials

		Truth		
		$\Delta < MCID$	$\Delta \geq MCID$	
Decision	Stop	0.65	0.01	0.66
	Pause	0.12	0.02	0.14
	Go	0.05	0.14	0.19
		0.82	0.17	

*Probabilities do not sum to 1.00 due to rounding

Table 7.4 Estimated unconditional probabilities for LPDAT trial design from 10,000 simulated trials

		Truth		
		$\Delta < MCID$	$\Delta \geq MCID$	
Decision	Stop	0.81	0.02	0.83
	Pause	0.01	0.03	0.04
	Go	0.00	0.14	0.14
		0.82	0.19	

*Probabilities do not sum to 1.00 due to rounding

Table 7.5 Estimated unconditional probabilities for TV trial design from 10,000 simulated trials

		Truth		
		$\Delta < MCID$	$\Delta \geq MCID$	
Decision	Stop	0.78	0.08	0.86
	Go	0.05	0.10	0.15
		0.83	0.18	

*Probabilities do not sum to 1.00 due to rounding

Table 7.6 Estimated unconditional probabilities for TV$_{MCID}$ trial design from 10,000 simulated trials

		Truth		
		$\Delta < MCID$	$\Delta \geq MCID$	
Decision	Stop	0.82	0.08	0.90
	Go	0.00	0.10	0.10
		0.82	0.18	

Table 7.7 Estimated PPV and NPV values for five designs

	PPV	NPV
Traditional	0.84	1.00
ESoE	0.74	0.98
LPDAT	0.98	0.98
TV	0.68	0.90
TV$_{MCID}$	1.00	0.91

A simple comparison of PPV and NPV values shows that based on the PPV and NPV, the LPDAT design is likely to be regarded as the best among the five designs because it has the highest value for the average of PPV and NPV without either value being much inferior to the best achieved by the other designs. Such a comparison does not, however, take into account the different sample sizes and thus the resources required. The LPDAT design has a smaller sample size than the traditional design and virtually the same sample size as the TV$_{\text{MCID}}$ design. So given its performance, LPDAT would likely be preferred to either design. The ESoE design has a much smaller sample size and a good NPV value so might be preferred especially if considered as a screening design and the PPV and Pause probabilities are deemed acceptable. The TV design has a very small sample size (22 per group). Considering its comparatively low PPV and NPV, it may be worthwhile to invest more resources when an effect size like MCID is enough to move the new drug forward.

We will next discuss the situation when the true treatment effect needs to be at least equal to or greater than the target value for a correct Go decision. The target value is set to be an effect size of 0.5. Tables 7.8, 7.9, 7.10, 7.11, 7.12 and 7.13 repeat the computations in Tables 7.2, 7.3, 7.4, 7.5, 7.6 and 7.7 except that now the true treatment value needs to be equal to or greater than the target value for a correct Go decision.

As before, a simple comparison of PPV and NPV values suggests that of these options the TV$_{\text{MCID}}$ design is likely to be a strong design candidate if the choice is based on PPV and NPV alone. The traditional and LPDAT designs have notably inferior PPV values compared to the TV$_{\text{MCID}}$ design. So, given their similar or bigger sample size, they are unlikely to be preferred to the TV$_{\text{MCID}}$ design. The TV and ESoE designs have similar PPV and NPV values, so between these two designs the TV design would probably be preferred given its smaller sample size.

Again, it is important to keep in mind the assumptions behind the comparisons. In this case, the requirement on the treatment effect is quite strong (effect size has

Table 7.8 Estimated unconditional probabilities for traditional trial design from 10,000 simulated trials

		Truth		
		$\Delta < TV$	$\Delta \geq TV$	
Decision	Stop	0.79	0.00	0.79
	Go	0.11	0.10	0.21
		0.90	0.10	

Table 7.9 Estimated unconditional probabilities for ESoE trial design from 10,000 simulated trials

		Truth		
		$\Delta < TV$	$\Delta \geq TV$	
Decision	Stop	0.66	0.00	0.66
	Pause	0.14	0.01	0.15
	Go	0.10	0.09	0.19
		0.90	0.10	

Table 7.10 Estimated unconditional probabilities for LPDAT trial design from 10,000 simulated. Trials

		Truth		
		$\Delta < TV$	$\Delta \geq TV$	
Decision	Stop	0.83	0.00	0.83
	Pause	0.03	0.01	0.04
	Go	0.04	0.09	0.13
		0.90	0.10	

Table 7.11 Estimated unconditional probabilities for TV trial design from 10,000 simulated trials

		Truth		
		$\Delta < TV$	$\Delta \geq TV$	
Decision	Stop	0.83	0.03	0.86
	Go	0.07	0.07	0.14
		0.90	0.10	

Table 7.12 Estimated unconditional probabilities for TV_{MCID} trial design from 10,000 simulated trials

		Truth		
		$\Delta < TV$	$\Delta \geq TV$	
Decision	Stop	0.88	0.02	0.90
	Go	0.02	0.08	0.10
		0.90	0.10	

Table 7.13 Estimated PPV values and NPV values for required truth of $\Delta \geq TV$

	PPV	NPV
Traditional	0.48	1.00
ESoE	0.49	1.00
LPDAT	0.68	1.00
TV	0.47	0.96
TV_{MCID}	0.80	0.98

to be equal to or greater than 0.5). As a result, an approach that has a more stringent Go-criterion will likely fare better in the comparisons.

It is also important to look at the row marginals in Tables 7.2, 7.3, 7.4, 7.5 and 7.6 (and Tables 7.8, 7.9, 7.10, 7.11 and 7.12). The probability of a Go decision is the highest for the traditional design and the lowest under the TV_{MCID} design. The decreasing Go-probabilities from the traditional and ESoE to the TV and TV_{MCID} designs reflect the more stringent criteria placed on the Go decision for the latter.

Table 7.14 Estimated probabilities for ESoE trial design with amended decision criteria from 10,000 simulated trials

		Truth		
		$\Delta < TV$	$\Delta \geq TV$	
Decision	Stop	0.654	0.003	0.657
	Pause	0.232	0.046	0.278
	Go	0.014	0.051	0.065
		0.900	0.100	

The analyses above can be repeated with changed decision criteria and if desired, a changed sample size. For example, a developer may wonder if a better trade-off between PPV and NPV values could be achieved for the ESoE design with the same sample size, but a modified criterion. Suppose, the developer considers accelerating development when the test statistic is significant at the one-sided 0.001 level instead of at the one-sided 0.05 level while leaving the decision of when to Kill a compound the same as in the original design. Using the amended decision criterion, one can obtain the results in Table 7.14. The PPV of the amended rule is 0.78 and the NPV is still 1.00 (with rounding error). But the Go probability has now decreased to 6.5%!

It can be seen that the PPV value is now close to that for the TV_{MCID} design and the NPV has remained at 1.00 to two decimal places. Given that the sample size for the amended ESoE design (50 per group) is less than half that for the TV_{MCID} design (136 per group), it seems that this amended design could be a viable alternative to the TV_{MCID} design if the probability of a Pause decision (about 28%) is acceptable. By allowing a Pause decision that has an acceptable probability in this case, one is able to improve the PPV and keep the NPV basically intact.

7.7 Sensitivity Analyses for the Choice of Prior Distribution

The choice of prior distribution for the unconditional evaluation of trial designs may not be clear-cut. For a subjective prior, different experts may have different opinions, which may lead to different prior distributions. Similarly, there may be disagreement about which standard distribution to use. In these cases, it seems reasonable to evaluate designs with respect to each of the possible prior distributions and seek designs that perform reasonably well for all of the possible priors.

7.8 Binary Data

For binary data, provided that the Normal approximation to the binomial distribution is reasonable, we can replace the test statistic in (7.1) by

$$Z = \frac{\hat{p}_{\text{drug}} - \hat{p}_{\text{control}}}{\sqrt{\frac{2\hat{p}(1-\hat{p})}{n}}} \tag{7.3}$$

where $\hat{p}_{\text{drug}}$ is the observed proportion of responders in the drug treatment group, $\hat{p}_{\text{control}}$ is the observed proportion of responders in the control group, $\hat{p}$ is the observed overall proportion of responders, and n represents the common number of patients in each treatment group.

Three of the five decision-making approaches for continuous data, those described in Sects. 7.2.1, 7.2.2 and 7.2.4 can be applied to binary data using the test statistic given by (7.3). For the LPDAT approach, the expression for a confidence interval for the difference in proportions (as used in (7.4) in Sect. 7.8.1) can be used. For TV$_{\text{MCID}}$, the same expression for a confidence interval can be used together with (7.3) adapted to have the same standard error as used for the confidence interval. Similarly, the sample sizing methods of Sects. 7.3.1 to 7.3.5 can be used. The true treatment difference Δ is the difference in the true proportion of responders between drug and control treatments. When deciding upon the sample size, the observed proportions in the variance formula will be replaced by the assumed true values.

When the Normal approximation to the binomial distribution is considered inadequate, exact methods could be used for the construction of significance tests and confidence intervals.

7.8.1 An Example

To illustrate the use of the decision-making approaches with binary data, we consider a case where we wish to test a new drug for rheumatoid arthritis and the primary endpoint of interest is the binary endpoint ACR20. The ACR20 is a composite measure defined as improvement of at least 20% in the number of tender and number of swollen joints, accompanied by at least 20% improvement in three of the following five criteria (Felson et al., 1995):

- Patient global assessment;
- Physician global assessment;
- Functional ability measure (most often assessed by the Health Assessment Questionnaire);
- Visual analog pain scale;
- Erythrocyte sedimentation rate or C-reactive protein (CRP).

The parameter of interest is the percentage of patients who achieved ACR20 at the time point of interest. These patients are often called ACR20 responders.

We assume that the true ACR20 response proportion in the control group is 0.3, the minimum clinically important difference (equal to the minimum acceptable value) is 0.2 and that the target value is an improvement in the response proportion of 0.3 (i.e., the ACR20 response proportion in patients receiving the new drug is 0.6).

Table 7.15 Sample sizes per group for five different approaches for the ACR20 example

Approach	Sample size
Trad	$n = 91$
ESoE	$n = 31$
LPDAT (MAV = MCID)	$n = 124$
TV	$n = 14$
TV$_{MCID}$	$n = 122$

Sample sizes were obtained using the Normal approximation to the binomial distribution with the same assumptions as described in Sect. 7.6. Under the Normal approximation, the variance of the observed proportion was calculated using the true response proportion as we stated above.

For the LPDAT approach, we want a sample size that would result in a Stop probability closest to 50% when the true response proportion is 0.3 in the control group and $\Delta = 0.2$. As a reminder, a Stop decision under the LPDAT in Sect. 7.6 is defined by the upper one-sided 95% confidence interval for Δ being less than TV (i.e., 0.3). The required sample size could be estimated by solving the equation in (7.4) . One could refine the estimate by checking if a value in the neighborhood of the estimate from (7.4) would produce a Stop probability closer to 50%. However, this extra step will not likely change the estimate by much.

$$Pr(\hat{p}_{drug} - \hat{p}_{control} + 1.645$$
$$\times \sqrt{\frac{0.5 \times 0.5 + 0.3 \times 0.7}{n}} < 0.3 \mid p_{drug} = 0.5, \, p_{plaebo} = 0.3) = 0.5 \qquad (7.4)$$

The sample sizes needed for the five approaches are given in Table 7.15.

We can adapt the programs for the example in Sect. 7.6 to calculate the probabilities of Go, Stop and Pause for the ACR20 examples. These results are displayed in Figs. 7.5, 7.6 and 7.7.

7.9 Bayesian Approaches to Decision Making

The five Frequentist approaches described in Sects. 7.2.1–7.2.5 can be adapted to allow the use of Bayesian methods by incorporating prior distributions and making use of posterior probabilities and posterior credible intervals.

For example, the traditional hypothesis-testing approach in Sect. 7.2.1 can be adapted so that the decision to continue is made when the posterior probability that the true treatment difference is greater than zero is greater than $(1-\alpha)$.

For the ESoE approach in Sect. 7.2.2, a Kill decision can be taken if the posterior probability that the treatment difference is greater than zero is less than some pre-specified probability. Similarly, an Accelerate decision can be taken if the posterior

Fig. 7.5 Probability of a Go decision for five different approaches for the binary data example

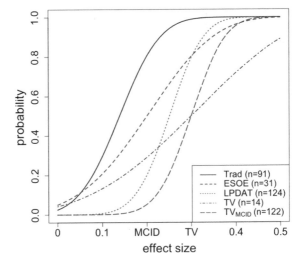

Fig. 7.6 Probability of a Stop decision for five different approaches for the binary data example

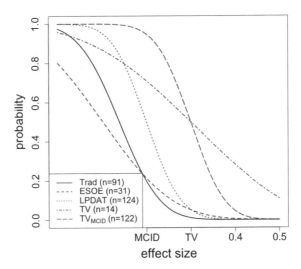

probability that the treatment difference is greater than Δ_{ESoE} is greater than another pre-specified probability. The pre-specified probabilities are chosen such that there is a region between the Kill and Accelerate regions which allows a Pause decision.

The LPDAT approach in Sect. 7.2.3 can be implemented using a Bayesian approach by replacing confidence intervals with posterior credible intervals.

Lastly, the TV and TV_{MCID} approaches can be implemented as Bayesian procedures by first requiring that the posterior probability of the true effect being bigger than the target value TV to be greater than 0.5. In addition, the posterior probability that the true treatment difference is greater than 0 has to be greater than $(1-\alpha)$ for

Fig. 7.7 Probability of a
Pause decision for two
different approaches for the
binary data example

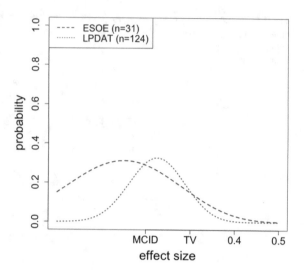

the TV approach while the posterior probability that the true treatment difference is greater than the MCID has to be greater than $(1-\alpha)$ for the TV_{MCID} approach.

Even though the decision criteria are Bayesian, we can evaluate the Frequentist operating characteristics of the decisions. For example, we can calculate the probabilities of Go, Stop and Pause under different assumed true treatment effects. We will illustrate the evaluation of Frequentist operating characteristics for a Bayesian approach to decision making in Sect. 7.10.2.

7.10 The Use of Historical Control Data

In Chap. 5, we discussed how prior data on a control group could be used in future trials. We will discuss two examples of how these data could be used in designing and designing/analyzing a POC trial. The first example is to set a threshold for treatment effect in a single-arm study. The second example is to use the historical data to augment data from the concurrent control in a POC study.

7.10.1 Setting Thresholds on Treatment Effect

When a concurrent control is ethically not possible or undesirable, historical information could be used to identify an efficacy threshold (treated as a target value) and a futility threshold (treated as a minimum acceptable value). With these thresholds, the five approaches outlined in Sect. 7.2 can be adapted so that the results from the single treatment group will be compared against the identified thresholds. For example, the statistic in (7.1) would be changed to that in (7.5). For the ESoE approach Stop, Pause and Go regions could be identified for values of the same test statistic.

$$Z = \frac{\overline{X}_{drug}}{\sqrt{\frac{\sigma^2}{n}}} \qquad (7.5)$$

Similarly, we can change the test statistic in (7.3) to focus on only the result from a single arm and use the Normal approximation to the binomial distribution, if the approximation is appropriate. Alternatively, exact methods for single group data on a binary endpoint can be used to assess the strength of the evidence against the identified thresholds.

7.10.2 Augmenting the Control Data with Historical Information

In this section, we consider an example of applying a robustified meta-analytic predictive (MAP) prior to the control group in a POC study and illustrate how metrics of interest can be evaluated. Most of the materials in this section come from Baeten et al. (2013) and Weber et al. (2019). In particular, Weber et al. developed the R package RBest (R Bayesian Evidence Synthesis Tools) that implements the MAP approach and was used in our evaluation.

As a reminder, for a continuous endpoint, the MAP approach for the control (see Sect. 5.10.2) assumes that the model parameters for the control group in all historical trials and the current trial are exchangeable and drawn from the same Normal distribution as described in (7.6).

$$\theta_{C_{H_k}} = \mu_\theta + \eta_K, \ k = 1, \dots K \text{ and } \theta_{C_D} = \mu_\theta + \eta_{K+1} \qquad (7.6)$$

where $\theta_{C_{H_k}}$ is the response for the kth historical control arm, θ_{C_D} is the response for the concurrent control arm, μ_θ is the population mean for these parameters, and η_k ($k = 1,\dots, K + 1$) is distributed as

$$\eta_k \sim N\left(0, \sigma_\eta^2\right)$$

In the above formulation, σ_η represents between trial variability (heterogeneity). The MAP prior is derived from the meta-analysis of the historical trials using the above model and is a predictive distribution for θ_{C_D}, the response for the control arm and not the population mean μ_θ itself.

We will consider a robust MAP approach proposed by Schmidli et al. (2014). This particular robust MAP approach adds a less informative component to the MAP prior to offer additional protection against the situation when the actual trial data strongly differ from the MAP prior. The mixture prior takes the form in (7.7),

$$w * \pi_{\text{MAP}} + (1 - w) * \pi_{\text{robust}} \qquad (7.7)$$

where w is a weight between 0 and 1, π_{MAP} is the MAP prior and π_{robust} is a weakly informative component. The weight w is given an initial value which, once data are observed, is adapted to support the prior that provides the best prediction for the observed data (Lunn et al., 2013). The greater the consistency between historical control data and the concurrent control data is, the larger the value of the updated w will be.

We take as our example the study described in Weber et al. (Weber et al., 2019). This is a POC study of 28 weeks to compare secukinumab with placebo for the treatment of ankylosing spondylitis (Baeten et al., 2013). The study was designed to use historical data on placebo to "augment" data on the concurrent placebo in a Bayesian analysis. Because of this, the number of placebo patients in the study was purposely kept low with the use of a 4:1 randomization ratio to allow more patients to be assigned to secukinumab. Treatments were to be administered on days 1 and 22 with the primary efficacy comparison conducted at week 6.

Efficacy assessment was done using the Assessment in ankylosing spondylitis response criteria ASAS20 defined as an improvement of at least 20% and an absolute improvement of at least 10 units on a 0–100 scale in at least three of the following domains:

- Patient global assessment;
- Pain assessment;
- Function measured by Bath Ankylosing Spondylitis Functional Index;
- Inflammation (morning stiffness duration and morning stiffness severity on Bath Ankylosing Spondylitis Disease Activity Index).

The primary efficacy endpoint is the percentage of patients meeting the ASAS20 criteria at week 6. Consistent with a planned Bayesian analysis, the sponsor chose a Bayesian decision rule which would declare the study positive if the posterior probability that the ASAS20 response rate for secukinumab patients is greater than that for placebo patients is at least 95%.

The sample size for the study was determined to have 90% chance that the above POC criterion at the final analysis will be met if the true response rates for placebo and secukinumab are 25% and 60%, respectively. The calculations were done by simulation. It was determined that the study would need 20 patients on secukinumab and 5 on placebo. The sample size was increased by 5 to allow for early dropout, resulting in a target enrollment of 30.

Historical control data to be used in the analysis come from 8 trials as shown in Table 7.16.

Baeten et al. (2013) assumed exchangeable response rates and performed a random effect meta-analysis (Spiegelhalter et al., 2004) on the logit scale to obtain the MAP prior. To be more specific, they fit random effects logistic regression model using a half-Normal distribution as the prior for the between trial standard deviation σ_η. They used a Normal distribution with mean 0 and standard deviation of 2 for the one parameter for the intercept in the logistic regression model.

Table 7.16 Summary of eight historical control trial results for the ankylosing spondylitis example

Study	1	2	3	4	5	6	7	8
Patients (n)	107	44	51	39	139	20	78	35
Number of responders	23	12	19	9	39	6	9	10

We reproduce in Fig. 7.8 the forest plot corresponding to the meta-analysis they used to derive the MAP prior. We used the RBest package described in Weber (2019) to reproduce this analysis. Per-trial estimates are shown as light dots, 95% Frequentist intervals as dashed lines, model-derived medians as dark points and 95% credible intervals as dark lines. The dark points display the shrinkage which results from the random effects meta-analysis. The 95% credible interval for the MAP prior is given by the line at the bottom of the graph. As a comparison, we include the 95% credible interval for μ_θ from the random effects meta-analysis in the second row from the bottom. As can be seen from Fig. 7.8, the credible interval from the MAP prior is much wider.

For ease of use and interpretation, Baeten et al. (2013) approximated the predictive distribution by a beta distribution Beta(11,32) which has the same mean and standard deviation as the predictive distribution.

We considered a robustified MAP prior by adding a vague mixture component Beta(1,1) to Beta(11,32) as described in (7.7). We chose an initial weight of 0.2 for the vague prior.

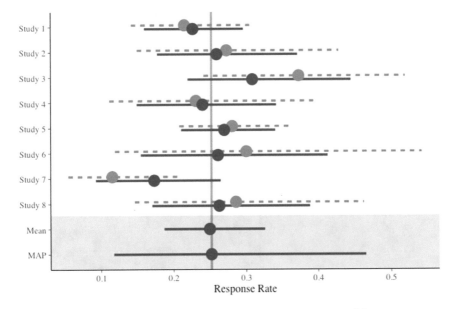

Fig. 7.8 Forest plot augmented with meta-analytic shrinkage estimates per trial

Following Baeten et al. (2013), we take the prior for the response on treatment to be a beta distribution with shape parameters 0.5 and 1 (i.e., Beta(0.5,1)). This prior is used in the Bayesian analysis of the trial results.

We conduct a conditional evaluation for a true treatment effect in the range of 0.25–0.75 in increments of 0.05. We assume a placebo response of 0.25 which is a likely value from the MAP analysis. With 24 patients for secukinumab and 6 for placebo, we can calculate the probability of a positive trial outcome using the RBesT R package. This probability is shown in Fig. 7.9. For comparison, we also include the probability of a positive result when the placebo response is assumed to be 0.40. Full details about the package and how to use it for this particular example can be found in Weber et al. (2019).

The Type I error rates in Fig. 7.9 are 0.018 when the placebo response is assumed to be equal to 0.25 and 0.125 when the placebo response rate is assumed to be equal to 0.40. In both cases the nominal Type I error rate is 0.05. The Type I error rate when the placebo response is equal to 0.40 reflects the general finding of Kopp-Schneider et al. (2020) that for Uniformly Most Powerful or Uniformly Most Powerful Unbiased tests, borrowing from external information cannot improve power while controlling Type I error rate at the same time. They point out, though, that this should not discourage the use of such methods in POC trials, but it does mean that the desire for strict control of the Type I error rate has to be given up.

Fig. 7.9 Probability of a positive result for the ankylosing spondylitis POC trial using a Bayesian approach

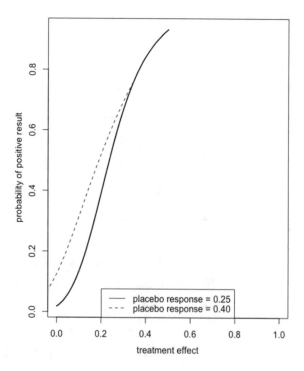

7.11 Discussion

In this chapter, we described a number of Frequentist approaches to decision making for POC studies. Together with choice of a type of experimental design (e.g., parallel or crossover) and desired values for the metrics at the POC stage, we can determine the needed sample size. We considered the case of a two-group parallel group study when the responses are Normally and independently distributed with possibly different means for the two groups and known constant variance. Results for other experimental designs and other endpoints can be derived using similar principles. We illustrated the extension to the case of a binary response.

We looked at a specific scenario for Normal data and showed how trial designs for the five approaches to decision making could be evaluated conditional on the true treatment effect and unconditionally, given a prior distribution for the treatment effect in terms of their PPV and NPV. These metrics are likely to be important at this stage of drug development. Further details of the approaches used in this chapter and conditional evaluation of designs for another scenario can be found in Kirby and Chuang-Stein (2017). We also considered an example for binary data and conducted a conditional evaluation of the trial designs.

For comparison purpose, we assumed the same target value for the ESoE, LPDAT, TV and TV_{MCID} approaches. This assumption could be relaxed. However, a common definition of a correct decision would be needed if we want to compare various trial designs using the concept of a target value.

We briefly considered Bayesian versions of the decision rules in Sect. 7.9 and illustrated the use of one of these in the robust MAP example in Sect. 7.10.2. We assessed the operating characteristics of the Bayesian approach from a Frequentist perspective.

A natural question in evaluating the unconditional operating characteristics of the Bayesian rule described above is whether the distribution assumed for the treatment effect in simulating the trial data should be the same as the prior used in calculating the posterior distribution. While using the same prior will produce consistency between data generation and analysis, in the case of a new drug for a medical condition with no treatment options, the prior may come completely from expert opinions or from a general reference distribution. In these cases, we recommend, as described in Sect. 7.7, to also use other prior distributions to generate the trial data and examine the impact of different data-generating priors. One can then choose a sample size that provides good coverage for a range of plausible data-generating priors for the treatment effect in the trial.

References

Baeten, D., Baraliakos, X., Braun, J., et al. (2013). Anti-Interleukin-17A Monoclonal antibody secukinumab in treatment of ankylosing spondylitis: A randomised, double-blind, placebo-controlled trial. *The Lancet, 382*(9906), 1705–1713.

Brown, M. J., Chuang-Stein, C., & Kirby, S. (2012). Designing studies to find early signals of efficacy. *Journal of Biopharmaceutical Statistics, 22*(6), 1097–1108.

Cohen, J. (1988). *Statistical power analysis for the behavioral sciences* (2nd ed.). Laurence Erlbaum Associates.

Emerson, J. D., & Tritchler, D. (1987). The three-decision problem in medical decision making. *Statistics in Medicine, 6*(2), 101–112.

Felson, D. T., Anderson, J. J., Boers, M., et al. (1995). American College of Rheumatology preliminary definition of improvement in rheumatoid arthritis. *Arthritis and Rheumatism, 38*(6), 727–735.

Fleming, T. R. (1982). One-sample multiple testing procedures for phase II clinical trials. *Biometrics, 38*(1), 143–151.

Hay, M., Thomas, D. W., Craighead, J. L., et al. (2014). Clinical development success rates for investigational drugs. *Nature and Biotechnology, 32*(1), 40–51.

Hong, S., & Wang, Y. (2007). A three-outcome design for randomized comparative phase II clinical trials. *Statistics in Medicine, 26*(19), 3525–3534.

Kinnersley, N., & Day, S. (2013). Structured approach to the elicitation of expert beliefs for a Bayesian-designed clinical trial: A case study. *Pharmaceutical Statistics, 12*, 104–113.

Kirby, S., & Chuang-Stein, C. (2017). A comparison of five approaches to decision making for a first clinical trial of efficacy. *Pharmaceutical Statistics, 16*(1), 37–44. https://doi.org/10.1002/pst.1775

Kopp-Schneider, A., Calderazzo, S., & Wiesenfarth, M. (2020). Power gains by using external information in clinical trials are typically not possible when requiring strict type I error control. *Biometrical Journal, 62*, 361–374.

Lunn, D., Jackson, C., Best, N., et al. (2013). *The BUGS book: A practical introduction to Bayesian analysis*. Chapman & Hall/CRC Press.

Matthews, J. N. S. (2000). *An introduction to randomized controlled clinical Trials*. Arnold.

O'Hagan, A., Beck, C. E., Daneshkhah, A., et al. (2006). *Uncertain judgements: Eliciting experts' probabilities*. Wiley.

Sargent, D. J., Chan, V., & Goldberg, R. M. (2001). A three-outcome design for Phase II clinical trials. *Controlled Clinical Trials, 22*(2), 117–125.

Schmidli, H., Gsteiger, S., Roychoudhury, S., et al. (2014). Robust meta-analytic-predictive priors in clinical trials with historical control information. *Biometrics, 70*(4), 1023–1032.

Shuster, J. (2002). Optimal two-stage designs for single arm Phase II cancer trials. *Journal of Biopharmaceutical Statistics, 12*(1), 39–51.

Spiegelhalter, D. J., Abrams, K. R., & Myles, J. P. (2004). *Bayesian approaches to clinical trials and health-care evaluation*. John Wiley & Sons.

Storer, B. E. (1992). A class of Phase II designs with three possible outcomes. *Biometrics, 48*(1), 55–60.

Thall, P. F., Simon, R. M., & Estey, E. H. (1995). Bayesian sequential monitoring designs for single-arm clinical trials with multiple outcomes. *Statistics in Medicine, 14*(4), 357–379.

Walley, R. J., Smith, C. L., Gale, J. D., & Woodward, P. (2015). Advantages of a wholly Bayesian approach to assessing efficacy in early drug development: A case study. *Pharmaceutical Statistics, 14*, 205–215.

Weber, S., Li, Y., Seaman, J.W., et al. (2019). Applying meta-analytic-predictive priors with the R Bayesian evidence synthesis tools. *Journal of Statistical Software*. https://doi.org/10.18637/jss.v000.i00.

Chapter 8
Designing Dose–Response Studies with Desired Characteristics

The dose makes the poison.
—*Paracelsus*

8.1 Introduction

As described in Chap. 6, "elucidation of the dose–response function" is regarded as a key stage in drug development (ICH E4, 1994). Consequently, designing a dose–response study with the desired characteristics is an important activity in drug development. Sacks et al. (2014) found in a review of reasons for delay and denial of FDA approval of initial applications for new drugs from 2000–2012 that 16% of unsuccessful first time applications included uncertainties related to dose selection. Further back in time for the period 1980–1999, Cross et al. (2002) found that dosage changes in indicated populations occurred in 21% of new molecular entities considered to be evaluable in their assessment.

In this chapter, we focus on examples using the Emax model, but application to other dose–response models or in the case of MCP-Mod (Bornkamp et al., 2009; Bretz et al., 2005) to a collection of models could be extended easily. We start by briefly reviewing the Emax model as background. We then consider the design of a dose–response study covering both practical constraints and optimal designs proposed by various researchers.

Three metrics for assessing a dose–response design were introduced in Chap. 6 (see Sect. 6.3). We recap these metrics before discussing examples in which they are calculated.

Similarly to a POC design, it may be the case that only a conditional assessment of the metrics (conditional on fixed values for the parameters in a dose–response model) is thought to be appropriate for a particular dose–response design. We consider a common way that such a conditional approach can be carried out by specifying a

C. Chuang-Stein and S. Kirby, *Quantitative Decisions in Drug Development*, Springer Series in Pharmaceutical Statistics,
https://doi.org/10.1007/978-3-030-79731-7_8

number of interpretable scenarios. We apply this approach using maximum likelihood fits of the 3-parameter Emax model and a test for trend.

To assess a dose–response design unconditionally, a prior distribution is needed for the unknown model parameters. We describe how such a prior distribution can be derived given POC study results and PK-PD modeling which gives a projection of compound potency. We again apply the approach using the maximum likelihood analysis method and a test for trend. We also use a Bayesian method of analysis with the same prior as used for the evaluation of the design and a Bayesian assessment of the significance of the Emax model fit.

In the penultimate section, we look at fitting an Emax model to binary data using the example of two studies conducted for the development programme for tofaci-tinib. This example is of particular interest because it illustrates the need to include sufficiently low doses and a sufficient dose range in a dose–response study.

We conclude with a general discussion of designing dose–response studies and related issues.

8.2 The Emax Model

The 4-parameter Emax model was introduced in Chap. 6 and is reproduced below.

$$E(Y_i|d_i) = E_0 + E_{\max} \times \frac{d_i^\lambda}{\left(ED_{50}^\lambda + d_i^\lambda\right)} \tag{8.1}$$

We focus on the Emax model because Thomas et al. (2014) and Thomas et al. (2014b) found that for the small molecule compounds with continuous endpoints they studied, assuming the errors for the Emax model to be Normally and independently distributed with constant variance, "compound-specific estimates and Bayesian hierarchical modeling showed that dose–response curves for most compounds can be approximated by Emax models with "Hill" parameters close to 1.0." Here, the Hill parameter is another name for the λ parameter in model (8.1). Setting λ equal to 1 gives a rectangular hyperbola shape for the dose–response curve as shown in Fig. 8.1. The resulting model is the 3-parameter Emax model. Wu et al. (2018) examined placebo-controlled dose–response studies for biologics and found that the majority of the biologics they investigated conformed to a consistent dose–response relationship that could be described by the Emax model

Model (8.1) is usually used with continuous dose–response data. Binary data can be modelled using the same model with a binomial distribution for the response at each dose and constraints on the parameters to ensure that the modelled response is in the range 0 to 1. An alternative is to fit the model

$$E(Y|d_i) = F\left(E_0 + E_{\max}x\frac{d_i^\lambda}{ED_{50}^\lambda + d_i^\lambda}\right) \tag{8.2}$$

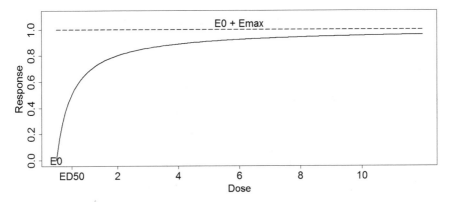

Fig. 8.1 Example of a model (8.1) with $\lambda = 1$

with a binomial distribution for each dose and F being the cumulative Normal or cumulative logistic distribution. The latter model is one of the class of generalized nonlinear models (Turner & Firth, 2020).

8.3 Design of a Dose–Response Study

When designing a dose–response study, there are a number of practical constraints that need to be considered. Perhaps primary among these is the existence of an upper limit for the dose that can be given. This is likely to have been established in a preceding multiple ascending dose study. The upper limit for dose is the highest dose that is regarded as safe and can be tolerated by subjects. It is conventionally referred to as the maximum tolerated dose (MTD).

Another key practical consideration for solid dosage forms is that usually only certain doses are manufactured and therefore available. This comes about because of constraints on the number and particular doses that pharmaceutical sciences can provide.

Given the above constraints, it is unlikely that we will be able to routinely implement the optimal unconstrained design according to some optimality criterion. Nevertheless, we review below some optimality criteria that have been suggested for designing a study (Atkinson et al., 2007; Fedorov & Leonov, 2013).

1. D-optimality: minimizing the determinant of the variance–covariance matrix for the parameter estimates for a model
2. A-optimality: minimizing the average of the variances of the parameter estimates
3. E-optimality: minimizing the variance of the least well-estimated linear combination of parameters.

Of the above optimality criteria, D-optimality tends to be the most frequently used because it is interpretable as minimizing the generalized variance of the estimated parameters in a model and because D-optimal designs often perform well according to other optimality criteria (Atkinson & Donev, 1992).

As an example, for the 3-parameter Emax model, assuming independent and identically distributed observations with constant variance, the D-optimal unconstrained design would put one third of the subjects on each of the following doses: 0, the ED_{50} and the (theoretical) dose required to achieve the maximum response (Dette et al., 2010). The constraint of a maximum dose can be easily incorporated into the minimization problem, and this leads to another dose (instead of the ED_{50}) between 0 and the ED_{50} being allocated one third of the subjects. The resulting design may not be used for a number of reasons, however, including

1. The ED_{50} dose or other identified "middle" dose not being available
2. A desire to have more doses in case the 3-parameter Emax model is not appropriate
3. A desire to have more doses to collect safety data.

An optimal design can be used, though, to measure the relative efficiency of other designs to see how far they depart from the optimum.

It should be noted that the above criteria lead to locally optimal designs, i.e., designs that are optimal when the true values for the unknown parameters are close to those used to derive the design. This is because the information matrix used in the above optimality criteria depends on knowing the values of the parameters. It should also be noted that the optimality criteria above are not directly related to the metrics for dose–response designs described in Chap. 6 and recapped below. However, we expect a D-optimal design that minimizes the generalized variance of the estimated parameters in a model to have good properties with respect to minimizing the average prediction error (i.e., Metric #3 in Sect. 8.4).

Bayesian optimal designs can be derived by integrating an optimality criterion over a prior distribution and selecting the design that has the lowest/highest value for a criterion that is to be minimized/maximized. This approach thus takes into account the uncertainty in the parameter values.

8.4 Metrics for Dose-Ranging Studies

Three metrics were introduced in Chap. 6 and are repeated here for convenience. The metrics are as follows:

Metric #1   Probability to correctly detect a positive dose–response relationship.

Metric #2   Probability to correctly identify a target dose, given that a positive dose–response relationship has been concluded. A target dose could be a dose with a minimum treatment effect or a dose that has a desired effect from the commercial perspective.

Metric #3   Relative average prediction error obtained by averaging the absolute differences between the estimated and the true dose–response values at each of the doses included in the study and dividing the average by the absolute target effect.

It was noted in Chap. 6 (see Sect. 6.3) that Metrics #1 and #2 above could be combined to create a joint metric requiring detection of a dose–response relationship and correct identification of a target dose. A further metric that has been proposed is the probability of detecting any dose with at least the minimum treatment effect (Bornkamp et al., 2007). We do not advocate this metric because we think that Metric #2 or the combination of Metrics #1 and #2 are more likely to give better assessments of a dose–response design. This is because the ultimate goal of a Phase 2 dose-ranging design is to select a target dose or doses for confirmatory testing in Phase 3.

8.5 Conditional Evaluation of a Dose–Response Design

One way to conduct a conditional evaluation of a dose–response design is to consider a number of plausible scenarios for which we hope to have a design that has good characteristics. For example, we can consider Base, Pessimistic and Optimistic scenarios as frequently hypothesized by pharmaceutical companies. While such scenarios usually consider more than just efficacy, we will only focus on differences in efficacy between the scenarios in this chapter. The Base case is taken to be the dose–response if the compound performs as expected. The Pessimistic case is when the compound does not perform as well as expected but would still make the compound minimally interesting. Finally, the Optimistic case corresponds to a situation when the dose–response is better than expected and probably represents as good a dose–response as one could hope for. To check the false positive error rate for detecting a positive dose–response, the null scenario of no dose–response can also be included.

To illustrate this approach, we adapt the example scenario used by Bornkamp et al. (2007). The example is a 6-week dose-ranging study for neuropathic pain in which the primary endpoint is the change from baseline at 6 weeks on a visual analogue scale (VAS) of pain. The VAS takes values between 0 (no pain) and 10 (highest pain) on a continuous scale and is assumed to be Normally distributed. Weekly VAS measurements are collected for each patient.

Let VAS_k denote the VAS measurement at the kth Week, $k = 1, \ldots, 6$ and with $k = 0$ representing baseline. The primary endpoint is defined as $Y = VAS_6 - VAS_0$. Following Bornkamp et al., we assume that Y is Normally distributed with variance $\sigma^2 = 4.5$. Negative values of Y give indication of efficacy in reducing the neuropathic pain. It is assumed that the available doses are 0, 1, 2, 3, 4, 5, 6, 7 and 8 units.

We consider three possible dose–response curves corresponding to the Base, Pessimistic and Optimistic scenarios. For the Base case, we consider that the true dose–response curve is

$$E(Y|d_i) = -1.5 \times \frac{d_i}{(0.79 + d_i)} \tag{8.3}$$

while for the Pessimistic case, we have

$$E(Y|d_i) = -1.2 \times \frac{d_i}{(0.79 + d_i)} \qquad (8.4)$$

and for the Optimistic case, we have

$$E(Y|d_i) = -1.8 \times \frac{d_i}{(0.79 + d_i)} \qquad (8.5)$$

We follow the assumption adopted by Bornkamp et al. that the placebo response is zero (i.e., the expected change from baseline at week 6 for the placebo group is 0). In all three dose–response curves, ED_{50} is assumed to be 0.79 which is what Bornkamp et al. used to linearize the Emax model. The three assumed dose–response curves are displayed in Fig. 8.2 for a dose range from 0 to 10 units.

We suppose that the design we wish to evaluate is one with five equally spaced doses of 0, 2, 4, 6 and 8 units where a dose of 8 units is the MTD. We choose five doses because they are generally sufficient to allow the fit and assessment of a 4-parameter Emax model if required while not being so many as to be considered impractical. From our experience, a design with equally spaced doses or log doses is among the most commonly used design. We assume that 30 subjects are randomized to each dose. The use of 30 subjects per dose reflects another common approach of having an equal number of subjects given each dose, while the total of 150 subjects reflects a plausible constraint on the number of subjects for the neuropathic pain indication. We assume that the target minimum treatment effect is a reduction of at least 1 point compared to placebo.

Using the "LDOD" package in the R software (R Core Team, 2020; Masoudi et al., 2013), we found the relative efficiency of the above design to the D-optimal design with a maximum dose of 8 units to be 61% for all three possible values for E_{max} (i.e., -1.2, -1.5 and -1.8) in (8.3)–(8.5).

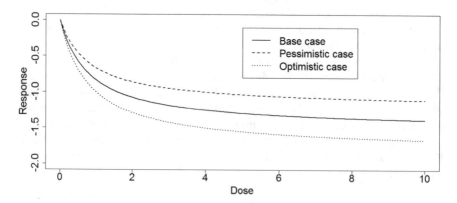

Fig. 8.2 Scenarios for conditional evaluation of designs for a 3-parameter Emax model

The metrics described in Sect. 8.4 are implemented as follows. The detection of a positive dose–response is assessed using a trend test defined as the t-test for a negative slope when a linear regression model with dose as the explanatory variable is fitted. The test is conducted using the one-sided 5% significance level. To assess whether a target dose is correctly identified, we define a target dose interval as all doses which give an effect within 10% of the target effect of a 1-point reduction in VAS score using the true dose–response model. For a given target effect, the target dose for a 4-parameter Emax model is given by

$$\text{target dose} = \frac{ED_{50}}{\left(\frac{E_{\max}}{\text{target}} - 1\right)^{1/\lambda}} \tag{8.6}$$

provided that $\frac{E_{\max}}{\text{target}} > 1$.

For the three scenarios, the target dose intervals are given in Table 8.1

Correctly identifying the target dose is defined as identifying a dose that is within the target dose interval. For simplicity, the estimated dose is allowed to be continuous and to lie outside the range of the doses used. The framework of evaluation is equally applicable when additional conditions are imposed on the estimated target dose. Finally, the relative average prediction error is defined using the five doses included in the study.

To evaluate the design, we use a maximum likelihood fit of a 3-parameter Emax model with parameter values bounded to avoid numerical overflow (Brain et al., 2014). The parameter bounds we use are $-1000,000$ to $1,000,000$ for the parameter E_0, -10 to 10 for $\log(ED_{50})$ and $-1,000,000,$ to $1,000,000$ for $E_{\max}$. Simulating 10,000 data sets for each scenario and measuring Metrics #1 to #3 gave the results shown in Table 8.2.

Table 8.1 Target dose intervals for three scenarios (target defined as 1-point reduction in pain score from baseline compared with placebo)

Scenario	Target dose interval
Pessimistic	(2.37, 8.69)
Base	(1.19, 2.17)
Optimistic	(0.79, 1.24)

Table 8.2 Results for 10,000 simulated trials for maximum likelihood fit of a 3-parameter Emax model with 30 subjects per dose for doses 0, 2, 4, 6 and 8 units

Metric	Scenario		
	Pessimistic	Base	Optimistic
#1 probability to correctly detect a positive dose–response relationship	0.61	0.77	0.89
#2 probability to correctly identify a target dose given that a positive dose–response has been declared	0.44	0.18	0.13
#3 relative (to target effect) average prediction error	0.21	0.21	0.22

It can be seen immediately from Table 8.2 that correctly identifying a target dose given evidence of a positive dose–response can be a difficult problem. The probabilities for correctly detecting a dose–response for all of the scenarios might be viewed as reasonable, bearing in mind that the Pessimistic scenario is of minimal interest. The relative average prediction error is estimated to be just over 20% for all three scenarios.

To see if the probability of correctly identifying a target dose can be improved, we consider the effect of doubling the sample size per dose or widening the interval allowed around the target effect for a correct decision on the target dose.

Doubling the number of subjects per dose, we obtained the results in Table 8.3.

From Table 8.3, it can be seen that doubling the number of subjects per dose has some impact on the probability of correctly identifying a target dose given that a positive dose–response relationship has been declared for the Optimistic and Base scenarios but actually lessens the corresponding probability for the Pessimistic scenario. By comparison, the probability of correctly detecting a positive dose–response relationship is now virtually 100% for the Base and Optimistic scenarios.

We next examine the effect of varying the allowed interval around the target effect for the original design. We display the results for allowing the interval around the target effect to be ±15%, ±20%, ±25% and ±30% in Table 8.4.

Table 8.3 Results for 10,000 simulated trials for maximum likelihood fit of a 3-parameter Emax model with 60 subjects per dose for doses 0, 2, 4, 6 and 8 units

Metric	Scenario		
	Pessimistic	Base	Optimistic
#1 probability to correctly detect a positive dose–response relationship	0.94	0.99	1.00
#2 probability to correctly identify a target dose given that a positive dose–response has been declared	0.33	0.23	0.21
#3 relative (to target effect) average prediction error	0.16	0.16	0.17

Table 8.4 Probability of correctly identifying a target dose given a positive dose–response has been declared for results from 10,000 simulated trials for the maximum likelihood fit of a 3-parameter Emax model with 30 subjects per dose for doses 0, 2, 4, 6 and 8 units

Allowed interval around target effect for a correct decision	Scenario		
	Pessimistic	Base	Optimistic
±15%	0.54	0.27	0.20
±20%	0.61	0.35	0.26
±25%	0.65	0.45	0.32
±30%	0.67	0.54	0.39

Table 8.5 Results for 10,000 simulated trials for maximum likelihood fit of a 3-parameter model with 40 subjects per dose for doses 0, 1 and 8 units and 15 subjects per dose for doses 2 and 5 units

Metric	Scenario		
	Pessimistic	Base	Optimistic
#1 probability to correctly detect a positive dose–response relationship	0.65	0.81	0.92
#2 probability to correctly identify a target dose given that a positive dose–response has been declared	0.39	0.20	0.17
#3 relative (to target effect) average prediction error	0.21	0.22	0.22

We can see from Table 8.4 that widening the allowed interval about the target effect generally increases the probability of correctly identifying a target dose. The probabilities are biggest for the Pessimistic scenario because the dose–response is flattest for this scenario and a larger interval around the target effect translates to a large target dose interval. Correspondingly, the dose–response is steepest for the Optimistic scenario, and the larger target effect interval does not translate into a similarly larger target dose interval for this scenario.

It is of interest to compare the first dose–response design (i.e., 30 subjects on each of five equally spaced doses of 0, 2, 4, 6 and 8 units) with one that is closer to the local D-optimal design. We thus consider a design with still a total of 150 subjects and five doses but with the following allocation to doses: 40 subjects to placebo, 40 subjects to a dose of 1, 15 subjects to a dose of 2, 15 subjects to a dose of 5 and 40 subjects to a dose of 8. This design places more subjects at the two ends of the dose range. It also uses different doses (doses 0, 1, 2, 5 and 8) compared to the first design.

The estimated metrics obtained for 10,000 simulations for the new design are shown in Table 8.5. It is worth noting that the efficiency of this design relative to the local D-optimal design, as given by the "LDOD" package in R, is 89% for all three assumed values for E_{max}.

From Table 8.5, it can be seen that the estimated metric for detecting a positive dose–response is improved somewhat but the probability of correctly identifying a target dose given a positive dose–response has been declared is estimated to be lower for the Pessimistic scenario. The relative prediction error is similar. A disadvantage of this design is the reduction in the amount of safety data for the two middle doses.

8.6 Unconditional Evaluation of a Dose–Response Design

We proceed to consider unconditional evaluation of a dose–response design using a design prior distribution. We will first describe one way to obtain such a distribution, given the results of a POC study and the projected potency of a compound in the next section.

8.6.1   Obtaining a Prior from POC Study Results and a Projection of Compound Potency

For an Emax model, a prior is needed for the model parameters. We consider the fit of the 4-parameter Emax model so require a prior for the parameters E_0, E_{max}, ED_{50} and λ. One approach is to combine independent prior distributions for each of these parameters to obtain a joint distribution.

For E_0, there is often some information about the placebo response in the POC study. There may also be other studies in the literature that can be used to help derive a prior distribution for E_0. A prior distribution for the ED_{50} can be obtained by using a PK/PD prediction of potency and placing a distribution around it. In practice, Normal distributions are frequently assumed for E_0 and the response for a particular dose.

As for a prior for the E_{max} parameter, we can first define a prior for the response to a particular dose used in a POC study. This prior together with prior distributions for E_0, and λ defines a prior distribution for the E_{max} parameter. Under this approach, the prior distribution for the E_{max} parameter is derived indirectly.

For the λ parameter, in the absence of other information, Thomas et al. (2014) suggested using a beta distribution scaled to (0,6) with parameters 3.03 and 18.15 as a prior. Thomas et al. derived this distribution and a t_3 distribution with mean 0.79 and scale parameter 0.6 for $\log(ED_{50}/P_{50})$, where P_{50} is a preliminary prediction of the ED_{50}, by fitting a Bayesian hierarchical model to the mean response $E(Y_{jk}|D)$ at dose D based on data from studies of 27 small molecule compound-indication combinations. Thomas et al. normalized the data so that the overall mean was 0 and the overall standard deviation was 1 for each compound before their investigations. Thomas et al. included only compounds that differentiated from placebo.

$$E(Y_{jk}|D) = E_{0jk} + \frac{E_{\max j} D^{\lambda_j}}{ED_{50j}^{\lambda_j} + D^{\lambda_j}} \qquad (8.7)$$

In (8.7), j denotes the jth compound and k the kth study for compound j. Residual errors were assumed Normally distributed with a constant variance for a compound.

The t_3 distribution with mean 0.79 and scale parameter 0.6 and the rescaled beta distribution are approximate posterior predictive distributions for $\log(ED_{50}/P_{50})$ and λ, obtained from the fitted Bayesian hierarchical model using a more informative prior for the ED_{50} and a scaled beta prior for λ. The approximate scaled beta distribution was the most diffuse of the predictive distributions obtained for λ considered by Thomas et al., and the t_3 distribution with mean 0.79 and scale parameter 0.6 was the corresponding approximate predictive distribution obtained for $\log(ED_{50}/P_{50})$.

For a more detailed discussion on the derivation and use of the rescaled beta and the t$_3$ distributions, see Thomas et al. (2014).

8.6.2 An Example

We consider the same example as introduced in Sect. 8.5, but instead of assuming particular sets of values for the parameters in a 3-parameter Emax model, we now assume that we have a 4-parameter Emax model with a design prior distribution for the four parameters.

The design prior distribution we shall use is the product of four independent prior distributions for the parameters as follows:

1. For E_0, we assume a $N(0; 0.1^2)$ distribution.
2. For E_{max}, we assume a $N(1.5; 0.2^2)$ distribution.
3. For ED_{50}, we assume a t_3 distribution with mean 0.79 and scale parameter 0.6 for $\log(ED_{50}/P_{50})$ as described in Sect. 8.6.1. We use the value 0.79 for P_{50}. (Please see Sect. 8.5 on the origin of this assumption for P_{50}.)
4. For λ, we assume a beta distribution with parameters 3.03 and 18.15 scaled to (0.6) as described in Sect. 8.6.1.

The assumed prior distribution for each parameter is shown in Fig. 8.3.

To give an idea of the corresponding joint prior distribution obtained by combining the independent priors for each parameter in terms of the dose–response curves, we generate 50 Emax curves by taking random samples from the prior distributions for E_0, E_{max}, ED_{50} and λ. The curves are shown in Fig. 8.4.

We also give in Table 8.6 six point summaries for the prior distribution for dose effects relative to placebo from 10,000 random samples.

To illustrate the evaluation of designs using the above design prior we use the two designs discussed in Sect. 8.5 and repeated in Table 8.7.

Using each of the designs and taking 10,000 samples from the design prior distribution, we can, as before, examine the estimated metrics for the design from a maximum likelihood fit and the use of the test for trend. We want to make it clear

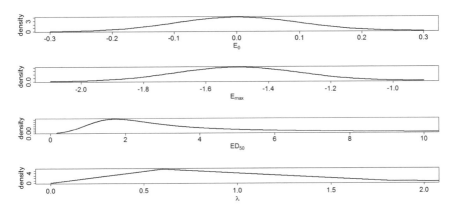

Fig. 8.3 Prior distributions for the four parameters for unconditional evaluation of designs for a 4-parameter Emax model

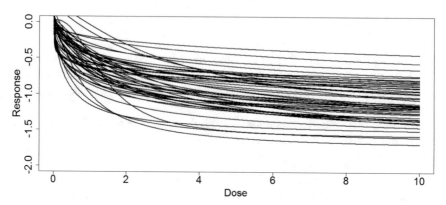

Fig. 8.4 Fifty simulated 4-parameter Emax model dose–response curves using priors for parameters displayed in Fig. 8.3

Table 8.6 Summary statistics for dose effects for 10,000 simulated dose–response curves using prior distributions displayed in Fig. 8.3

Dose	Min	Q1	Median	Mean	Q3	Max
1	−1.83	−0.75	−0.60	−0.60	−0.44	0.00
2	−1.97	−0.94	−0.78	−0.79	−0.64	0.00
3	−2.01	−1.06	−0.89	−0.90	−0.74	0.00
4	−2.02	−1.14	−0.96	−0.98	−0.80	0.00
5	−2.02	−1.20	−1.02	−1.03	−0.85	0.00
6	−2.04	−1.24	−1.06	−1.07	−0.89	0.00
7	−2.06	−1.28	−1.09	−1.10	−0.92	0.00
8	−2.07	−1.30	−1.12	−1.12	−0.94	0.00

Table 8.7 Designs to be evaluated using prior distributions displayed in Fig. 8.3

Design 1		Design 2	
Dose	Number of subjects	Dose	Number of subjects
0	30	0	40
2	30	1	40
4	30	2	15
6	30	5	15
8	30	8	40

that we use the design prior distribution to generate data but use maximum likelihood to fit the Emax model to the resulting data. In other words, we are not conducting any Bayesian analysis of the simulated data.

Given the use of the design prior distribution, we can further split the metrics obtained by whether or not the truth of a 1-point difference from placebo is satisfied

Table 8.8 Results for 10,000 simulated trials from maximum likelihood fit of a 4-parameter model under Design 1 in Table 8.7

Metric	True effect for highest dose		Overall
	<1.0	≥1.0	
#1 probability to correctly detect a positive dose–response relationship	0.14	0.49	0.63
#2 probability to correctly identify a target dose given that a positive dose–response has been declared	0.03	0.21	0.24
#3 relative (to target effect) average prediction error	0.23	0.23	0.23

Table 8.9 Results for 10,000 simulated trials from maximum likelihood fit of a 4-parameter Emax model under Design 2 in Table 8.7

Metric	True effect for highest dose		Overall
	<1.0	≥1.0	
#1 probability to correctly detect a positive dose–response relationship	0.16	0.52	0.68
#2 probability to correctly identify a target dose given that a positive dose–response has been declared	0.03	0.17	0.20
#3 relative (to target effect) average prediction error	0.22	0.23	0.23

at the highest dose. Doing this, we obtain the results in Tables 8.8 and 8.9 for the first and second designs, respectively.

The probability of detecting a dose–response is only moderate for both designs although it is slightly higher for the Design 2. Again we can see that the probability of correctly identifying a target dose given that a positive dose–response has been declared is quite low.

The use of a design prior distribution allows us to estimate the probability that the top dose has an effect of at least 1 point if a positive dose–response is declared. Here, this is equal to

$$\frac{0.49}{0.63} = 0.78$$

for Design 1 and 0.76 for Design 2. Thus, the detection of a dose–response using either design would give a reasonably high probability that the true treatment effect at the highest dose is greater than or equal to 1 point.

We can also assess the metrics for a Bayesian fit of the Emax model that uses the same analysis prior distribution as the design prior distribution. The posterior probability distribution for the E_{max} parameter is now used to test if there is a positive dose–response relationship. For example, if the posterior probability that the E_{max} parameter is <0 is greater than 0.95, we consider that there is sufficient evidence of a positive dose–response relationship. We use the posterior means for each dose to assess the probability of correctly identifying a target dose and to calculate the relative average prediction error.

To fit the Bayesian model using WinBUGS, 50,000 samples were used as the burn in before a further 50,000 samples were obtained from the assumed converged posterior distribution. A gamma prior distribution was used for the inverse of the residual variance with shape and size parameters both equal to 0.001.

The estimated results for the two designs obtained for 1000 simulations are shown in Tables 8.10 and 8.11.

The Bayesian analysis yields an estimated probability of 100% of detecting a positive dose–response. This means that the probability that the top dose has an effect of at least 1 point if a positive dose–response is declared is simply the probability that the true treatment effect at the highest dose is at least 1 point. This probability is estimated to be 0.69 for Design 1 and 0.67 for Design 2. These are less than their counterparts for the use of the maximum likelihood fit of the 4-parameter Emax model. We note that the conditional probability of correctly identifying a target dose

Table 8.10 Results for 1000 simulated trials for Bayesian fit of a 4-parameter Emax model under Design 1 in Table 8.7

Metric	True effect for highest dose		Total
	<1.0	≥1.0	
#1 probability to correctly detect a positive dose–response relationship	0.31	0.69	1.00
#2 probability to correctly identify a target dose given that a positive dose–response has been declared	0.11	0.30	0.41
#3 relative (to target effect) average prediction error	0.13	0.13	0.13

Table 8.11 Results for 1000 simulated trials for Bayesian fit of a 4-parameter model under Design 2 in Table 8.7

Metric	True effect for highest dose		Total
	<1.0	≥1.0	
#1 probability to correctly detect a positive dose–response relationship	0.33	0.67	1.00
#2 probability to correctly identify a target dose given a positive dose–response has been declared	0.12	0.29	0.41
#3 relative (to target effect) average prediction error	0.13	0.13	0.13

is, however, estimated to be far bigger than that for the maximum likelihood analysis, and the relative average prediction error is also noticeably improved.

It is important to note that the use of the same prior in the analysis and in generating the data contributes to a better result on the conditional probability of correctly identifying a target dose. We expect this probability to decrease if the data behave quite differently from the prior distributions assumed for analysis.

8.7 Fitting an Emax Model to Binary Data—Two Tofacitinib Dose–Response Studies

In this section, we look at fitting an Emax model to binary data for two of the dose–response studies conducted for the compound tofacitinib.

The first dose–response study for tofacitinib was a randomized, double-blind, placebo-controlled, multicenter study to compare doses of 5, 15 and 30 mg BID of tofacitinib versus placebo for 6 weeks in subjects with acute rheumatoid arthritis (ClinicalTrials.gov identifier NCT00147498). The primary endpoint was the ACR20 response—the percentage of subjects achieving greater than or equal to 20% improvement in, tender joints count, swollen joints count and in at least three of the remaining ACR core measures (participant assessment of pain, participant global assessment of disease activity, physician global assessment of disease activity, self-assessed disability assessed using the disability index of the Health Assessment Questionnaire and C-Reactive Protein). Detailed definition of ACR20 can be found in Sect. 7.8.1 in Chap. 7 or in Felson et al. (1995).

The results for ACR20 are displayed in Table 8.12.

We consider fitting model (8.2) using the cumulative logistic distribution and with the parameter λ set equal to 1. To fit this model, we use the R software package clinDR (R Core Team, 2020; Thomas, 2020) with the maximum likelihood method of fitting.

The model fit transformed back to the scale of proportion of responders is shown in Fig. 8.5. The asterisks denote observed proportions, the black bars 90% confidence intervals for the means and the gray bars 90% prediction intervals.

It can be seen from Fig. 8.5 that the fit is reasonable but that the proportion of responders rises very steeply between 0 and 5 mg. To obtain more information about this portion of the curve between 0 and 5 mg, a second dose–response study was run.

Table 8.12 ACR20 response rate (%) by treatment group for first tofacitinib dose–response study

	Treatment group			
	5 mg	15 mg	30 mg	Placebo
N	61	69	69	65
# of Responders	43	56	53	19
%	70.49	81.16	76.81	29.23

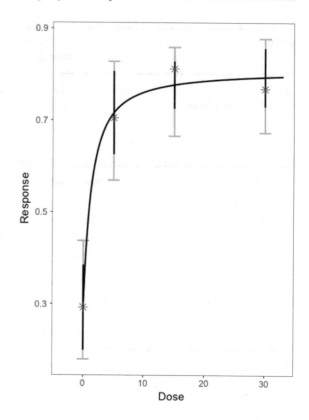

Fig. 8.5 Transformed fit of model (8.2) with λ = 1 for first tofacitinib dose–response study

The second dose–response study for tofacitinib was a randomized, double-blind, placebo-controlled, multicenter study to compare six dose regimens of tofacitinib versus placebo for six weeks in subjects with inadequate response to methotrexate treatment alone (ClinicalTrials.gov identifier NCT00413660). The dose regimens were 1, 3, 5, 10 and 15 mg, all given BID, with a background of stable methotrexate treatment and 20 mg tofacitinib given once a day with a background of stable methotrexate treatment. The primary endpoint was again the ACR20 response rate in each group. Here, we consider just the results for the BID tofacitinib treatment and placebo (Table 8.13).

Table 8.13 ACR20 response rate (%) by treatment group for second tofacitinib dose–response study

	Treatment group					
	1 mg	3 mg	5 mg	10 mg	15 mg	Placebo
N	70	68	71	74	75	69
# of Responders	33	38	40	43	42	25
%	47.14	55.88	56.34	58.11	56.00	36.23

Fig. 8.6 Transformed fit of model (8.2) for second tofacitinib dose–response study

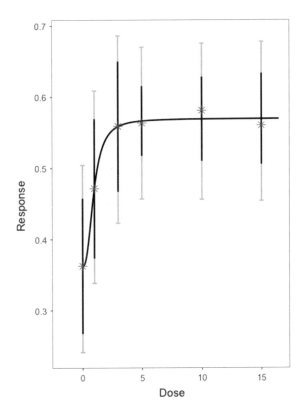

We again fit model (8.2) using the maximum likelihood method but this time without constraining the λ parameter to be equal to 1. The transformed fit with 90% confidence and prediction intervals is shown in Fig. 8.6.

It can be seen from Fig. 8.6 that although the result for 3 mg lies close to that for 5 mg, the inclusion of the 1 mg dose fills in a result for the curve between 0 and 5 mg, hence better characterizing the dose–response curve for low doses.

This example from the development of tofacitinib is instructive because it illustrates the potential importance of including sufficiently low doses and a sufficient dose range. The FDA approved the 5 mg BID dose, but the elucidation of the dose–response curve below a dose on or near the plateau of response likely helped in their evaluation and gave reassurance that a much lower dose would not have the same efficacy. An alternative approach that might have been taken in the development of tofacitinib is to use an adaptive dose-ranging design. We describe an example of such an adaptive dose-ranging design in Chap. 13 (see Sect. 13.5).

8.8 Discussion

In this chapter, we focus on the design and analysis of a dose–response study using an Emax model because of the findings by Thomas et al. (2014), Thomas et al. (2014b) and Wu et al. (2018). The approaches to evaluating designs based on other dose–response models or collections of dose–response models could proceed similarly.

In this chapter, we looked at using D-optimal designs as well as pragmatic designs often used in practice. While use of a D-optimal design may not be practical, comparison of other designs against a D-optimal design gives a yardstick to assess their efficiency. An optimality criterion other than D-optimality could alternatively be chosen as a reference.

In practice, there are likely to be a number of key constraints in the design of a dose–response study. We have considered constraints given by a maximum possible dose, the doses available and the desire to have a minimum number of subjects for a minimum number of doses. It is possible that there are other additional constraints that need to be taken into account as well.

The Emax model assumes a monotone dose–response relationship. Some may be concerned that a true dose–response relationship may not be monotonic in some situations. The evidence, however, suggests that this is not a common occurrence. For example, Thomas et al. (2014) found just one compound-indication combination out of a portfolio of 33 compound-indications with evidence of a non-monotone dose–response. If there is a good rationale for a non-monotone response, then flexible models that do not assume monotonicity should be used to model the dose–response relationship. Two possible models are the normal dynamic linear model (Smith et al., 2006) and smoothing splines (Kirby et al., 2009). One caution here is that a true monotonic dose–response may produce observed mean responses that are not monotonic. For the Base case scenario for the first example in Sect. 8.5, the probability of getting any non-monotonic configuration of sample means is estimated to be 92% from simulating 10,000 trials. The probability of getting a configuration where the top dose shows a smaller reduction from baseline than the next highest dose is estimated to be 47% from the same simulations. In other words, approximately half of the time we would expect the observed effect for the highest dose to be less than that for the next highest dose.

In addition to sampling variability, a higher dropout rate at the highest dose together with the analytical method chosen to handle missing data (e.g., baseline observation carried forward, an approach that was commonly used at the turn of the century) could lead to the appearance of a non-monotone dose–response relationship in the observed mean response. Therefore, unless there are biologic rationales or repeat precedents about a class of drugs, we recommend using the Emax model as the starting point to design and analyze a dose–response study.

In Sect. 8.5, we illustrated the conditional evaluation of a dose–response design using three scenarios under a 3-parameter Emax model. If it is suspected that the dose–response curve takes a different shape from the hyperbola shown in Fig. 8.1, an

Emax model with $\lambda \neq 1$ can be used. What we illustrated in Sect. 8.5 is a framework for conducting the evaluation.

In this chapter, we considered a dose range where the highest dose was eightfold of the lowest dose. We adopted this choice because it was used in Bornkamp et al. (2007) and Pinheiro et al. (2010). Thomas et al. (2014a) suggested from their investigation that a dose range less than 20-fold was dubious in its ability to well characterize a dose–response relationship given the uncertainty in the ED_{50} at the initiation of dose-finding studies and the nearly 100-fold range in doses between minimal and maximal response predicted by the hyperbolic Emax model. We recommend readers to consider a wider dose range than the one used in this chapter chosen primarily for illustrative purposes.

We have not considered modeling exposure–response in this chapter. Modeling exposure–response can have advantages in certain situations compared with modeling dose–response, as described by Pinheiro et al. (2010). Pinheiro et al. concluded that modeling exposure–response could provide more accurate target dose selection and characterization of the response profile when the pharmacokinetic variability was high (e.g., individual clearances for the scenarios they considered), when the gradient of the underlying response profile was large within the region of greatest interest and when the exposure assessment error variability (e.g., error in the assessment of the clearances for their scenarios) was relatively low. Pinheiro et al. noted that for any real drug development program the value of exposure–response versus dose–response should be assessed via simulations that consider the available knowledge about the compound and disease state.

We have not considered cost or economic considerations in this chapter either. These and the possible use of adaptive designs will be covered in Chaps. 11 and 13. We note here that the use of an adaptive design may offer the possibility of more accurately detecting a target dose. For example, Pinheiro et al. (2010) described the DcoD method in which D-optimality was applied for a design for a 4-parameter Emax model in a first stage of a trial and then C-optimality, the minimization of the variance of a linear combination of parameters, was used to maximize the precision of estimation of the minimum effective dose under the assumed sigmoid Emax model in a second stage. We include an adaptive dose-ranging study in Sect. 13.5 in Chap. 13.

Finally, we will discuss joint modeling of efficacy and safety in Chap. 14 (see Sect. 14.2).

References

Atkinson, A. C., & Donev, A. N. (1992). *Optimum experimental designs.* Clarendon Press.

Atkinson, A. C., Donev, A. N., & Tobias, R. D. (2007). *Optimum experimental designs, with SAS.* Oxford University Press.

Bornkamp, B., Bretz, F., Dmitrienko, A., et al. (2007). Innovative approaches for designing and analyzing adaptive dose-ranging trials. *Journal of Biopharmaceutical Statistics, 17*(6), 965–995.

Bornkamp, B., Pinheiro, J., & Bretz, F. (2009). MCPMod: An R Package for the design and analysis of dose-finding Studies. *Journal of Statistical Software, 29*(7), published in February.

Brain, P., Kirby, S., & Larionov, R. (2014). Fitting Emax models to clinical trial dose-response data when the high dose asymptote is ill defined. *Pharmaceutical Statistics, 13*(6), 364–370.

Bretz, F., Pinheiro, J. C., & Branson, M. (2005). Combining multiple comparisons and modeling techniques in dose-response studies. *Biometrics, 61*(3), 738–748.

Cross, J., Lee, H., Westelinck, A., et al. (2002). Postmarketing drug dosage changes of 499 FDA-approved new molecular entities, 1980–99. *Pharmacoepidemiology and Drug Safety, 11*(6), 439–446.

Dette, H., Kiss, C., Bevanda, M., & Bretz, F. (2010). Optimal designs for the emax, log-linear and exponential models. *Biometrika, 97*(2), 513–518.

Felson, D. T., Anderson, J. J., Boers, M., et al. (1995). American College of Rheumatology preliminary definition of improvement in rheumatoid arthritis. *Arthritis and Rheumatism, 38*(6), 727–735.

Fedorov, V. V., & Leonov, S. L. (2013). *Optimal design for nonlinear response models.* Chapman Hall/CRC Press.

ICH E4 (1994). Dose-response information to support drug registration.

Kirby, S., Colman, P., & Morris, M. (2009). Adaptive modelling of dose-response relationships using smoothing splines. *Pharmaceutical Statistics, 8*(4), 346–355.

Masoudi, E., Sarmad, M., & Talebi, H. (2013) Package LDOD. Available at https://cran.r-project.org/web/packages/LDOD/index.html

Pinheiro, J., Sax, F., Antonijevic, Z., et al. (2010). Adaptive and model-based dose-ranging trials: Quantitative evaluation and recommendations. *Statistics in Biopharmaceutical Research, 2*(4), 435–454.

R Core Team. (2020). R: A language and environment for statistical computing. R Foundation for Statistical Computing, Vienna, Austria. ISBN 3-900051-07-0. URL http://www.R-project.org/

Sacks, L. V., Shamsuddin, H. H., Yasinskaya, Y. I., et al. (2014). Scientific and regulatory reasons for delay and denial of FDA approval of initial applications for new drugs, 2000–2012. *Journal of the American Medical Association, 311*(4), 378–384.

Smith, M. K., Jones, I., Morris, M. F., et al. (2006). Implementation of a Bayesian adaptive design in a proof of concept study. *Pharmaceutical Statistics, 5*(1), 39–50.

Thomas, N. Package clinDR. Available at https://cran.r-project.org/web/packages/clinDR/index.html

Thomas, N., Sweeney, K., & Somayaji, V. (2014). Meta-analysis of clinical dose–response in a large drug development portfolio. *Statistics in Biopharmaceutical Research, 6*(4), 302–317.

Thomas, N., Roy, D., Somayaji, V., & Sweeney, K. (2014b). Meta-analyses of clinical dose response. Presentation at the European Medicines Agency/European Federation of Pharmaceutical Industries and Associations workshop on the importance of dose finding and dose selection for the successful development, licensing and lifecycle management of medicinal products. Available at http://www.ema.europa.eu/docs/en_GB/document_library/Presentation/2015/01/WC500179795.pdf (accessed 15 February 2021).

Turner, H., & Firth, D. (2020) Generalized nonlinear models in R: An overview of the gnm package. Available at https://cran.r-project.org/web/packages/gnm/vignettes/gnmOverview.pdf

Wu, J., Banerjee, A., Jin, B., et al. (2018). Clinical dose-response for a broad set of biological products: A model-based meta-analysis. *Statistical Methods in Medical Research, 27*(9), 2694–2721.

Chapter 9
Designing Confirmatory Trials with Desired Characteristics

Chance favors the prepared mind.
—Louis Pasteur

9.1 Introduction

By the time a new drug moves into the confirmatory stage, its developer should in theory have a reasonable amount of information on the effect of the drug on several efficacy endpoints. After all, a primary objective of a confirmatory trial is to confirm a treatment effect with the use of tightly controlled and rigorously pre-specified hypothesis tests.

Ideally, one of the above efficacy endpoints is the endpoint needed for regulatory approval and information on the treatment effect is available at the time point required by the regulatory agencies. Unfortunately, this is not always the case. For example, tumor response is often the primary endpoint for Phase 2 cancer studies of solid tumors while progression-free survival or overall survival is typically the primary endpoint in Phase 3 studies.

There are also situations that while the endpoint is the same, the available information on treatment effect is at an earlier time point. For example, a developer of a new drug for chronic obstructive pulmonary disease may have information pertaining to the drug effect on FEV_1 (forced expiratory volume in the first second after taking a deep breath) at the end of a 2-week treatment period instead of 26 weeks. Similarly, the developer of a drug to treat the primary infection of the human immunodeficiency virus may have viral suppression data at the end of a 16-week treatment period instead of 48 weeks from its Phase 2 trials.

As a result, the developer may need to translate the available information from Phase 2 trials to an estimate of the drug effect on the endpoint at the time point of interest for Phase 3. This may require building a model to predict the drug effect on one endpoint from another. It may also require building a longitudinal model that predicts a patient's response at a later time point from their earlier ones. We mentioned how some of this could be done in Chap. 5 (see Sect. 5.9). As we emphasized in Sect. 5.9, building these models requires close collaboration among scientists from multiple disciplines such as statistics, pharmacometrics, clinical pharmacology and medicine.

In this chapter, we assume that some treatment effect information on the primary endpoint and for the appropriate patient population is available for planning a Phase 3 trial. We will review how this information can be used to assess the probability of success of the study (POSS) and discuss how POSS can in turn help a sponsor assess the effectiveness of the sample size calculated from the hypothesis-testing perspective. In addition, we will discuss factors that could affect POSS and how these factors should be incorporated into the planning of the confirmatory program. We hope the discussion will help explain why a robust investment in Phase 2 trials is important for a desirable level of POSS at the Phase 3 stage.

9.2 Useful Metrics at the Confirmatory Stage

In this chapter, we use the axitinib example in Chuang-Stein et al. (2011) to illustrate useful metrics at the confirmatory stage. These metrics are discussed in detail in Chap. 6 (see Sect. 6.4).

Axitinib is an oral, potent and selective tyrosine kinase inhibitor of vascular endothelial growth factor receptors 1, 2 and 3. Based on signs of clinical activity observed in single-agent Phase 2 studies in renal cell carcinoma, non-small-cell lung carcinoma, and thyroid cancer, a randomized, open-label Phase 2 study (NCT00219557) in patients with locally advanced or metastatic pancreatic cancer was initiated in July 2005. Locally advanced or metastatic pancreatic cancer is one of the deadliest forms of cancer with limited treatment options to improve survival.

The Phase 2 study had overall survival as its primary endpoint. The study planned to enroll 102 patients and follow them for at least one year from randomization or until death. The number of deaths was planned to be 68. The study randomized patients in a 2:1 ratio to axitinib combined with gemcitabine or to gemcitabine alone. The study, with the planned number of events, would have 80% power to detect a hazard ratio (combination vs gemcitabine alone) of 0.6 or less based on a log-rank test and a one-sided 10% significance level (Spano et al., 2008).

The Phase 2 study randomized 103 patients, 69 to the combination treatment and 34 to gemcitabine alone. The Cox proportional hazards model analysis yielded an estimated hazard ratio (HR) for the death of 0.71 with a 95% confidence interval of (0.44, 1.13) (Spano et al., 2008). Since the analysis of HR is typically done on the natural logarithmic scale and then converted back to the HR scale for reporting purpose, one can calculate the standard error of the $\ln(HR)$ estimate from the reported confidence interval. The latter is found to be 0.24. Thus, the $\ln(HR)$ estimate has approximately a Normal distribution $N(\ln(0.71); 0.24^2)$.

Based on the Phase 2 results, the developer planned a double-blind Phase 3 study to compare the same combination of axitinib plus gemcitabine against gemcitabine plus placebo in the same patient population. The primary endpoint is again the overall survival. One proposal under consideration was to enroll approximately 600 patients. Under the assumption of an accrual period of 14 months, a non-uniform accrual of roughly 40% of patients by 7 months, a minimum 9-month follow-up on all subjects (or until death), and an assumed 36.7% improvement in median overall survival from 6 months to 8.2 months in patients receiving axitinib plus gemcitabine, this would give rise to approximately 460 events (deaths).

Assuming an exponential distribution for time to death, the above design would have approximately 90% power to detect a hazard ratio of 0.73. Denoting HR by λ and defining the trial success as rejecting the null hypothesis of H_0: $\lambda \geq 1$ versus the alternative hypothesis of H_A: $\lambda < 1$ at the one-sided 2.5% significance level, the developer would like to know the probability that the trial would be successful, or the POSS.

Using the sampling distribution for the HR estimate to reflect our uncertainty about the true λ, we can estimate the POSS using the expression in (9.1). The same expression was first discussed in Chap. 5 (see Eq. (5.2)).

$$\text{POSS} = \int \text{Pr}\,(\text{Significant Result} \mid \lambda)\,p(\lambda)\,d\lambda \qquad (9.1)$$

In (9.1), $p(\lambda)$ represents the density function of the sampling distribution of $\ln\left(\hat{\lambda}\right)$ obtained from the Phase 2 data, i.e., the density function of the Normal distribution $N(-0.34; 0.24^2)$.

One way to explain the calculation in (9.1) to non-statisticians is to use Table 9.1. In Table 9.1, the range for λ (column 1) is first divided into intervals of width 0.1 except for the two end intervals. Statistical power (column 2) is then calculated at the midpoint of each interval for λ except for the two end intervals where statistical power is calculated at 0.35 for $\lambda < 0.4$ and at 1.05 for $\lambda > 1.0$. The probability that λ is within an interval (c_1, c_2) is given by the area under the Normal density curve $N(-0.34; 0.24^2)$ between $\ln(c_1)$ and $\ln(c_2)$ (column 3). Multiplying numbers in the second column by the corresponding numbers in the third column gives the entries in the fourth column. Finally, adding the products together yields an approximation to the POSS in (9.1). In this example, the sum is 0.73. This number is an approximation to the POSS and is substantially lower than the 90% statistical power planned for the study.

Breaking down the calculation in Table 9.1 sheds some interesting insight on what makes up the POSS. First, the distribution for $\ln(\lambda)$ suggests that there is an almost 50% chance that the true λ is ≤ 0.7, and these low λ values contribute to approximately 64% (=0.47/0.73) of the overall POSS.

Considering that the sampling distribution is based on a small number of deaths and therefore has a high dispersion parameter, the low λ values could well be due to the high dispersion and represent an overestimation of the truth. Low λ values are

Table 9.1 Approximation to POSS of a design with 460 planned events when $\ln(\lambda)$ Is assumed to follow a Normal distribution $N(-0.34; 0.24^2)$

True λ	Statistical power at the midpoint of the λ-interval[a]	Probability that λ is in the interval in the first column	Product of column 2 and column 3
<0.4	1.00	0.01	0.01
0.4–0.5	1.00	0.06	0.06
0.5–0.6	1.00	0.17	0.17
0.6–0.7	1.00	0.23	0.23
0.7–0.8	0.87	0.21	0.19
0.8–0.9	0.41	0.15	0.06
0.9–1.0	0.08	0.09	0.01
>1.0	0.01	0.08	<0.001
			0.73[b]

[a] Power is calculated at $\lambda = 0.35$ for the first interval ($\lambda < 0.4$) and at $\lambda = 1.05$ for the last interval (>1.0). The calculation applies Normal approximation of $N(\ln(\lambda); 4/460)$ to the distribution of the estimate $\ln\left(\hat{\lambda}\right)$ in the Phase 3 trial.

[b] Obtained by adding the entries in column 4 before rounding

suspicious considering that locally advanced or metastatic pancreatic cancer is an extremely hard to treat disease. This is further supported by a review conducted by Zhang (2013) over a broad range of cancer treatments. Zhang obtained an empirical prior for the HR for progression-free survival. He estimated that overall, only about 16% of cancer drugs had a HR for progression-free survival ≤ 0.7. We will return to this topic in Chap. 12. These observations should caution us to view the POSS reported in Table 9.1 with care.

For the time being, we will assume a Normal prior $N(-0.34; 0.24^2)$ for $\ln(\lambda)$. Suppose that the treatment is only of interest if the true HR λ is ≤ 0.75. A decision to continue or to stop, based on whether the Phase 3 study yields a statistically significant result at the one-sided 2.5% level, will lead to the estimated probabilities in Table 9.2. The results in Table 9.2 are based on 10,000 random samples from the prior distribution.

Table 9.2 Estimated probabilities of various decisions assuming a design of 460 deaths, a prior distribution $N(-0.34; 0.24^2)$ for $\ln(\lambda)$ and a decision to continue if the result is significant at the one-sided 2.5% level

		Truth		Total
		$\lambda > 0.75$	$\lambda \leq 0.75$	
Decision	Discontinue	0.26	0.01	0.27
	Continue	0.15	0.58	0.73
	Total	0.41	0.59	

From Table 9.2, we see that the probability of making a correct decision is 0.84 ($= 0.26 + 0.58$). The PPV is 0.79 (=0.58/0.73), and the NPV is 0.96 ($= 0.26/0.27$). The probability of continuing (i.e., 0.73) includes 0.15 which is the probability of continuing and $\lambda > 0.75$ (an incorrect decision to continue). The near-perfect NPV gives strong assurance that should the study fail to reject the null hypothesis of $\lambda \geq 1$ at the one-sided 2.5% level, we can be quite confident that the true hazard ratio is greater than 0.75.

We note that although the derivation of the POSS in Table 9.1 used the midpoint of each interval to calculate the statistical power as an approximation to the numerical integration required in (9.1) for this example, the probability of continuing in Table 9.2 is the same as that obtained in Table 9.1 from simulation with a large number of runs.

9.3 Relationship Between Sample Size and Metrics

In this section, we will use two examples to illustrate how sample size, or sample size together with a set of rules, affects the metrics at the confirmatory stage.

Example 1 Under the Frequentist hypothesis-testing approach, a developer can increase the power of a test by increasing the sample size. This property has led to examples where a treatment effect, while statistically significant at a pre-specified level, is not clinically meaningful. A question is whether a substantial increase in sample size could lead to a sizeable increase in the POSS.

Consider the axitinib example with twice the number of events planned, i.e., 920 events instead of 460. One can construct a table like Table 9.1 with the second column replaced by the corresponding statistical power with 920 events. The results are shown in Table 9.3.

With 920 events, statistical power to detect a HR of 0.73 is 99.8%. (A study with 920 events has at least 80% power to detect a HR as high as 0.83.) By comparison, the increase in POSS, from 73 to 80%, is only modest. A developer needs to decide if this increase in POSS is worthy of doubling the number of events, especially after taking into consideration the rarity of $\lambda \leq 0.7$ as discussed in Sect. 9.2.

It is worth pointing out that because the prior distribution places 8% weight on λ being greater than 1, the POSS for the planned trial can never achieve 100%.

Example 2 We return to the example about SC-75416 discussed in Chap. 5 (see Sect. 5.5). For illustration purposes, we assume that we are planning a confirmatory trial (instead of a POC trial) and a prior exists for the difference in mean responses in TOTPAR6 between SC-75416 and ibuprofen. The prior has a Normal distribution $N(3.27; (0.6)^2)$. The standard deviation of the endpoint TOTPAR6 is assumed known and equals to 7 units. This assumption is used in all of the calculations.

Suppose that SC-75416 is of interest only if its true mean benefit over ibuprofen measured by TOTPAR6 (and denoted by Δ) is at least 3 units. Because of this

Table 9.3 Approximation to POSS of a design with 920 planned events when $\ln(\lambda)$ is assumed to follow a Normal distribution $N(-0.34; 0.24^2)$

True λ	Statistical power at the midpoint of the λ-interval[a]	Probability that λ Is in the interval in the first column	Product of column 2 and column 3
<0.4	1.00	0.01	0.01
0.4–0.5	1.00	0.06	0.06
0.5–0.6	1.00	0.17	0.17
0.6–0.7	1.00	0.23	0.23
0.7–0.8	0.99	0.21	0.21
0.8–0.9	0.69	0.15	0.10
0.9–1.0	0.12	0.09	0.01
>1.0	<0.01	0.08	<0.001
			0.80[b]

[a]Power is calculated at $\lambda = 0.35$ for the first interval and at $\lambda = 1.05$ for the last interval. The calculation applied Normal approximation of $N(\ln(\lambda); 4/920)$ to the distribution of the estimate $\ln\left(\hat{\lambda}\right)$.

[b]Obtained by adding the entries in column 4 before rounding

condition, a team is considering two designs and associated decision rules for a parallel group study of SC-75416 against ibuprofen.

Design A   Randomize 225 patients to each treatment group. Continue the development if the null hypothesis of no benefit of SC-75416 over ibuprofen is rejected at the one-sided 2.5% level and the observed mean benefit of SC-75416 over ibuprofen is at least 3 units. Otherwise, discontinue the development.

Design B   Randomize 150 patients to each treatment group. Continue the development if the null hypothesis of no benefit of SC-75416 over ibuprofen is rejected at the one-sided 2.5% level and the observed mean benefit of SC-75416 over ibuprofen is at least 2.5 units. Otherwise, discontinue the development.

The operating characteristics of these two designs obtained by 10,000 simulations are given in Tables 9.4 and 9.5, respectively. For both designs, the requirement on the observed mean benefit dominates that on rejecting the null hypothesis of no benefit under the assumption of a known variance.

The PPV for Design A and Design B is 84% and 76%, respectively. The corresponding NPV is 61% and 67%. Since the requirement on the observed mean benefit dominates that on rejecting the null hypothesis (again, assuming a known variance), it is understandable that Design A has a higher PPV because it has a more stringent criterion to continue. So, when Design A leads to a Continue decision, it is more likely that the true benefit Δ is indeed ≥ 3 than when Design B leads to a Continue decision. On the other hand, since it is harder to discontinue under Design B (21%

Table 9.4 Operating characteristics of Design A under the assumption that Δ has a prior distribution $N(3.27;(0.6)^2)$

		Truth		Total
		$\Delta < 3$	$\Delta \geq 3$	
Decision	Discontinue	0.23	0.15	0.38
	Continue	0.10	0.52	0.62
	Total	0.33	0.67	

Table 9.5 Operating characteristics of Design B under the assumption that Δ has a prior distribution $N(3.27; (0.6)^2)$

		Truth		Total
		$\Delta < 3$	$\Delta \geq 3$	
Decision	Discontinue	0.14	0.07	0.21
	Continue	0.19	0.60	0.79
	Total	0.33	0.67	

compared with 38% for Design A), it is more likely that Δ is <3 when a Discontinue decision is made under this design.

One way to contrast between the two designs is to construct Table 9.6 that displays clearly how the two designs differ with respect to the metrics.

Table 9.6 shows that the estimated probability for making a correct decision is very similar under the two designs. The difference is how the probability is broken down into those for correct Continue and correct Discontinue decisions. Which design to choose depends on the impact of incorrect Continue and incorrect Discontinue in a particular application. Other factors to consider in selecting a design include budget and the need for more safety data at this stage of development.

Table 9.6 Comparisons between design A and design B

	Design A	Design B
Pr(Correct Continue decision)	0.52	0.60
Pr(Correct Discontinue decision)	0.23	0.14
Pr(Correct decisions)	0.75	0.74
Pr(Incorrect Continue decision)	0.10	0.19
Pr(Incorrect Discontinue decision)	0.15	0.07
Pr(Incorrect decisions)	0.25	0.26
Pr(Continue)	0.62	0.79

Table 9.7 Approximation to POSS of a design with 460 planned events when $\ln(\lambda)$ is assumed to follow a Normal distribution $N(-0.34; 0.17^2)$

True λ	Statistical power at the midpoint of the λ-interval[a]	Probability that λ Is in the interval in the first column	Product of column 2 and column 3
<0.4	1.00	<0.001	<0.001
0.4–0.5	1.00	0.02	0.02
0.5–0.6	1.00	0.14	0.14
0.6–0.7	1.00	0.30	0.30
0.7–0.8	0.87	0.29	0.25
0.8–0.9	0.41	0.16	0.07
0.9–1.0	0.08	0.06	0.01
>1.0	0.01	0.03	
			0.79[b]

[a]Power is calculated at $\lambda = 0.35$ for the first interval and at $\lambda = 1.05$ for the last interval
[b]Obtained by adding the entries in column 4 before rounding

9.4 The Impact of Prior Data on POSS

In the first example in Sect. 9.3, the estimated HR is based on a small number of events. Suppose the HR estimate is based on twice the number of events and the point estimate for $\ln(\lambda)$ remains the same. The standard error of the estimate $\ln\left(\hat{\lambda}\right)$ will be roughly $0.24/\sqrt{2}$, or 0.17. Using $N(-0.34; (0.17)^2)$ as the prior, we can reconstruct Table 9.1 and obtain the POSS for a design with 460 planned events as shown in Table 9.7. The POSS is now around 79%.

The 79% POSS is very close to the 80% figure shown in Table 9.3 under a design with 920 planned events. This means that for the same point estimate for λ, obtaining twice as many events as observed in the Phase 2 trial has approximately the same effect on the POSS for the Phase 3 trial as an additional 460 events in the Phase 3 trial. This example illustrates that obtaining a more reliable estimate can be a more cost-effective way to ensure future trial success. This concept is not new, but having a way to quantify the differential benefit of additional data in Phase 2 versus Phase 3 trials is a useful communication tool.

9.5 Sample Size Consideration Based on POSS

So far, we have focused on prior information about the parameter that summarizes the differential mean response to two treatments, while assuming that the standard deviation associated with the response is known. Chuang-Stein and Yang (2010) proposed to take into account the uncertainty around the standard deviation of the endpoint as well as that around the comparative mean response.

Assume that the endpoint follows a Normal distribution with a standard deviation of σ. Let Δ denote the difference in the mean response between the new drug and a control. Chuang-Stein and Yang (2010) began with a non-informative prior $p(\Delta, \sigma) \propto 1/\sigma$ which was proposed by Jeffrey (1961) and advocated by other researchers (e.g., Berger & Bernardo, 1992; Yang, 1995).

Suppose that a Phase 2 study produced sample mean responses $\overline{X}_{\text{drug}}$ and $\overline{X}_{\text{control}}$ based on m patients in each group. The observed difference $D = \overline{X}_{\text{drug}} - \overline{X}_{\text{control}}$ has a Normal distribution $N(\Delta; 2\sigma^2/m)$. The pooled sum of squares (SS) has a distribution $\sigma^2 \chi^2_{2m-2}$ where χ^2_{2m-2} is a chi-square distribution with $(2m-2)$ degrees of freedom. The posterior distribution $p(\Delta, \sigma | \text{Phase 2 data})$ has a density function proportional to

$$\frac{1}{\sigma^{2m}} \times \exp\left\{-\frac{(d-\Delta)^2}{4\sigma^2/m}\right\} \times \exp\left\{-\frac{SS}{2\sigma^2}\right\} \qquad (9.2)$$

Chuang-Stein and Yang (2010) used the distribution in (9.2) as the prior to calculate the POSS for a Phase 3 trial. They found that the loss in POSS by incorporating the uncertainty in σ was very minor (<1% on the POSS scale) compared to the loss due to the uncertainty in Δ.

Chuang-Stein and Yang (2010) discussed planning sample size to reach a desirable level for the POSS using the distribution in (9.2) as the prior. The sample size required per group in the Phase 3 study to obtain 80% or 90% POSS varies substantially as a function of the sample size m and the observed treatment effect d in the Phase 2 trial. Table 9.8 contains select results from Table 1 in Chuang-Stein and Yang (2010). In some instances, the POSS cannot reach the 90% level no matter how large the sample size is (e.g., the first row in Table 9.8). In other instances, the sample size is clearly too large to be practical. As a comparison, Table 9.8 also includes the sample size needed to detect an effect size equal to the observed effect size d using the traditional sample size formula (e.g., see (2.4) in Chap. 2). Because the traditional method does not take into consideration the sample size of the source data, it produces the same sample size for the new study whether the sample size (per group) in the Phase 2 study is 25, 50 or 75.

Table 9.8 is not the only instance when no sample size, no matter how large it is, could yield a 90% POSS. This can occur when the prior evidence is weak or is based on very limited data to allow reasonable precision for the estimate of the treatment effect. This finding could help a sponsor judge whether there is adequate information on the treatment effect prior to initiating a confirmatory trial. For example, if the sample size needed to have a reasonable POSS (e.g., 80%) is impractically large, this would signal the lack of precision of the prior evidence or a minimal treatment effect if precision is adequate.

Table 9.8 shows that the sample size based on the POSS consideration is uniformly higher than that based on the traditional method. The difference is the most pronounced when the source data come from smaller studies with a small observed treatment effect.

Table 9.8 Sample size per group calculated from the traditional sample size method and from the need to have 80% or 90% POSS

Phase 2 sample size per group	Observed effect size in Phase 2	80% Power based on traditional method	80% POSS	90% Power based on traditional method	90% POSS
25	0.30	174	2262	233	–
	0.40	98	343	131	8384
	0.50	63	139	84	525
	0.60	44	76	58	188
	0.70	32	48	43	98
50	0.30	174	511	233	4660
	0.40	98	180	131	474
	0.50	63	93	84	183
	0.60	44	57	58	99
	0.70	32	39	43	63
100	0.30	174	295	233	699
	0.40	98	132	131	233
	0.50	63	76	84	120
	0.60	44	50	58	75
	0.70	32	35	43	51

9.6 Other Applications of the Concept of POSS at the Confirmatory Stage

The idea of POSS has other applications beyond sample size planning at the confirmatory stage. Chuang-Stein and Yang (2010) discussed two such applications in helping make interim decisions about a confirmatory trial. One relates to futility stopping and the other relates to sample size re-estimation.

9.6.1 Conditional POSS

Spiegelhalter et al. (1986) raised the question of whether to use conditional or predictive power to monitor clinical trials. Given interim data, conditional power is calculated by assuming that the future data follow a certain distribution with specific values for the parameters of interest. Spiegelhalter et al. (1986) defined predictive power as the quantity obtained by averaging the conditional power with respect to the current belief about the population parameters of interest.

At present, conditional power is often used to make futility decisions following an interim analysis (Dmitrienko et al., 2005). Instead of fixing the parameters of interest at specific values, a developer can use the interim data to update the prior distribution about the parameters and use the posterior distribution to calculate the probability of obtaining a positive outcome. This idea is the same as the predictive power.

To be specific, let Z_m represents the test statistic at an interim analysis based on m patients per group and Z_N the final test statistic based on N subject per group. Let (Δ, σ) denotes the treatment effect and standard deviation applicable to future patients after the interim analysis. Let $P_m(\Delta, \sigma)$ denotes the probability of obtaining a positive final outcome at the one-sided $100 \times \alpha\%$ level, conditioning on Z_m. When σ is assumed known, $P_m(\Delta, \sigma)$ has the closed-form expression in (9.3) (Dmitrienko et al., 2005):

$$P_m(\Delta, \sigma) = \Pr(Z_N > Z_\alpha | Z_m = z_m \text{ and the treatment effect in future data is } \Delta)$$

$$= \Phi\left(\frac{\sigma\sqrt{m}z_m + \frac{(N-m)\Delta}{\sqrt{2}} - \sigma\sqrt{N}Z_\alpha}{\sigma\sqrt{N-m}}\right) \tag{9.3}$$

In (9.3), Z_α is the upper $100 \times \alpha^{\text{th}}$ percentile of the standard Normal distribution. For a confirmatory trial, α is typically set at 2.5%.

Instead of calculating the conditional power $P_m(\Delta, \sigma)$, one can average $P_m(\Delta, \sigma)$ with respect to the density function $p(\Delta, \sigma | \text{all available data})$ of the posterior distribution of Δ and σ obtained by adding the interim data to the prior distribution of Δ and σ before the trial began. The average takes the form in (9.4). For consistency with our terminology, we will call the average in (9.4) the conditional POSS. The idea behind the conditional POSS is the same as that behind the predictive power.

$$\int P_m(\Delta, \sigma) p(\Delta, \sigma | \text{all prior data}) d\Delta\, d\sigma \tag{9.4}$$

One can use the conditional POSS to make a futility decision. If the conditional POSS is substantially lower than the POSS calculated at the beginning of the trial, it may be worthwhile to consider terminating the trial for futility. A major advantage of the conditional POSS over $P_m(\Delta, \sigma)$ is that we do not need to rely on a fixed Δ (and σ) to make the futility decision.

9.6.2 Sample Size Re-estimation

When there is much uncertainty about the population parameters at the design stage, a common approach is to include a pre-planned sample size re-estimation (SSR) at an appropriate interim time while the trial is ongoing.

SSR methods have been developed since the 1990s. They fall into two main categories, depending on whether treatment information is used (unblinded SSR) or not (blinded SSR) (Chuang-Stein et al., 2006). A blinded SSR is typically used to assess the accuracy of our assumptions about the key nuisance parameters such as the standard deviation of the endpoint or the accrual rate of a time-to-event endpoint. Unblinded SSR, on the other hand, typically uses a revised estimate of the treatment effect to re-estimate the sample size. Since the Type I error (false positive) rate is often affected when using unblinded interim data to effectuate trial adaptations, adjustment is necessary for the final analysis on such occasions.

A common approach to control the Type I error rate adopts the combination test principle that combines stage-wise p-values using a pre-specified combination function (Bauer and Köhne, 1994). The key idea is to calculate separate test statistics for different stages of the trial (e.g., before and after an interim analysis if there is only one interim analysis) and combine them in a pre-specified manner for the final decision. Examples of P-value combination functions include Fisher's product test, and the inverse Normal method (Fisher, 1998; Lehmacher and Wassmer, 1999; Cui et al., 1999). Another unblinded SSR method that has received increasing attention in recent years is the promising zone design advocated by Mehta and Pocock (2011). While some researchers have criticized the promising zone design as not being the most efficient (Jennison & Turnbull, 2015), the design has some nice features as described in Mehta and Pocock (2011).

Suppose we have decided to conduct an unblinded SSR when 50% of the planned information becomes available and use a combination test for the final analysis. We have also decided that the final statistic Z_F will be a weighted average of the test statistics before and after the interim analysis with equal weights. One option to determine the number of additional patients per group is to have enough patients so that the conditional power $\Pr(Z_F > Z_{\alpha/2}|Z_m)$ at the observed treatment effect (for a two-sided significance level α) is at an acceptable level (Fisher, 1998). Cui et al. (1999) recalculated the sample size by using the treatment effect and the standard deviation observed at the interim in the traditional sample size formula.

Instead of using the conditional power, Chuang-Stein and Yang (2010) proposed to re-estimate the sample size so that the conditional POSS in (9.5) was at an acceptable level.

$$\int \Pr(Z_F > Z_\alpha|z_m, \Delta, \sigma)p(\Delta, \sigma|\text{all prior data})d\Delta d\sigma \qquad (9.5)$$

Let $\alpha = 0.025$, the one-sided significance level for testing the hypothesis in the trial. Assuming a non-informative prior $p(\Delta, \sigma) \propto 1/\sigma$ and using the interim data to formulate a posterior distribution $p(\Delta, \sigma|\text{prior data})$ similar to that in (9.2), Chuang-Stein and Yang calculated the sample size needed per group after the interim analysis so that the conditional POSS in (9.5) was 80% for various treatment effects observed at the interim analysis. We include in Table 9.9 results pertaining to the situation when 100 patients per group were originally planned for the study and an SSR is planned when 50 patients per group (50%) have reached the time point of interest. With 100 patients per group, the trial as originally planned has 80% power to detect an effect size of 0.40.

Table 9.9 Additional sample size (per group) after an interim SSR conducted when 50% information is available in a study planned with 100 patients per group initially

Interim observed effect size	Fisher's method[a]		Cui et al.'s method[b]		Conditional POSS approach[c]
	Number per group	Conditional POSS	Number per group	Conditional POSS	
0.25	179	0.65	201	0.67	825
0.30	99	0.68	124	0.72	250
0.35	57	0.72	78	0.76	103
0.40	33	0.74	48	0.80	48
0.45	18	0.76	28	0.82	23
0.50	10	0.78	13	0.81	11

[a] Targeting 80% conditional power
[b] Setting power to 80% in the traditional sample size calculation
[c] Requiring the conditional POSS to be 80%

Table 9.9 also includes the number of additional patients needed by the methods of Fisher and Cui et al. For completeness, we include in Table 9.9 the conditional POSS under the sample size determined by these two other methods. Results in Table 9.9 are sourced from Table 2 in Chuang-Stein and Yang (2010). In general, the conditional POSS approach leads to the largest sample size postinterim analysis, except for when the observed interim effect size is large.

Chuang-Stein and Yang (2010) allowed the sample size to decrease in their example. When the observed interim treatment effect is favorable, all three methods lead to a smaller sample size. The decrease can be substantial in some cases, e. g., when the observed interim effect size is at least 0.45.

One can structure the sample size re-estimation in such a way that the final sample size stays the same as originally planned or meets a pre-specified minimum requirement in the case of a favorable interim result. The latter allows a developer to verify that the favorable efficacy results observed during the earlier part of the trial remain strong in the remainder of the trial.

9.7 The Application of POS to Binary Data

The probability of success (POS) for binary data for the two-group case can be calculated by using the Normal approximation to the binomial distribution for a prior distribution for the difference in proportions together with a Beta distribution for the prior distribution for the control group proportion. The POS for sample size n in each group can then be calculated by repeating the following steps a large number (e.g., 10,000) of times:

1. Draw a random value from the prior distribution for the difference in treatment proportion minus control proportion and denote this value by d.

2. Draw a random value from the beta prior distribution for the control group proportion and denote the value obtained by p_C.
3. Calculate the treatment proportion as $p_T = d + p_C$. If p_T is > 1.0, set $p_T = 1.0$. If p_T is < 0, set $p_T = 0$.
4. Draw a random value from the binomial distribution with parameters n and p_T.
5. Draw a random value from the binomial distribution with parameters n and p_C.
6. Calculate the test statistic and record if statistical significance is achieved at the required significance level.

The value of POS is given by the proportion of simulations which achieve the required level of significance.

An example of calculating the POS for a binary endpoint as part of a program-level success assessment is described in Sect. 14.1. That example includes multiple parts of (i) deriving a prior distribution for the control group proportion based on historical trials; (ii) deriving a prior distribution for the difference in proportions between the control and the treatment groups; (iii) repeating the above for two aspects of treatment effect (induction and maintenance); (iv) estimating the correlation coefficient between the induction and maintenance treatment effects; (v) calculating the probability of program success when the program consists of 2 induction trials and one maintenance trial, all of which need to demonstrate a statistically significant effect at the one-sided 2.5% level. We refer readers to Sect.14.1 for details.

9.8 Summary

In the case of axitinib, the developer initiated a Phase 3 study designed to detect a reduction in the hazard rate for mortality that was of the magnitude observed in the Phase 2 study. The planned number of deaths was 460. Based on a 1:1 randomization, a planned accrual period of 14 months, and a follow-up of approximately 9 months, it was estimated that 596 patients would be needed to provide 460 events. Interim analyses for futility and efficacy were planned as described in Kindler et al. (2011).

Between July 27, 2007, and Oct 31, 2008, 632 patients were randomized with 316 patients assigned to each treatment group. Three hundreds and five (305) patients in the gemcitabine plus axitinib group and 308 in the gemcitabine plus placebo group received study medications. At a planned interim analysis in January 2009, the independent Data Monitoring Committee (DMC) concluded that the futility boundary had been crossed. The DMC recommended terminating the study. The developer accepted the recommendation and stopped the trial in the same month. The developer ended its development program of axitinib in pancreatic cancer altogether. The development was continued for other types of cancer. Axitinib was approved in January 2012 for the treatment of advanced renal cell carcinoma (RCC) in patients after failure of one prior systemic therapy. It was subsequently approved as a first-line therapy for patients with advanced RCC.

The idea of using a predictive approach to size a study is not new. For example, Spiegelhalter and Freedman (1986) advocated using a predictive approach and clinical input to plan the sample size. In this chapter, we apply basically the same idea for a confirmatory trial, using data available before a study or in the case of a pre-planned SSR, using interim results plus prior information.

The work by Chuang-Stein and Yang (2010) suggests that incorporating uncertainty surrounding the variability parameter in the calculation of POSS has minimal effect on POSS in the case of Normal distributions. Consequently, for the ease of calculation, we suggest calculating POSS including only uncertainty about the estimated treatment effect. This simplification leads to a closed-form expression for the POSS when a Normal prior is used for a Normally distributed endpoint.

When using a prior for the treatment effect to calculate the POSS of a new study, it is important that the population that gives rise to the prior is similar to the population intended in the new study. It is not unusual for the effect of a treatment to be a function of certain pre-treatment covariates such as disease state or a patient's gender. If the new study is enriched to have a higher representation of certain subgroups of the patient population, then the prior needs to be adjusted to describe likely treatment effect in the enriched population. One way to approach this is to consider the prior as a mixture of distributions that reflect treatment effects in various subgroups. The mixture proportions are determined by the percentages of patient subgroups targeted in the new study.

So, even if the Phase 2 population is not the same as the Phase 3 population, but as long as major subgroups intended for Phase 3 were reasonably represented in Phase 2, we can still obtain treatment effect estimates in these subgroups and standardize the overall effect relative to the target population planned for Phase 3. However, if these major subgroups were not included in Phase 2 trials, we will have difficulty in developing a prior for the likely treatment effect in Phase 3 trials.

In addition to patient populations, how data were analyzed in the past trials will also impact treatment effect estimate. For example, many trials completed before the end of the first decade in the twenty-first century used the last-observation-carried-forward method to handle missing data (National Research Council, 2010). Since then, many new trials have been analyzed with mixed models for repeated measurements that assume missing data to be missing at random. How to handle missing data has become an integral part of the design and analysis of clinical trials since the publication of the ICH E9(R1) document. If a sponsor has access to individual patient data from past trials that give rise to the prior, it will be beneficial for the sponsor to reanalyze the data using the same analytical methods planned for the new trial. If accessing individual patient data is not possible, a sponsor should consider using slightly different prior distributions in a sensitivity analysis to assess the operating characteristics of the new design.

Pinheiro et al. (2010) cautioned the risk of accelerating market entry of a product candidate by reducing the time and investment dedicated to dose finding. We have illustrated in this chapter, through POSS, how critically important the precision in the treatment effect estimate could be to the success probability of a Phase 3 study.

We echo a recommendation by Pinheiro et al. that a developer should strive for a suitable balance in resource allocation between the dose–response and the confirmatory phases in order to optimize the overall likelihood of success of a development program.

References

Bauer, P., & Köhne, K. (1994). Evaluation of experiments with adaptive interim analyses. *Biometrics, 50*(4), 1029–1041.

Berger, J., Bernardo, J. M. (1992). On the development of reference priors. In J. M. Bernardo, J. O. Berger, Dawid, A. P., & A.F.M. Smith (Eds.), *Bayesian Statistics 4*. Clarendon Press.

Chuang-Stein, C., Anderson, K., Gallo, P., & Collins, S. (2006). Sample size reestimation: A review and recommendations. *Drug Information Journal, 40*(4), 475–484.

Chuang-Stein, C., & Yang, R. (2010). A revisit of sample size decisions in confirmatory trials. *Statistics in Biopharmaceutical Research, 2*(2), 239–248.

Chuang-Stein, C., Kirby, S., French, J., et al. (2011). A quantitative approach for making go/no-go decisions in drug development. *Drug Information Journal, 45*(2), 187–202.

Cui, L., Hung, H. M. J., & Wang, S. J. (1999). Modification of sample size in group sequential clinical trials. *Biometrics, 55*(3), 853–857.

Dmitrienko, A., Molenbergs, G., Chuang-Stein, C., & Offen, W. (2005). *Analysis of clinical trials using SAS®: A practical guide*. SAS Institute.

Fisher, L. D. (1998). Self-designing clinical trials. *Statistics in Medicine, 17*(14), 1551–1562.

ICH E9(R1). (2019). Estimands and sensitivity analysis in clinical trials.

Jeffrey, H. (1961). *Theory of Probability* (3rd ed.). Oxford University Press.

Jennison, C., & Turnbull, B. W. (2015). Adaptive sample size modification in clinical trials: Start Small then ask for more? *Statistics in Medicine, 34*(29), 3793–3810.

Kindler, H. L., Ioka, T., Richel, D. J., et al. (2011). Axitinib plus gemcitabine versus placebo plus gemcitabine in patients with advanced pancreatic adenocarcinoma: A double-blind randomized phase 3 study. *Lancet Oncology, 12*(3), 256–262.

Lehmacher, W., & Wassmer, G. (1999). Adaptive sample size calculations in group sequential trials. *Biometrics, 55*(4), 1286–1290.

Mehta, C. R., & Pocock, S. J. (2011). Adaptive increase in sample size when interim results are promising: A practical guide with examples. *Statistics in Medicine, 30*(28), 3267–3284.

National Research Council - Panel on Handling Missing Data in Clinical Trials. (2010). *The Prevention and Treatment of Missing Data in Clinical Trials*. National Academies Press.

Pinheiro, J., Sax, F., Antonijevic, Z., et al. (2010). Adaptive and model-based dose-ranging trials: Quantitative evaluation and recommendations. *Statistics in Biopharmaceutical Research, 2*(4), 435–454.

Spano, J. P., Chodkiewicz, C., Maurel, J., et al. (2008). Efficacy of gemcitabine plus axitinib compared with gemcitabine alone in patients with advanced pancreatic cancer: An open-label randomized phase II study. *Lancet, 371*(9630), 2101–2108.

Spiegelhalter, D. J., & Freedman, L. S. (1986). A predictive approach to selecting the size of a clinical trial, based on subjective clinical opinion. *Statistics in Medicine, 5*(1), 1–13.

Spiegelhalter, D. J., Freedman, L. S., & Blackburn, P. R. (1986). Monitoring clinical trials: Conditional or predictive power? *Controlled Clinical Trials, 7*(1), 8–17.

Yang, Y. (1995). Invariance of the reference prior under reparametrization. *TEST, 4*(1), 83–94.

Zhang, J. (2013). Evaluating regression to the mean of treatment effect from phase II to phase 3. https://www.amstat.org/meetings/jsm/2013/onlineprogram/AbstractDetails.cfm?abstractid=309685. Accessed 12 Feb 2021.

Chapter 10
Designing Phase 4 Trials

Generalization is the essence of knowledge.
—Swami Vivekananda

10.1   Introduction

As described in Chap. 1, Phase 4 trials can be of a number of different types. These trials are conducted to (1) further investigate the drug in the indicated population(s) or in pediatric patients with the indicated disorder(s); (2) compare the drug head-to-head with an approved drug for the same disorder(s); (3) investigate the effect of the drug at a lower/higher dose or with different administration schedules (e.g., once a day instead of twice a day); (4) study the drug in combination with other drugs or (5) test the drug for other indications.

In this chapter, we cover the design of Phase 4 trials from the point of view of obtaining a prior distribution for the treatment effect from past trials but focus primarily on assessing the design of a trial for comparative effectiveness. By comparative effectiveness, we mean the comparison of different treatments for a condition to determine which work best in patients. We adopt this focus because trials for comparative effectiveness are of increasing importance given the increasing competitiveness in the market place and the need for reimbursement justification.

We start with an outline of network meta-analysis using a proposed model and proceed to consider the design of a trial against a comparator using the information obtained from a network meta-analysis. Network meta-analysis gives a potential way to assess prospective trial designs without requiring much or any data on direct comparisons. We consider which metrics are likely to be important in assessing a trial design for Phase 4 trials.

We then review how prior distributions for treatment effects might be obtained by other means such as PK/PD modeling.

10.2   Network Meta-Analysis

Network meta-analysis combines different sources of pairwise comparisons across trials. It combines direct comparisons from trials that test both treatments of interest with indirect comparisons from trials that test only one of the two treatments but are connected through other treatments in other trials (Lumley, 2002). An artificial example network is displayed in Fig. 10.1.

In Fig. 10.1, letters represent treatments and the studies that compared pairs of treatments are written alongside the treatments. In the network in Fig. 10.1, trials have been conducted to compare treatment A with treatments C and D and to compare treatment B with treatments C and D. The lines connect treatments compared in the same trial. From this network, it can be seen that treatments A and B are not compared directly but can be compared indirectly. The indirect comparison can be calculated via two routes through the network. One route is to subtract the difference of B minus C from the difference of A minus C. The other route is to subtract the difference of B minus D from the difference of A minus D. These two routes through the network give two estimates of the A minus B difference. These two estimates can be combined, provided that it is reasonable to do so as discussed below, to give a single estimate of the A minus B difference.

The above network is relatively simple. Networks depicting treatment comparisons for a set of treatments can be much more complex. To analyze a network, we consider a model that has been proposed for network meta-analysis by Piepho

Fig. 10.1 Example of an artificial treatment network

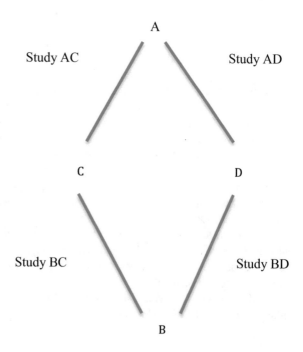

Table 10.1 Treatment designs as used in model (10.1) for four treatments when every pair of treatments is compared in a trial

Design	Treatments compared in trial
1	A and B
2	A and C
3	A and D
4	B and C
5	B and D
6	C and D

(2014). This model is structured in terms of treatment means rather than contrasts with a reference or baseline treatment as used by some authors (Higgins et al., 2012; Lu & Ades, 2004; White et al., 2012). Piepho et al. (2012) showed that analyses using a mean model can produce identical or essentially the same results as a model that uses baseline/reference contrasts.

The model for the mean response written in terms of a linear predictor is

$$\eta_{hij} = \alpha_h + \beta_{hi} + \gamma_j + v_{hj} + u_{hij} \tag{10.1}$$

where α_h is a main effect for the hth design, β_{hi} is an effect for the ith trial nested within the hth design, γ_j is the main effect of the jth treatment, v_{hj} is an interaction effect for the hth design and the jth treatment ,and u_{hij} is an interaction effect for the ith trial and jth treatment nested within the hth design. In the above formulation, "design" means the classification of groups of trials according to the treatments used. For example, possible designs for trials comparing pairs of treatments among A, B, C and D are shown in Table 10.1.

The interaction effect v_{hj} represents inconsistency in the treatment mean for the jth treatment and hth design. The term u_{hij} represents heterogeneity within the hth design.

The above model can be used with individual patient data or with treatment summaries from the trials. When summary measures are analyzed, it is common to use a linear model or linear mixed effects model with the assumption of normality and deal with any heterogeneity in precision by weighting. We consider the analysis of summary measures below.

The model may be fitted using maximum likelihood or restricted maximum likelihood (REML) or in the Bayesian framework with software such as WinBUGS (WinBUGS). If the Bayesian approach is used, then a separate distribution and vague prior is needed for each trial if the principle of concurrent control is to be respected. This corresponds to the estimation of a separate fixed effect for each trial using maximum likelihood or REML.

For model (10.1), one can consider all of the terms as fixed effects for a fixed effects model or treat the interaction effect u_{hij} representing heterogeneity as random with the remaining terms as fixed effects for a mixed effects model. If the mixed effects model is fitted using REML, one can test for heterogeneity by comparing the variance for u_{hij} with the residual variance using an F test. If heterogeneity is detected, one can use the effect for heterogeneity to test for inconsistency represented by v_{hj} with an F test using the Kenward–Roger adjustment (Kenward & Roger, 2009) for the denominator degrees of freedom.

If the fixed effects model is fitted using maximum likelihood, one can test for heterogeneity by using a Wald-type chi-squared statistic for the term u_{hij}. If heterogeneity is detected, however, there is no basis for testing for inconsistency because of the nesting of heterogeneity effects in relation to inconsistency. If this were the case, one could look for subsets of trials that do not display heterogeneity. Both Piepho (2014) and Senn et al. (2013) prefer treating u_{hij} as random whenever appropriate to treating the term as fixed.

If heterogeneity is detected using either a mixed effects model or a fixed effects model, it is important in practice to consider possible explanations for heterogeneity. If inconsistency is detected in a network meta-analysis, this should also be investigated. Bafeta et al. (2014) recommended that estimates from direct comparisons, indirect comparisons and mixed comparisons be reported for review in all cases.

To illustrate the use of network meta-analysis, we look at the diabetes example published by Senn et al. (2013) and re-analyzed by Piepho (2014). The network is displayed in Fig. 10.2.

Twenty-six studies were selected after a systematic literature search for the additional effect of oral glucose-lowering treatments added to a background sulfonylurea therapy on HbA1c change in patients with Type 2 diabetes. One study had three

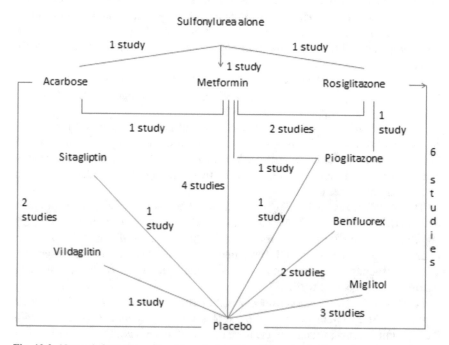

Fig. 10.2 Network for a network meta-analysis of the effect of oral glucose-lowering treatments added to a baseline sulfonylurea therapy on HbA1c change

Table 10.2 Treatment abbreviations for the diabetes network meta-analysis example

Four-letter abbreviation of treatment	Treatment
acar	acarbose
benf	benfluorex
metf	metformin
migl	miglitol
piog	pioglitazone
plac	placebo
rosi	rosiglitazone
sita	sitagliptin
SUal	sulfonylurea alone
vild	vildagliptin

treatment arms, and the remaining studies compared two treatments (Fig. 10.2). The treatments identified were acarbose, benfluorex, metformin, miglitol, pioglitazone, placebo, rosiglitazone, sitagliptin, sulfonylurea alone and vildagliptin. The study with three treatment arms compared the treatments acarbose, metformin and placebo.

For each study and treatment arm, mean change from baseline or mean outcome was used in the analysis. Up to three estimates of the standard deviation were available so if more than one was recorded, the median value was used after checking for consistency. Assuming homoscedasticity within trials, overall variances were calculated by weighting variances by their degrees of freedom. Finally, the variance of the mean for each arm was obtained by dividing the pooled estimate of variance by the number of patients per arm.

The treatments are abbreviated as shown in Table 10.2 when referenced in the designs required by model (10.1).

The designs for use in model (10.1) are shown in Table 10.3.

Piepho (2014) fitted model (10.1) using PROC MIXED within SAS (SAS Institute) with all effects fixed and found the chi-squared test for heterogeneity corresponding to the u_{hij} parameters to be significant ($p < 0.0001$). When he included the interaction effect for heterogeneity as random, however, there was no evidence of inconsistency represented by the v_{hj} parameters ($p = 0.9268$). Senn et al. (2013) explored the nature of the heterogeneity further, but for our purposes we take the mixed effects model as adequate for estimating the treatment effects. Welton et al. (2015) discussed the modeling of heterogeneity in relative treatment effects.

10.3 Example Evaluation of a Design Using the Results of a Network Meta-Analysis

To illustrate how results from such a network meta-analysis may be used to help design a new study, we suppose that there is interest in conducting a superiority

Table 10.3 Designs for the diabetes network meta-analysis example

Design	Design number
acar:plac	1
acar:SUal	2
benf:plac	3
metf:plac	4
metf:acar:plac	5
metf:SUal	6
migl:plac	7
piog:plac	8
piog:metf	9
piog:rosi	10
rosi:plac	11
rosi:metf	12
rosi:SUal	13
sita:plac	14
vild:plac	15

study of metformin versus acarbose. Before designing the study, we briefly consider the metrics likely to be of interest in the evaluation of a Phase 4 design for comparative effectiveness.

The metrics identified of interest for confirmatory trials in Chap. 6 are likely to also be the primary ones of interest for Phase 4 trials that assess comparative effectiveness, i.e., the metrics (1) the probability of study success (POSS); (2) the PPV and NPV and (3) the probability of a correct decision.

Piepho (2014) obtained a difference in mean reduction of HbA1c for metformin versus acarbose of 0.287 (with standard error equal to 0.250) in favor of metformin by using model (10.1) with the term v_{hj} omitted and modeling heterogeneity as random. We suppose that a parallel group study is sized using this difference with an assumed known standard deviation of 1.0. Using the expression for sample size per group (n) given by

$$n = \frac{2\sigma^2\left(Z_\alpha + Z_\beta\right)^2}{\Delta^2}$$

with $\alpha = 0.025$, $\beta = 0.20$, $\sigma = 1$ and $\Delta = 0.287$ gives n = 191 when rounded up to the nearest integer. Here, Z_γ represents the upper $(100 \times \gamma)\%$ percentile of the standard Normal distribution.

We take as our prior a Normal distribution with mean equal to the estimated difference between metformin and acarbose and standard deviation equal to the associated standard error. A positive result is taken to be significance at a one-sided 2.5% significance level. We obtained the results shown in Table 10.4 by simulating 10,000 trials.

Table 10.4 Results for 10,000 simulations of a Phase 4 parallel group trial using a prior distribution for the treatment effect obtained from a network meta-analysis

	True difference in HbA1c reduction (metformin minus acarbose)		
	≤ 0	>0	
Negative result	0.13	0.25	0.38
Positive result	0.00	0.62	0.62
	0.13	0.87	

Table 10.5 POSS and PPV values obtained from 10,000 simulated Phase 4 parallel group trials using a prior distribution for the treatment effect obtained from a network meta-analysis

Sample size per group	POSS	PPV
191	0.62	1.00
250	0.67	1.00
400	0.72	1.00
600	0.75	1.00
800	0.77	1.00
1000	0.79	1.00

We see immediately from the results that although the probability of compound success (POCS) is 0.87, the probability of study success (POSS) is just 0.62. This suggests that we may be able to achieve a better trade-off between POSS and sample size (and hence cost). We also note that a positive result has a PPV of 1.0, i.e., we can essentially be sure that the real difference is in favor of metformin if we obtain a positive result. We give below some possible trade-offs between POSS and sample size per group together with PPV, estimated again in each case by simulating 10,000 trials (see Table 10.5).

We see that it is possible to increase the POSS to approximately 80% which is the targeted statistical power used in the sample size calculation. However, this increase requires a sample size approximately five times that given by the traditional sample size calculation. This requirement for a much greater sample size to achieve a POSS equal to a planned power probability was also noted in Chap. 9 (see Sect. 9.4) when a small Phase 2 trial may cause the POSS for a Phase 3 trial to be small.

We can evaluate how much information the network meta-analysis result is equivalent to by considering its worth in terms of an effective sample size for a parallel group trial. The standard error for the estimated treatment effect given above is 0.250. Using the assumed standard deviation of 1 and the expression for the standard error of a difference for a parallel group trial given by

$$\sqrt{\frac{2\sigma^2}{n}}$$

we can equate 0.250 to this expression and solve for n to obtain an effective sample size per group for a parallel group trial. Doing this we obtain 32 for n. Thus, the precision of the network meta-analysis result corresponds to the result of a small clinical trial comparing metformin with acarbose with 32 subjects per group. This illustrates another caution about the use of a network meta-analysis. Although a network may be of reasonable size, it is possible that there is not much information about the comparison between two particular treatments.

The acarbose versus metformin comparison used here as an example has been studied more extensively by Gu et al. (2015). Gu et al. found no significant difference based on direct comparisons with an estimated difference in favor of metformin of 0.06 and a standard error of 0.13. For indirect comparisons through placebo and sulfonylurea, however, there were significant differences. The indirect comparison of acarbose versus metformin through placebo yielded a mean difference of 0.38 in favor of metformin with a standard error of 0.18. The indirect comparison of acarbose versus metformin through sulfonylurea gave a mean difference of 0.34 in favor of metformin with a standard error of 0.16. Thus, Gu et al. found a lack of consistency between direct and indirect comparisons of acarbose and metformin which would suggest further exploration of the results to understand the possible cause of the lack of consistency.

10.4 Pediatric Study Designs

The FDA draft guidance on General Clinical Pharmacology Considerations for Pediatric Studies for Drugs and Biological Products (2014) identifies two main approaches to providing substantial evidence to support the safe and effective use of drugs in pediatric populations for the same indication as in adults. One approach relies on evidence from adequate and well-controlled investigations in pediatric populations. The second approach relies on evidence in adequate and well-controlled investigations in adults together with additional information in the specific pediatric population.

The first approach is easy to understand. For example, antidepressants were typically studied in children and adolescents in controlled clinical trials before approval for these populations. Designing a clinical trial in a pediatric population generally involves the use of prior disease and exposure–response knowledge from studies in adults and relevant pediatric information. If a PK-PD disease model can be developed with appropriate inclusion of sources of variability, then this can be used to simulate results for pediatric patients, which can in turn be used to simulate results for the pediatric trial under planning. An example is given by Mouksassi et al. (2009) who looked at the potential use of teduglutide in neonates and infants with short-bowel syndrome (SBS). Teduglutide was approved for adult patients with SBS who were dependent on parenteral support. Mouksassi et al. (2009) explored developing a dosing regimen with the goal of obtaining an exposure greater than the target efficacy level in > 90% of the population while ensuring that the exposure in pediatric patients did not exceed the highest level previously observed in adult patients. A randomized trial was ultimately conducted in pediatric patients aged 1 year through 17 years. The trial compared teduglutide to the standard of care. Teduglutide was approved for pediatric patients in May 2019.

For the second approach, it is possible that a PK study may be considered sufficient additional information. To design such a study, a PK model specific to the pediatric population can be developed and used to assess a study design. One of the metrics for assessing such a study design is likely to be, as above, the probability of a dose achieving the target exposure.

Extrapolating clinical information from adults to pediatrics has received increasing attention in recent years. This is because pediatric drug development needs to be efficient and flexible with an overarching objective to expose the least number of children to an investigational drug while still producing valid and persuasive evidence necessary for approval. The extrapolation has been facilitated by the applications of Bayesian methods that decide the amount of borrowing from the adult population to the pediatric population based on the actual data. A case study was presented by Xia (2020) for cinacalcet HCI (Sensipar™). Cinacalcet HCI was approved in 2004 in the USA for the treatment of secondary hyperparathyroidism (SHPT) in adult patients with chronic kidney disease and receiving dialysis. Xia (2020) applied a three-level Bayesian hierarchical model to adult and limited pediatric clinical trial data to estimate the effect of cinacalcet in pediatric patients. Cinacalcet was approved for SHPT for the pediatric population in 2019 in the European Union. As of March 2021, cinacalcet was still awaiting approval for SHPT in children in the USA.

10.5 Designs to Investigate the Effect of the Drug at a Lower/Higher Dose or with Different Administration Schedules

If the dose–response relationship has been well characterized as described in Chaps. 6 and 8, then one can obtain a distribution for the treatment effect at a new dose and use it as a prior distribution for a further study.

If a different administration schedule is to be studied, however, then a PK/PD model relating the different exposure to the PD endpoint of interest needs to be developed to obtain a prior distribution for the treatment effect in the evaluation of study designs. For example, Katsube et al. (2008) proposed a PK/PD modeling strategy to simulate in vivo bactericidal effects for three carbapenem antibiotics that could be used for deciding an optimal dosing regimen.

10.6   Studies in New Populations

If the new population is a reasonably sized subpopulation of a more general population already studied and there are sufficient data for the general population, then it may be possible to analyze the subset of data corresponding to the new population to derive a prior distribution for a treatment effect.

On the other hand, if a new population represents a mostly different population from the patients already studied, it may still be possible to model the likely treatment effect in the new population using a PK/PD model or a model-based meta-analysis of the new drug and other drugs with a similar mode of mechanism that have been studied both in the new population and the other populations.

An example of the use of a PK/PD model in new populations for the treatment of venous thromboembolism (VTE) is given by Leil et al. (2014). Venous thromboembolism is a serious and potentially fatal complication after total knee replacement (TKR) or total hip replacement (THR) surgery. New oral anticoagulants such as apixaban offer the possibility of improved efficacy, lower bleeding risk and more convenient formulations. Leil et al. used a model-based approach to integrate PK and bleeding data from clinical trials of apixaban to predict bleeding risk in TKR and THR patients and subpopulations of these populations. Clinical trial simulations were used to predict the range of bleeding probabilities to be expected in various TKR and THR populations for clinically relevant scenarios. Here, bleeding is regarded as a safety endpoint, and the level of exposure is assumed to give the required level of efficacy in prevention of VTE. We include many aspects of these considerations in an adaptive dose-ranging study in Chap. 13 (see Sect. 13.5). Additional discussion of how to model efficacy and safety endpoints jointly can be found in in Chap. 14 (see Sect. 14.2).

10.7   Studies to Test a Drug in Combination with Other Drugs

The likely effect of a combination of two drugs can be modeled by adding the effects of the individual drugs and including an interaction term to represent synergism or antagonism. Information about the interaction term may be obtainable from other similar drug combinations. If such information is not available, it may be preferable to assess designs conditionally for different plausible interaction effects instead of assuming a particular prior distribution for the interaction effect. An example of the investigation of a drug combination is the COMPASS-1 study (Gruenig et al., 2009). The study investigated the effects of the combination of bosentan and sildenafil versus sildenafil alone on morbidity and mortality in symptomatic patients with pulmonary arterial hypertension.

10.8   Studies in New Indications

As for new populations, it may be possible to bridge to the likely effect of a treatment in a new indication by using a model-based meta-analysis of the treatment of interest and other treatments considered to act similarly that have been studied in the new indication and the existing indications.

10.9   Discussion

We have seen in this chapter that network meta-analysis presents a possible way of making indirect comparisons with other drugs. This is important in the consideration of whether to proceed with a study comparing a drug with a competitor because of the risk of finding a drug to be inferior to a comparator and the cost involved. Forming a prior distribution for a treatment effect from a network meta-analysis allows a possible design to be assessed for its likely outcome. Network meta-analysis is not necessarily straightforward, however, and care needs to be taken in the modeling of heterogeneity and the assessment of consistency of results. For example, Carroll and Hemmings (2016) made the case for increased rigor and care in the conduct and interpretation of network meta-analyses. They noted a number of assumptions that underpin network meta-analysis. In particular and in common with standard meta-analysis, is an assumption of similarity of trials and also an assumption of consistency. They recommended that the following be reported for the proper assessment of a network meta-analysis: A full reference list of all trials is involved; a list of the characteristics of each trial; a separate presentation of direct and indirect estimates for each comparison along with 95% confidence intervals or credible intervals and the weights applied for combining direct and indirect estimates along with the estimated correlation between the two.

The head-to-head comparisons in some of the Phase 4 studies could have great impact on treatment policy recommendations. An example is the study PROVE-IT that was conducted between November 2000 and December 2001 comparing 40 mg of pravastatin daily with 80 mg of atorvastatin daily. Prior to the study, medical understanding on the relationship between high cholesterol and increased risk for cardiovascular events had led to treatment guidelines on reducing cholesterol (NCEP, 1994), especially the low-density lipoprotein cholesterol (LDL-C). At the turn of the twenty-first century, the guidelines recommended a target LDL-C of less than 100 mg per deciliter for patients with established coronary artery disease or diabetes (NCEP, 2001). Even so, questions remained on the optimal level of the LDL-C and whether LDL-C should be aggressively managed in some patients beyond the 100 mg per deciliter level.

In PROVE-IT, the pravastatin treatment represented a standard therapy in managing LDL-C per the guidelines. Atorvastatin, at the highest dose approved (i.e., 80 mg per day), represented an aggressive LDL-C lowering therapy. PROVE-IT was designed as a non-inferiority trial where non-inferiority would be declared if the upper limit of a one-sided 95% confidence interval of the relative risk for a pre-specified composite cardiovascular endpoint at two years between pravastatin and atorvastatin is less than 1.17.

In PROVE-IT, the median LDL-C achieved during treatment was 95 mg per deciliter in the pravastatin group and 62 mg in the atorvastatin group. Kaplan–Meier estimates of the rates of the pre-specified composite cardiovascular endpoint at two years were 26.3% in the pravastatin group and 22.4% in the atorvastatin group (Cannon et al., 2004), reflecting a 16% reduction in the hazard rate in favor of atorvastatin. The non-inferiority criterion was not met.

Results in PROVE-IT and other contemporary studies led to the revision of the guidelines (Stone et al., 2014). The new guidelines state that for individuals that warrant guideline-recommended statin therapy, they should be treated with the maximum appropriate intensity of a statin that does not cause adverse effects.

PROVE-IT was a major undertaking. While it contributed greatly to the question on the value of intensively managing LDL-C level in at-risk patients, the results nevertheless were a surprise to the sponsor. It will be of interest to explore retrospectively if an analysis including all statins and a model linking LDL-C level to the risk for cardiovascular events could help the sponsor assess the probability of study success at the design stage, when the idea of the trial was first conceived.

For a number of other types of Phase 4 trial considered in this chapter, modeling based on available data of the drug or available data of other drugs with a similar mode of mechanism offers an opportunity to obtain a distribution for the treatment effect that may be used as a prior distribution to evaluate a design. The modeling is essentially an extrapolation from existing data to new situations. We have discussed the extrapolation of adult clinical data to pediatric data in Sect. 10.4. The latter is also included in a framework developed by the EMA on extrapolation approaches that would be considered scientifically valid and reliable to support medicine authorization in pediatric patients (2018).

References

Bafeta, A., Trinquart, L., Seror, R., & Ravaud, P. (2014). Reporting of results from network meta-analyses: methodological systematic review. *British Medical Journal, 348*, g1741.

Cannon, C. P., Braunwald, E., McCabe, C. H. et al. (2004). Intensive versus moderate lipid lowering with statins after acute coronary syndromes. *New England Journal of Medicine, 350*(15), 1495–1504.

Carroll, K., & Hemmings, R. (2016). On the need for increased rigour and care in the conduct and interpretation of network meta-analyses in drug development. *Pharmaceutical Statistics, 15*(2), 135–142.

EMA Reflection paper on extrapolation of efficacy and safety in paediatric medicine development. (2018).

Gruenig, E., Michelakis, E., Vachiéry, J.-L., et al. (2009). Acute hemodynamic effects of single-dose sildenafil when added to established bosentan therapy in patients with pulmonary arterial hypertension: Results of the COMPASS-1 study. *Journal of Clinical Pharmacology, 49*(11), 1343–1352.

Gu, S., Shi, J., Tang, Z., et al. (2015). Comparison of glucose lowering effect of metformin and acarbose in type 2 diabetes mellitus: A meta-analysis. *PLoS ONE, 10*(5), e0126704. https://doi.org/10.1371/journal.pone.0126704.

Higgins, J. P. T., Jackson, D., Barrett, J. K., et al. (2012). Consistency and inconsistency in network meta-analysis: Concepts and models for multi-arm studies. *Research Synthesis Methods, 3*(2), 98–110.

Katsube, T., Yamano, Y., & Yano, Y. (2008). Pharmacokinetic-Pharmacodynamic modelling and simulation for in vivo bactericidal effect in murine infection model. *Journal of Pharmaceutical Sciences, 97*(4), 1606–1614.

Kenward, M. G., & Roger, J. H. (2009). An improved approximation to the precision of fixed effects from restricted maximum likelihood. *Computational Statistics and Data Analysis, 53*(7), 2583–2595.

Leil, T. A., Frost, C., Wang, X., et al. (2014). Model-based exposure-response analysis of Apixaban to quantify bleeding risk in special populations of subjects undergoing orthopaedic surgery. *CPT: Pharmacometrics & Systems Pharmacology, 3*, e136. https://doi.org/10.1038/psp.2014.34.

Lu, G., & Ades, A. E. (2004). Combination of direct and indirect evidence in mixed treatment comparisons. *Statistics in Medicine, 23*(20), 3105–3124.

Lumley, T. (2002). Network meta-analysis for indirect treatment comparisons. *Statistics in Medicine, 21*(16), 2313–2324.

Mouksassi, M. S., Marier, J. F., Cyran, J., & Vinks, A. A. (2009). Clinical trial simulations in pediatric populations using realistic covariates: Application to teduglutide, a glucagon-like peptide-2 analog in neonates and infants with short-bowel syndrome. *Clinical Pharmacology & Therapeutics, 86*(6), 667–671.

National Cholesterol Education Program (NCEP). (1994). Second report of the expert panel on detection, evaluation, and treatment of high blood cholesterol in adults (Adult Treatment Panel II). *Circulation, 89*(3), 1333–1445.

National Cholesterol Education Program (NCEP). (2001). Executive summary of third report of the expert panel on detection, evaluation, and treatment of high blood cholesterol in adults (Adult Treatment Panel III). *Journal of the American Medical Association, 285*(19), 2486–2497.

Piepho, H. P. (2014). Network-meta analysis made easy: Detection of inconsistency using factorial analysis-of-variance models. *BMC Medical Research Methodology, 14*, 61. http://www.biomedcentral.com/1471-2288/14/61.

Piepho, H. P., Williams, E. R., & Madden, L. V. (2012). The use of two-way mixed models in multitreatment meta-analysis. *Biometrics, 68*(4), 1269–1277.

SAS/SAT® Software. SAS Institute, Cary, North Carolina.

Senn, S., Gavini, F., Magrez, D., & Scheen, A. (2013). Issues in performing network meta-analysis. *Statistical Methods in Medical Research, 22*(2), 169–189.

Stone, N. J., Robinson, J. G., Lichtenstein, A. H. et al. (2014). 2013 ACC/AHA guideline on the treatment of blood cholesterol to reduce atherosclerotic cardiovascular risk in adults: A Report of the american college of cardiology/American Heart Association task force on practice guidelines. *Journal of the American College of Cardiology, 63*(25 Supp. 2), 2889–2934.

U.S. FDA Draft Guidance for Industry: General Clinical Pharmacology Considerations for Pediatric Studies for Drugs and Biological Products. (2014).

Welton, N. J., Soares, M. O., Palmer, S., et al. (2015). Accounting for heterogeneity in relative treatment effects for use in cost-effectiveness models and value-of-information analyses. *Medical Decision Making, 35*(5), 608–621.

White, I. R., Barrett, J. K., Jackson, D., & Higgins, J. P. T. (2012). Consistency and inconsistency in network meta-analysis: Model estimation using multivariate meta-regression. *Research Synthesis Methods, 3*(2), 111–125.

WinBUGS. Available at http://www.mrc-bsu.cam.ac.uk/software/bugs/.

Xia, A. (2020). *Bayesian applications for extrapolations from adult to pediatric data.* Presented at an NISS-Merck workshop on 27 April 2020. Available at https://www.niss.org/news/bayesian-statistics-focus-popular-nissmerck-meetup. Accessed 3 March 2021.

Chapter 11
Other Metrics That Have Been Proposed to Optimize Drug Development Decisions

All men by nature desire to know.
—Aristotle

11.1 Introduction

So far, we have focused on metrics that address specific goals of different stages of drug development. While each stage is designed to enable quality decision-making necessary at that stage, there is a common goal that underpins all stages of a drug development program and this common goal may sometimes be forgotten during stage-specific optimizations. The common goal is to get a safe and effective drug to the marketplace as soon as possible, and doing this at the lowest cost plausible. The emphasis on speed serves both the patients and the sponsor. A faster entry means that patients in need will have access to the medicine sooner. For the sponsor, this means a longer patent life remaining on the drug and an earlier start to recover the development costs. Keeping development costs low is easy to understand, especially at a time when the average cost of developing a successful drug is estimated to be around $2.56 billion USD in 2013 money (DiMasi et al., 2016; see also Sect. 1.1 in Chap. 1).

The quest for speed and cost is often at odds with the desire for quality. For example, we have learned from earlier chapters the need for replication before moving into the confirmatory stage and the need for a heavier investment in dose-ranging studies than the current practice. For Phase 3 studies, the metrics we have discussed in Chap. 9 will typically go up in value with a larger sample size. But, a heavier investment means higher costs and generally a longer development timeline, which in turn means a delayed market entry and a shorter patent life remaining at the product launch. In some cases, it makes a major difference commercially whether a drug is the first or the third of its class to enter into the marketplace.

C. Chuang-Stein and S. Kirby, *Quantitative Decisions in Drug Development*, Springer Series in Pharmaceutical Statistics,
https://doi.org/10.1007/978-3-030-79731-7_11

An important question is—how can we balance between quality, cost and speed? Are there reasonable ways to help us assess the combined effect of these three factors and optimize over these three in a quantitative manner?

In this chapter, we will discuss two approaches that incorporate costs in making strategic development decisions. The first approach uses an efficiency score proposed by Chen and Beckman (2009, 2014). Chen and Beckman argue that the exploratory nature of a proof-of-concept (POC) study gives a sponsor the liberty to choose the Type I error rate and statistical power for conducting a hypothesis test at this stage. They propose to make this choice by optimizing a benefit–cost efficiency score that measures the cost-effectiveness of the POC trial. The idea is to maximize the return on socioeconomic investment in trials and yield the greatest knowledge with the minimum patient exposure. They argue that the same concept can be applied to program-level and franchise-level decisions.

The second approach combines costs and potential commercial return to assess drug development strategies. Patel and Ankolekar (2007) propose to do this when designing clinical trials and assessing portfolios of drugs. Burman et al. (2007) use a decision-analytic approach to calculate sample size from the perspective of maximizing company profit. Mehta and Patel (2006) consider net present value (NPV) when considering sample size re-estimation. More recently, net present value together with the probability of success of the confirmatory program has been used by Patel et al. (2012), Antonijevic et al. (2013) and Marchenko et al. (2013) to optimize late-stage programs in three case studies involving neuropathic pain, Type 2 diabetes and oncology. The three case studies are extensions of the work published in Pinheiro et al. (2010) who also include net present value as an optimization criterion in addition to probability of Phase 3 success.

We will discuss the above two approaches in Sects. 11.2 and 11.3, respectively. We will briefly mention a couple of additional metrics in Sect. 11.4 and share our thoughts on the use of metrics in general in Sect. 11.5.

11.2   Benefit–Cost Efficiency Score

In most oncology development programs, a positive POC study will move a drug into the confirmatory stage. This is because the maximum tolerated dose estimated in Phase 1 is traditionally the dose investigated in the POC and the confirmatory trials. The POC to confirmatory pathway means that if a sponsor can be more efficient with their POC strategies, more drugs could be studied at the POC stage and consequently more in Phase 3 trials.

We discussed five POC designs in Chap. 7. One of them is the Early Signal of Efficacy (ESoE) approach, aimed at using smaller studies to identify compounds with great potential. The approach pre-specifies acceptable risks in moving an ineffective drug forward and stopping an effective drug from being progressed. These risks can differ in value from the traditional choices of the Type I error and Type II error rates.

Once the risks are specified, the sample size can be determined using the traditional sample size formula.

Chen and Beckman (2009, 2014) approached the POC strategy similarly, but using a different metric. To describe their metric, we first return to Table 6.2 which displays the unconditional probabilities of various actions when testing a null hypothesis H_0 of no clinically meaningful treatment effect (e.g., effect $< \delta$) against the alternative hypothesis H_A of a clinically meaningful effect (e.g., effect $\geq \delta$). Because the interest is in only one direction of the treatment effect Δ, we will work with the one-sided Type I error rate (and significance level) as in other chapters of this book and denote it by α.

Assuming that the probability that H_A is true is p, then Table 6.2 could be re-expressed as in Table 11.1. In Table 11.1, β is the Type II error rate.

If rejecting H_0 leads to a Go decision, then the probability of Go is $p \times (1 - \beta) + (1 - p) \times \alpha$. Within this Go probability is the probability of a correct Go, $p \times (1 - \beta)$, i.e., the probability of advancing an effective drug.

Denote the total sample size of the POC study by C_2 and the total sample size for the confirmatory trial following a positive POC by C_3. The design of the confirmatory trial typically follows the standard practice with a one-sided 2.5% significance level and 90% power. Occasionally, a sponsor may choose to use a lower power such as 80%. On the other hand, the POC design can be more flexible because of the exploratory nature of the study.

The expected sample size from the POC study and the confirmatory study combined is

$$C = C_2 + C_3 \times [p \times (1 - \beta) + (1 - p) \times \alpha] \tag{11.1}$$

Chen and Beckman (2014) proposed to maximize the ratio of $p \times (1 - \beta)$ to C. They called the ratio the benefit–cost ratio (BCR) with benefit measured by the probability of advancing a truly effective drug and cost measured by the total of the POC sample size and the expected sample size of the confirmatory trial. The ratio measures how much a patient contributes to the development of an active drug. The higher the ratio is, the more efficient the POC design is.

For example, assume that the Phase 3 study is set to have a total of 600 patients. If the POC study is designed to have 80% power to detect an effect size of 0.3 at the one-sided 5% significance level, then the POC study needs 138 subjects per group for a two-arm randomized study. Assume $p = 0.1$, then the BCR for this POC design is 2.3×10^{-4} as shown in (11.2). If one designs the study to have 50% power to

Table 11.1 Unconditional probabilities of various actions in testing H_0 versus H_A

	H_0 true	H_0 false	Total
Accept H_0	$(1 - p) \times (1 - \alpha)$	$p \times \beta$	$(1 - p) \times (1 - \alpha) + p \times \beta$
Reject H_0	$(1 - p) \times \alpha$	$p \times (1 - \beta)$	$(1 - p) \times \alpha + p \times (1 - \beta)$
Total	$1-p$	P	1

detect the same effect size at a one-sided significance level of 3%, then one needs 79 subjects per group. The BCR for this new design is 2.4×10^{-4}, which is slightly higher than 2.3×10^{-4}, the ratio for a more traditional POC design.

$$\frac{0.1 \times (1 - 0.2)}{2 \times 138 + 600 \times [0.1 \times (1 - 0.2) + (1 - 0.1) \times 0.05]} = 0.00023 \qquad (11.2)$$

For the same α, β and sample size for the POC study, a higher p will lead to a higher BCR. For example, for the study with α (one-sided) $= 0.03$, $\beta = 0.50$ and 79 subjects per group, $p = 0.5$ will produce a BCR of 7.9×10^{-4}, higher than the 2.4×10^{-4} figure associated with $p = 0.1$. This is intuitive since the probability of moving an effective treatment is higher when $p = 0.5$ than when $p = 0.1$.

The benefit–cost ratio can be re-expressed as

$$\text{BCR} = \frac{1}{C_3} \frac{p \times (1 - \beta)}{\tau + [p \times (1 - \beta) + (1 - p) \times \alpha)]} \qquad (11.3)$$

In (11.3), $\tau = C_2/C_3$ is the ratio between the sample size of the POC trial and that of the confirmatory trial.

Chen and Beckman proposed to find α and β (and therefore the sample size C_2 for the POC study) that would maximize the BCR in (11.3). They considered such a design the most cost-effective from the perspective of maximizing each patient's contribution to the probability of identifying an active drug. For a given C_3 and p, maximizing BCR is equivalent to maximizing the second term on the right-hand side of (11.3). The optimization is not straightforward since τ is a function of α and β also.

To see the above, assume that the Phase 3 trial is sized with a one-sided significance level of 2.5% and power of 90%, Chen and Beckman express τ as the product of two terms λ and $(Z_\alpha + Z_\beta)^2/(Z_{0.025} + Z_{0.10})^2$ as shown in (11.4).

$$\tau = \frac{2 \times (Z_\alpha + Z_\beta)^2 / \delta_{\text{POC}}^2}{2 \times (Z_{0.025} + Z_{0.10})^2 / \delta_{\text{REG}}^2} = \frac{(Z_\alpha + Z_\beta)^2}{(Z_{0.025} + Z_{0.10})^2}$$

$$\times \frac{(Z_{0.025} + Z_{0.10})^2 / \delta_{\text{POC}}^2}{(Z_{0.025} + Z_{0.10})^2 / \delta_{\text{REG}}^2} = \frac{(Z_\alpha + Z_\beta)^2}{(Z_{0.025} + Z_{0.10})^2} \times \lambda \qquad (11.4)$$

In (11.4), δ_{POC} and δ_{REG} are the effect sizes that the POC study and the confirmatory trial are set to detect; λ is the ratio of the sample size of the POC trial and the Phase 3 study if the POC trial is also sized with a one-sided significance level of 0.025 and power of 0.90. This ratio reflects the difference in the endpoint (e.g., progression-free survival vs overall survival) and difference in the effect size to be detected. The term $(Z_\alpha + Z_\beta)^2/(Z_{0.025} + Z_{0.10})^2$ corresponds to the ratio between the POC sample size to have a (one-sided) Type I error rate of α and power of $1 - \beta$ and the sample size when one employs a one-sided significance level of 0.025 and power of 0.90. Z_γ is the upper $(100 \times \gamma)\%$ percentile of the standard Normal distribution.

Chen and Beckman (2014) approached this problem by varying λ and examining how α and β change as a function of λ. They found that for λ between 10 and 30% and p between 10 and 50%, the optimal α ranged from 2 to 8%. The power, on the other side, ranges from 48 to 60%. There is a trend for the optimal error rates (both α and β) to go up as p (between 0 and 50%) or λ increases.

Under the cost-effective optimal design, the Type I error rate does not differ very much from that under a traditional POC design. The power to detect a clinically meaningful effect, on the other hand, is substantially lower than that under a traditional POC design. The lower power leads to a reduced sample size. An immediate effect of this is that the treatment effect needs to be much higher for the study to have the kind of power (e.g., 80%) used in a more traditional POC design.

It is easy to see that if p is between 50 and 100%, the role of α and β reverses somewhat in optimizing the BCR metric. Suppose the historical success rate p is 60%, and we are looking at either setting $\alpha = 0.06$ and $\beta = 0.50$ (Choice #1) or $\alpha = 0.50$ and $\beta = 0.06$ (Choice #2). The effect size to detect is still 0.3. Sample sizes under these two choices are the same, i.e., 54 patients per group or a total of 108 patients in a two-arm study with equal randomization ratio, but Choice #1 has a BCR of 9.9×10^{-4} while Choice #2 has a BCR of 10.0×10^{-4}. The two BCRs are almost the same, with the BCR of Choice #2 just a bit higher than that of Choice #1. When p is over 50%, it becomes increasingly more important to be able to identify a Go opportunity.

Chen and Beckman applied the BCR concept to assess the efficiency of conducting multiple POC studies for different indications compared to one larger POC study for only one indication. Assume that resources are available to enroll 160 patients for a two-arm study (so that each arm will have 80 patients). A positive POC study (statistical significance at a pre-specified significance level) will be followed by a 600-patient Phase 3 study. Furthermore, assume that there are two competing options. One option (Option #1) is to devote all resources to a traditional POC study with $\alpha = 0.05$ and $\beta = 0.2$ for one indication. The second option (Option #2) is to divide the resources and devote 80 patients to a POC study for each of two indications. The false positive rate under Option #2 is stipulated to be at most 0.05 for both POC studies.

The sample size for the POC study under Option #1 is twice that under Option #2. This means that for the same effect size, the power of the POC study under Option #2, denoted by $1-\beta^*$, has to satisfy the relationship in (11.5).

$$\frac{(Z_{0.05} + Z_{0.20})^2}{(Z_{0.05} + Z_{\beta*})^2} = 2 \tag{11.5}$$

Solving for β^* in (11.5) leads to $\beta^* = 0.45$.

We assume that the prior experience in developing products for the two indications suggests a historical success rate of 0.3 for both indications. We also assume that the success in one indication has no impact on the chance of success for the other. The BCR under Option #1 is

$$\frac{0.3 \times (1 - 0.2)}{160 + 600 \times (0.3 \times (1 - 0.2) + 0.7 \times 0.05)} = 7.4 \times 10^{-4} \tag{11.6}$$

The BCR under Option #2 is

$$\frac{2 \times \{0.3 \times (1 - 0.45)\}}{2 \times \{80 + 600 \times (0.3 \times (1 - 0.45) + 0.7 \times 0.05)\}} = 8.3 \times 10^{-4} \tag{11.7}$$

The multiplier of 2 in (11.7) is due to the fact that there are two indications under consideration. Option #2 has a higher BCR than Option #1. So, dividing the resources available for POC investigation to explore two indications is more cost-effective according to the BCR metric in this instance.

The concept could also be used to assess the efficiency of different strategies to manage the portfolio. For the latter, a major advantage of the approach is that it is easy to understand and communicate. A disadvantage is that it treats all subjects across indications the same without addressing the potential return due to differences in the target patient populations associated with different indications.

11.3 Net Present Value

In economic terms, the net present value of an investment is the difference between the present value of the expected future cash flows from the investment and the amount of investment. Present value of the expected future cash flows is computed by discounting the expected future cash flows by an annual discount rate.

Developing a drug is an investment, and a highly risky one. The expected future cash flows from the investment come from the expected net revenue (gross revenue minus operating expenses) of the drug. The expected gross revenue depends on many factors such as the remaining patent life of the drug, trajectory of the sale before the patent expires and the rate of sale decline following patent expiration. Operating expenses include costs associated with raw materials, manufacturing, promotion, detailing, pharmacovigilance activities, conducting additional trials required by regulators, and liability lawsuits. Frequently, an estimate of the 5th-year net revenue is used as an anchor in this calculation. For convenience, we will denote the expected 5th-year net revenue by S5.

In this section, we will describe in some detail a case study for neuropathic pain by Patel et al. (2012) who used net present value as a metric to evaluate different program-level strategies when designing a Phase 2 dose–response study. We will focus on those aspects of the case study that relate to the calculation of net present value.

11.3.1 Present Value of Net Revenue

Patel et al. (2012) considered a net revenue model that projected the net return to increase linearly up to the 5th year, if more than 5 years remain on the patent life for the drug. After the 5th year, the rate of increase changes until the patent life runs out. From that point on, the expected revenue decreases following an exponential decay curve. If there are fewer than 5 years remaining on the patent life at the product launch, the net revenue will increase linearly toward the 5th year net revenue projection and decrease exponentially at the point of patent expiration.

Denote the net revenue in year t by $R(t)$, the remaining patent life at the time of product launch by TP, the rate of increase between the 5th year and TP in the case of TP > 5 by b per year, and the rate of exponential decline in net revenue per year after patent expiration by c. The above characterization of $R(t)$ could be described mathematically as follows:

If TP > 5 years,

$$R(t) = S5 \times t/5 \qquad\qquad\qquad\qquad\qquad\qquad\quad \text{if } t \leq 5 \text{ years}$$
$$= S5 \times [1 + b \times (t - 5)] \qquad\qquad\qquad\quad\ \text{if } 5 < t \leq \text{TP}$$
$$= S5 \times \big[1 + b \times (\text{TP} - 5)\big] \times \exp\big[-c \times (t - \text{TP})\big] \ \text{if } t > \text{TP}$$

If TP ≤ 5 years,

$$R(t) = S5 \times t/5 \qquad\qquad\qquad\qquad\qquad \text{if } 0 \leq t \leq \text{TP}$$
$$= S5 \times (\text{TP}/5) \times \exp[-c \times (t - \text{TP})] \ \text{if } t > \text{TP}$$

If the development of a drug is terminated prior to launch, then $R(t) = 0$ for all t.

We display, in Fig. 11.1, the net revenue $R(t)$ profile defined above for TP = 3, 7, 10, 13 years, S5 = $1B USD, $b = 0.1$, and $c = 0.5$.

Because a sponsor cannot expect revenue while a drug moves through Phase 2 and Phase 3 development, the net revenue occurs several years in the future and needs to be adjusted to reflect its present value.

Let TP2 denotes the anticipated duration of the Phase 2 dose–response study being planned, T23 the anticipated period between the completion of the dose–response study and the beginning of the Phase 3 program, TP3 the anticipated duration of the Phase 3 program and T3L the anticipated period between the completion of Phase 3 program and product launch. All durations are measured in years. Net revenue, if there is any, won't begin until after a period of (TP2 + TP23 + TP3 + T3L) years.

Let ρ be the annual discount rate when converting future money to its present-day value. Patel et al. used the expression in (11.8) to calculate the present value of the future net revenue (PVRev).

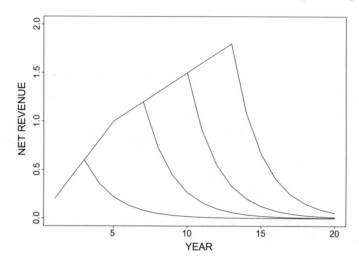

Fig. 11.1 Net revenue $R(t)$ profile ($B USD) over years, assuming a remaining patent life of 3, 7, 10 and 13 years at the product launch. Other assumptions in producing the curves include S5 = $1B, $b = 0.1$, and $c = 0.5$

$$\text{PVRev} = \int_{0}^{\infty} R(t) \times \exp\{-\rho(\text{TP2} + \text{TP23} + \text{TP3} + T3L + t)\}dt$$

$$= \exp\{-\rho(\text{TP2} + \text{TP23} + \text{TP3} + T3L)\} \int_{0}^{\infty} R(t) \times \exp\{-\rho t\}dt \quad (11.8)$$

11.3.2   Present Value of Development Cost

In Patel et al. (2012), the cost that has yet to be incurred includes the costs of the Phase 2 dose–response trial (C2), the costs of Phase 3 trials if the development moves into Phase 3 (C3), and startup costs of manufacturing and costs associated with the initial launch (CML). Patel et al. assumed that 2 identical confirmatory trials were to be conducted following a positive dose–response study. The framework developed by Patel et al. could be easily extended to allow more complicated scenarios. Patel et al. used the following notation in calculating C2, C3 and CML.

M2   Total number of sites in the Phase 2 trial.
AR2   Patient accrual rate per year per site in the Phase 2 trial.
M3   Total number of sites in each of the two Phase 3 trials.
AR3   Patient accrual rate per year per site in each of the two Phase 3 trials.

CS   Upfront cost per site (assumed to be the same for Phase 2 and Phase 3 trials for simplicity).

CP   Cost per patient (assumed to be the same for Phase 2 and Phase 3 trials for simplicity).

The costs of the Phase 2 trial consist of the upfront cost of $CS \times M2$ to initiate the sites plus the ongoing costs of enrolling/treating patients. The second part of the costs will be incurred on an ongoing basis in the future, so the associated cost needs to be adjusted to reflect their present value. Using the same principle as in (11.8), the present value of the Phase 2 costs (PVC2) can be estimated to be

$$PVC2 = CS \times M2 + \int_0^{TP2} CP \times AR2 \times \exp\{-\rho t\} dt \qquad (11.9)$$

Similarly, the costs of Phase 3 and manufacturing/initial launch will all be incurred at different times in the future if the development progresses to these milestones. Using the notation defined earlier, Phase 3 trials will not begin for a period of (TP2 + T23) years from now while manufacturing/launch will not begin for a period of (TP2 + T23 + TP3) years. Using the same principles behind (11.8) and (11.9), we can obtain the present value of the Phase 3 costs (PVC3) if the development moves to Phase 3 in (11.10) and the present value of the manufacturing/launch costs (PVCML) if launch is to take place in (11.11). The multiplier of 2 in (11.10) is due to the fact that two identical Phase 3 studies will be conducted.

$$PVC3 = 2 \times \exp\{-\rho(TP2 + T23)\} \left(CS \times M3 + \int_0^{TP3} CP \times AR3 \times \exp\{-\rho t\} dt \right)$$
$$(11.10)$$

$$PVCML = CML \times \exp\{-\rho(TP2 + T23 + TP3)\} \qquad (11.11)$$

11.3.3 Net Present Value

So, the expected net present value at the start of the Phase 2 dose–response study in the case study considered by Patel et al. is

$$NPV = PVRev - PVC2 - PVC3 - PVCML \qquad (11.12)$$

11.3.4   Fifth-Year Net Revenue

It should be clear by now that many assumptions are needed in the calculation of the NPV. Some of the assumptions such as the costs of initiating sites and treating patients come from years of experience in running similar trials. So, these figures are generally pretty close to the real costs. Patel et al. use an annual discount rate of 10% for the parameter ρ.

One factor that is critical to the calculations of the net revenue but subject to substantial uncertainty is the estimated 5th-year net revenue. The net revenue is obtained by subtracting the operating costs from drug sales. We discussed sources for operating costs earlier. As for drug sales, they depend heavily on the benefit–risk profile of the drug and the drug's order of market entry among drugs in the same class and drugs for the same indication. A sponsor often relies on market research to help forecast drug sale. Despite the advances in market research methodology, we have seen substantially missed predictions on product sales in both directions.

The efficacy of a drug for treating neuropathic pain can be measured by the reduction in pain intensity at the end of a treatment period (e.g., 12 weeks) from baseline. Pain intensity is frequently measured on a numerical rating scale (NRS) that ranges from 0 to 10. The minimum clinically important difference in the mean reduction in pain intensity between an investigational product and placebo is generally considered to be 1 unit on the NRS. Marketed products for neuropathic pain can generally achieve this level of efficacy. Lower efficacy may be acceptable to patients if the product has a better safety profile (i.e., more tolerable side effects) when compared with marketed products.

Common side effects (e.g., weight gain and decrease in sexual function) associated with neuropathic pain drugs are not serious, but are generally considered to be a nuisance. For these nuisance events, Patel et al. assumed a drug-related incidence rate between 0.2 and 0.3 for marketed products. A rate greater than 0.3 is worse than marketed products while a rate less than 0.2 is considered better than marketed products.

For the neuropathic pain case study, Patel et al. estimated 5th-year net revenue as a function of the drug's safety and efficacy profile. They sought input from experts familiar with pain research and management in developing the estimates. The estimates are given in Table 11.2.

11.3.5   Phase 2 Study Designs Considered

Patel et al. considered several design options. All the designs are fixed designs. They considered including 8 active doses (doses D_1 through D_8) or 4 active doses (doses D_2, D_4, D_6 and D_8). For the 8 active doses scenario, they considered a base design of assigning 30 patients to each of the 8 active doses and a placebo. This base design has $270 (= 9 \times 30)$ patients. They also considered 15, 25, 45, 60, 75 and 90 patients

Table 11.2 Estimates of the 5th-year net revenue (in billions of USD) for a new neuropathic pain drug (at a fixed dose) for various efficacy and safety profiles

Pain reduction on the NRS (compared to a placebo)	Rate of nuisance adverse events			
	<0.2	$0.2 \leq \cdots < 0.3$	$0.3 \leq \cdots \leq 0.5$	>0.5
<0.8	0.00	0.00	0.00	0.00
$0.8 \leq \cdots < 1.0$	1.00	0.75	0.25	0.00
$1.0 \leq \cdots < 1.5$	1.50	1.00	0.50	0.00
≥ 1.5	2.00	1.50	1.00	0.25

per group, resulting in a total of 135, 225, 405, 540, 675 and 810 patients for the design including 8 active doses.

For the 4 active doses scenario, the base design has 54 patients per group, resulting in a total of 270 patients ($= 5 \times 54$). Other sample sizes explored for the 4 active doses design by Patel et al. are 225 (45 per group), 405 (81 per group) and 675 (135 per group).

11.3.6 Range of Efficacy and Tolerability Considered

Patel et al. considered a range of dose–response relationships for the beneficial effect such as those described in Chap. 6 (see Sect. 6.3). These include a non-monotone dose–response like the quadratic (umbrella) curve in Fig. 6.2. The maximum efficacy in the base case is 1.1 on the NRS. A maximum efficacy of 0.55 and 1.65 was also considered. The latter represents 50% below or above the base case for efficacy.

As for the rate of the nuisance adverse events (AEs), they considered three dose–response relationships labeled as low, moderate and high. The rates associated with the 8 active doses under these three scenarios are given in Table 11.3.

Patel et al. simulated efficacy and safety data under various efficacy and safety profiles. For each simulated Phase 2 trial, they fitted a 4-parameter logistic model in (11.13) to the efficacy data and an isotonic regression model to the observed AE rates. Fitting an isotonic regression model involves pooling observed rates of adjacent doses that violate the monotonicity assumption for the AE rates (Robertson et al.,

Table 11.3 Three AE profiles considered by Patel et al. (2012)

Profile	Doses								
	Placebo	D_1	D_2	D_3	D_4	D_5	D_6	D_7	D_8
Low	0.1	0.1	0.1	0.1	0.1	0.1	0.125	0.15	0.175
Moderate	0.1	0.1	0.1	0.1	0.15	0.2	0.25	0.3	0.35
High	0.1	0.15	0.15	0.15	0.225	0.3	0.375	0.45	0.525

1988). Under the isotonic regression model, the fitted AE rates are non-decreasing as doses increase.

In (11.13), the parameter D represents dose on the (natural) log scale. For convenience, Patel et al. assumed that on the log scale, placebo was equivalent to a dose equal to $2 \times \ln(D_1) - \ln(D_2)$. In other words, placebo is of the same distance below D_1 as D_2 is above D_1 on the (natural) log scale. The 4-parameter logistic model in log dose is equivalent to a 4-parameter Emax model in the original dose. In addition, the best 4-parameter logistic model fit can approximate all the dose–response curves considered by Patel et al. to be within 0.1 on the absolute scale. The response Y in (11.13) is assumed to have a Normal distribution with variance σ^2. If $\delta > 0$, $E(Y|D)$ is monotonically increasing in D with minimum and maximum values of β and $\beta + \delta$.

$$E(Y|D) = \beta + \left(\frac{\delta}{1 + exp\left(\frac{\theta - D}{\tau}\right)} \right), \tau > 0 \qquad (11.13)$$

Patel et al. took a Bayesian approach when fitting (11.13). They used nearly flat priors to the 4 parameters in (11.13) and σ^2. They assigned Normal priors $N(0;10^2)$ and $N(1.1;10^2)$ for β and δ, respectively. The priors for θ and τ are discrete and uniform over a rectangular grid of 30 by 30 points. The prior for σ^2 is inverse gamma $(0.001, 1000)$ with a density function proportional to $(1/\sigma^2)^{1.001} exp(-1000/\sigma^2)$. Prior distributions are assumed to be independent of each other. Patel et al. obtained the joint posterior distribution for $(\beta, \delta, \theta, \tau, \sigma^2)$ from the dose–response study and used the Gibbs sampling algorithm to sample from this distribution when calculating the probability of success for Phase 3.

11.3.7   Selecting a Dose to Move to Phase 3

Patel et al. considered taking only one dose from the Phase 2 dose–response trial into Phase 3. They considered two methods for dose selection. However, before either method is applied, Patel et al. first conducted a linear trend test on the efficacy endpoint. If the trend test is significant at the one-sided 5% level, then the work proceeds to dose selection.

The first selection method chooses the dose estimated to provide efficacy over the placebo that is the closest to and above the target efficacy of 1 unit on the NRS. This method is called the target effect method. If no dose has an estimated efficacy of 1 unit over the placebo, development will not proceed to Phase 3.

The second method chooses the dose that will yield the highest 5th-year net return in Table 11.1 based on efficacy and AE rate estimated from the fitted efficacy and AE models. For convenience, we will call this method the maximum utility method. The word "utility" in this case refers to the net return at the 5th year. The maximum utility method does not impose any threshold for progressing to Phase 3 except for the obvious requirement that the net return needs to be positive.

11.3.8 Metrics Used to Evaluate Design Options

Patel et al. considered two primary metrics. One is the probability of Phase 3 success defined as the probability that both Phase 3 trials produce a statistically significant result. The second metric is the expected net present value of the drug at the start of the Phase 2 development.

As stated earlier, Patel et al. considered two identical Phase 3 studies. In theory, the Phase 3 study could be designed to have an adequate power (e.g., 90%) to detect a clinically meaningful treatment effect (e.g., 1 unit on the NRS) at the one-sided 2.5% significance level. Assuming a standard deviation of 2 units for the primary endpoint, this means the study needs only 84 patients per group or 168 patients per study. This suggests a pretty small Phase 3 program if a sponsor only needs to demonstrate efficacy for the new drug. The sample size per group will increase to 190 per group in a study if the standard deviation is assumed to be 3 units.

In this case, the sample size decision will be dominated by the requirement on the extent of pre-marketing exposure required by ICH E1 (1994). If neuropathic pain is the only indication sought for the new drug at the initial regulatory submission and the intent is to use the new drug for the condition chronically, then ICH E1 expects the total number of individuals treated with the drug at the dose intended for clinical use to be about 1500. Furthermore, there should be between 300 and 600 patients with at least 6 months of exposure and at least 100 patients with one year of exposure, all at the dose intended for clinical use.

Because of the above requirement on exposure, the sample size for the Phase 3 trials needs to be higher than what would have been necessary to demonstrate efficacy alone. For example, suppose 30 patients are randomized to each of 8 active dose groups in the Phase 2 study and 50% of the patients receiving the new drug will be rolled over to an extension study at the dose level to be confirmed in Phase 3. This means that the Phase 2 study will contribute a total of 120 patients ($= 50\% \times 30 \times 8$) toward the 1500-patient requirement. The remaining 1380 patients ($= 1500 - 120$) will have to come from the two identical Phase 3 studies if there are no other relevant exposure sources. In this case, each Phase 3 study will have 1380 patients, randomized in equal proportions to the new drug and a placebo so that a total of 1380 individuals will receive the new drug at the dose studied in the Phase 3 trials. The sample size requirement for the Phase 3 trials under other Phase 2 design scenarios can be determined similarly.

The framework set up by Patel et al. could be extended to situations where multiple indications are being sought simultaneously and exposure data will come from multiple programs. In the latter case, the total number of exposed patients for each indication could be substantially reduced.

Table 11.4 Optimal Phase 2 sample size in the 8-dose design as a function of the maximum efficacy and AE profile under the 4-parameter Emax efficacy model

Max efficacy	AE profile	Optimal Phase 2		Phase 2 sample size = 270		Phase 2 sample size = 405	
		Sample Size	Expected NPV ($B)	Expected NPV ($B)	Reduction from optimal (%)	Expected NPV ($B)	Reduction from optimal (%)
0.55	High	405	0.09	0.09	4	0.09	0
0.55	Moderate	540	0.27	0.25	5	0.26	5
0.55	Low	540	0.50	0.49	3	0.50	2
1.1	High	405	1.30	1.29	0	1.30	0
1.1	Moderate	270	2.32	2.32	0	2.23	4%
1.1	Low	270	3.57	3.57	0	3.36	6
1.65	High	135	2.77	2.71	2	2.55	8
1.65	Moderate	135	4.13	3.98	4	3.69	11
1.65	Low	135	5.80	5.54	5	5.13	11

11.3.9   High-Level Results

In the neuropathic pain case study, Patel et al. found that the maximum utility selection method typically yielded higher expected NPVs than the target effect method. This is not surprising considering that the maximum utility selection method aims to maximize the 5th-year net return, which is a critical building block for the expected NPV.

To see how Phase 2 sample size, efficacy and safety profiles, as well as the choice on the number of doses affect the probability of Phase 3 success and the expected NPV, we include in Tables 11.3 and 11.4 some select results from Patel et al. Results in these tables were obtained by simulation using the following assumptions. In general, Patel et al. carried out 500 simulations for each scenario.

Patent life remaining at start of the dose–response study = 15 years.
M2 (total number of sites in the Phases 2 trial) = 50.
AR2 (patient accrual rate per year per site in the Phase 2 trial) = 6.
M3 (total number of sites in each Phase 3 trial) = 80.
AR3 (patient accrual rate per year per site in each of the two Phase 3 trials) = 12.
CS (upfront cost per site) = $1,500 USD.
CP (cost per patient) = $3,500 USD.
CML (startup cost of manufacturing and launch cost) = $1 M USD.
T23 (period between Phase 2 completion and the beginning of Phase 3) = 6 months.
T3L (period between end of Phase 3 trials and product launch) = 12 months.
b (rate change in net revenue model in Sect. 11.3.1) = 0.1.

c (exponential decay function parameter in net revenue model in Sect. 11.3.1) = 0.5.

ρ (annual discount rate used in NPV calculation) = 10%.

One could argue that a higher cost per patient should be used for the Phase 3 studies because of the longer treatment duration (e.g., 1 year versus 12 weeks for the Phase 2 study). Patel et al. explored the impact of assuming a higher CP for Phase 3 trials and concluded that comparative results remained the same qualitatively.

For each (maximum efficacy, AE profile) combination and a dose–response model for efficacy, one can find the Phase 2 sample size among those investigated that yields the highest expected NPV. For example, under a 4-parameter Emax model, the optimal sample size for a maximum efficacy of 1.1 and a moderate AE profile (the base case) is 270 in a study with 8 active doses. These optimal sample sizes are given in the first block in Table 11.4 under the column heading of "Optimal Phase 2." One can calculate the reduction in expected NPV from the optimal value for other sample sizes. Two examples for this calculation are included for sample sizes of 270 and 405 in Table 11.4. Entries in Table 11.4 are extracted from Table 7 in Patel et al. (2012).

The probability of Phase 3 success for all cases included in Table 11.4 is between 56 and 72% when the maximum efficacy is 0.55. It is greater than 98% when the maximum efficacy is 1.1 or above. The relatively high probability of Phase 3 success when the maximum efficacy is only 0.55 is primarily due to the very large sample size for the Phase 3 trials. The low expected NPVs for this scenario, on the other hand, depict a less than desirable commercial picture for a drug with a maximum treatment efficacy of only 0.55 on the NRS.

Table 11.4 shows that the expected NPV associated with the sample size of 270 is always within 5% of the maximum expected NPV for the 9 (maximum efficacy, AE profile) combinations. Nevertheless, the optimal Phase 2 sample size does change as a function of the maximum efficacy and AE profile. If one thinks the 9 scenarios in Table 11.4 are equally likely, one can calculate the average expected NPV under the 9 scenarios and select the sample size that yields the largest average expected NPV. Alternatively, one can apply the minimax principle by selecting the sample size that minimizes the maximum reduction from the optimal expected NPV under the 9 scenarios.

One surprising finding in Patel et al. is that the 4-dose design performs pretty well when compared with the 8-dose design. For the 4-parameter Emax model, the optimal Phase 2 sample size for the 4-dose and 8-dose designs generally leads to a maximum or near maximum utility at dose D_6, making the design that includes doses D_2, D_4, D_6 and D_8 quite attractive. Similarly, for other dose–response curves, the optimal Phase 2 sample size often leads to the maximum or near maximum utility at or near a dose in the subset of doses D_2, D_4, D_6 and D_8.

We include in Table 11.5 select results from Patel et al. for the 4-dose versus 8-dose comparison under an exponential dose–response model for efficacy. We compare the two with respect to the optimal Phase 2 sample size under each design option. In all cases, the expected NPV for the optimal sample size for the 4-dose design is

Table 11.5 Impact of maximum efficacy, AE profile, number of doses on the optimal Phase 2 sample size, the probability of Phase 3 success and expected NPV under an exponential dose–response model for efficacy and two design options

Maximum efficacy	AE profile	4 Doses			8 Doses		
		Optimal Phase 2 sample size			Optimal Phase 2 sample size		
		Sample size	Prob of Phase 3 success	Expected NPV ($B USD)	Sample size	Prob of Phase 3 success	Expected NPV ($B USD)
0.55	High	675	0.66	0.07	675	0.58	0.06
0.55	Moderate	675	0.68	0.21	675	0.59	0.17
0.55	Low	675	0.72	0.49	675	0.62	0.42
1.1	High	405	0.97	0.68	405	0.91	0.59
1.1	Moderate	405	0.98	1.55	405	0.93	1.42
1.1	Low	405	0.98	3.28	405	0.94	3.03
1.65	High	225	0.99	1.95	270	0.99	1.80
1.65	Moderate	225	1.00	3.36	270	1.00	3.18
1.65	Low	225	1.00	5.49	270	1.00	5.30

higher than its counterpart for the 8-dose design. In addition, the probability of Phase 3 success is also higher under the 4-dose design. Patel et al. offered two possible explanations for this observation. First, the smaller number of patients per dose under the 8-dose design may make it harder to make a correct dose choice under this design. Second, the AE dose–response curve is generally steeper between D_6 and D_8 than the corresponding efficacy curve, contributing to the fact that dose D_7 contributes very little to the maximum utility selection method.

Once the framework is set up, one can assess the choice of doses and sample size on the Phase 3 success probability and the expected NPV under different scenarios. One can extend the idea of minimax or the average expected NPV to find a design that is optimal over a plausible group of possible dose–response curves for efficacy and nuisance AE incidence.

11.4 Other Metrics

The metric in (11.14) was once considered by a major pharmaceutical company as a possible measure for the productivity of its clinical development endeavor. The metric measures the average cost of a successful Phase 3 trial at the portfolio level. The metric is easy to understand since the success of the clinical development organization in an innovative pharmaceutical company can be measured by the percentage of positive Phase 3 trials. The metric, however, is sensitive to many factors including the makeup of the portfolio. Thus, it will be hard to compare the metric over time when there has been a major shift in the composition of the portfolio.

$$\text{Clinical Grant \$ in Phase 2\&3 Trials}/\text{Number of Successful Phase 3 Trials}$$
(11.14)

Götte et al. (2015) presented an approach to plan sample size for a Phase 2 trial in a time-to-event setting. Their approach selects a Go/No-Go decision boundary in such a way that the Phase 2 sample size or the expected sample size for the development program (one Phase 2 trial and one Phase 3 trial combined) is minimal while satisfying criteria on the probabilities of correct Go/No-Go decisions as well as the success probability of the Phase 3 trial. Simulations by Götte et al. show that unconditional probabilities of Go/No-Go decisions as well as the unconditional success probability for the Phase 3 trial are influenced by the number of events observed in the Phase 2 trial. Götte et al. (2015) concluded that requiring more than 150 events in the Phase 2 trial might not be necessary as the additional impact on the probabilities due to additional number of events in the Phase 2 trial became quite small.

The relationship between the amount of information provided by the Phase 2 trial and the probability of a successful Phase 3 trial was also discussed in Sect. 9.4 of this book. Through examining the change in the probability of a successful Phase 3 trial, one can assess the value of including additional information in the seeding Phase 2 trial.

11.5 Summary

Increasingly, researchers are looking for strategies that will optimize development at the program level. In this chapter, we review in some details the proposal by Chen and Beckman (2009, 2014) to use a benefit–cost efficiency score to assess the efficiency of a proof-of-concept study. For late-stage programs, literature has increasingly offered strategies that focus on exploiting the relationship between the Phase 2 dose-finding trial and the Phase 3 confirmatory trials.

Stallard et al. (2005) considered a situation common in oncology drug development where Phase 2 consisted of a single trial comparing an experimental treatment with a control. The Phase 2 trial, if successful, will be followed up by a single Phase 3 trial (or multiple trials, if needed). Because the Phase 2 trial often measures a short-term benefit (e.g., tumor response), a positive Phase 2 trial does not in itself provide sufficient evidence for the treatment's benefit on a longer-term clinical endpoint (e.g., progression-free survival or overall survival) required of the Phase 3 study. The goal of the Phase 2 trial is to decide if investment in the Phase 3 trial is worthwhile. Stallard et al. proposed to make this decision based on the posterior predictive probability of a statistically significant Phase 3 outcome, at the interim and final analyses of the Phase 2 trial. If the posterior predictive probability exceeds a pre-specified threshold at these decision points, the Phase 3 trial will be conducted. The Phase 2 trial itself may be terminated early for futility. This is another example where the Phase 2 trial is explicitly linked to the Phase 3 trial in making a program-level decision.

In the neuropathic pain example, Patel et al. (2012) investigated two methods to select one dose from the dose-finding study and compare the dose to placebo in each of exactly two trials. Bolognese et al. (2017) extended the work of Patel et al. by considering 1 or 2 doses in each of 2 Phase 3 trials and, if needed, 1 or 2 additional Phase 3 trials to substantiate the usefulness of the second dose. Dose selection was again based on program-level optimization using probability of Phase 3 success and the expected net present value. Bolognese et al. found that Phase 2 sample size could be optimized at small to modest size when allowing for the possibility of taking 2 doses to Phase 3. In addition, they found that choice between 1 or 2 doses depended on the magnitudes and shapes of the true underlying efficacy and nuisance AE dose–response curves.

There are other methods to select a dose or doses to bring into the Phase 3 stage. For example, Antonijevic et al. (2013) investigated a Phase 2b/Phase 3 drug development program for Type 2 diabetes. The program includes a single Phase 2b trial of five doses and a placebo. If the Phase 2b success criteria are met, one dose will be selected from the Phase 2b study and further tested in three pivotal Phase 3 trials. The three studies are to assess the new drug's effect as a monotherapy, an add-on to metformin, and an add-on to sulfonylurea.

The Phase 2b study considered by Antonijevic et al. (2013) employs a Bayesian adaptive design allocation, which updates treatment allocation algorithms every 4 weeks to target doses with the maximum utility values. The utility value of a dose is obtained by multiplying together two utility components corresponding to the change in the primary efficacy endpoint of HbA1c and the incidence of hypoglycemia (a common safety concern for antidiabetic medications).

For the HbA1c component, the utility function of a dose takes its largest value of 3 if the mean change in HbA1c from baseline compared to the placebo is $\leq -1.3\%$. The value of the utility function decreases linearly from 3 to 1 if the mean change in HbA1c (relative to the placebo) moves from -1.3% to -1.0%. It further decreases linearly from 1 to 0 if the mean change (relative to the placebo) moves from -1.0% to 0. If the placebo group experiences a greater mean decrease in HbA1c than a dose, then the HbA1c utility value for the dose is 0.

As for the hypoglycemic component, the utility function takes the largest value of 1 when the hypoglycemic incidence of a dose is less than 4% higher than the placebo. The utility function decreases linearly to 0 when the incidence is greater than the placebo but the excess amount is between 4 and 30%. If the excess incidence is greater than 30%, the utility function takes the value 0.

By multiplying the two components together, a sponsor obtains a utility score for each dose. Using the multiplicative metric, the sponsor signals that it would not be interesting at all in any dose that induces less mean change in the HbA1c than the placebo or has a greater than 30% higher incidence of hypoglycemia than the placebo. This utility value is a composite endpoint of efficacy and safety (or benefit and risk). In the example considered by Antonijevic et al., a utility score higher than 0.8 is considered to be clinically meaningful.

The idea of using a composite efficacy–safety endpoint to assess the desirability of a dose is not new. Ouellet et al. (2009) used a clinical utility index (CUI) to compare two calcium channel $\alpha2\delta$ ligands in development for treating insomnia. The CUI is made up of five measures of efficacy (wake after sleep onset, sleep quality, sleep latency and stage 1 and stage 3–4 in sleep architecture) and 2 measures of residual sedation (adverse effects). Peak CUI values were observed at doses that were not considered viable for both compounds, and the development of both compounds was subsequently discontinued.

We anticipate an increasing trend in using composite efficacy–safety endpoints to assess doses in dose–response studies. For one thing, composite endpoints incorporate the trade-off between efficacy and safety into the decision-making process. In addition, the increasing applications of the multi-criteria decision approach (Mussen et al., 2007a, 2007b) have raised awareness to the quantitative assessment of efficacy and safety jointly.

In our opinion, it makes sense to formally incorporate cost and speed into internal development program planning. Pinheiro et al. (2010) recommended balancing resource allocation between the learning and the confirmatory phases to optimize the probability of Phase 3 success and the expected NPV of a development program. We are in full agreement on the importance of examining these two metrics together. We feel it may be prudent to require that the probability of Phase 3 success exceed a certain threshold before progressing a drug candidate to the confirmatory stage. Otherwise, a sponsor may be lured by a large NPV figure which is solely due to an extremely large net revenue forecast and progress a development program that has little chance to succeed.

There are many different metrics that can be used to help us make study- or program-level decisions. The choice should be guided by a sponsor's development/business objectives while taking into consideration regulatory requirements. It is not unusual for dose selection criteria to be defined by personnel within the research and development department while the commercial team hopes to maximize the expected net returns. We recommend close collaboration between clinical, regulatory and commercial groups early in the development of a new pharmaceutical product to jointly identify strategies that could serve the needs of multiple groups.

Readers interested in learning more about design and investment strategies to optimize portfolio-level decisions are encouraged to read the book on "*Optimization of Pharmaceutical R&D Programs and Portfolios*" (2015) edited by Antonijevic and published by Springer.

If you want to go fast, go alone.
If you want to go far, go together.
—African proverb.

References

Antonijevic, Z., Kimber, M., Manner, D., et al. (2013). Optimizing drug development programs: Type 2 diabetes case study. *Therapeutic Innovation & Regulatory Science, 47*(3), 363–374.

Bolognese, J., Bhattacharyya, J., Assaid, C., & Patel, N. (2017). Methodological extensions of Phase 2 trial designs based on program-level considerations: Further development of a case study in neuropathic pain. *Therapeutic Innovation & Regulatory Science, 51*, 100–110.

Burman, C. F., Grieve, A., & Senn, S. (2007). Decision analysis in drug development. In A. Dmitrienko, C. Chuang-Stein, & R. D'Agostino (Eds.), *Pharmaceutical Statistics Using SAS®: A Practical Guide* (pp. 385–428). SAS Institute.

Chen, C., & Beckman, R. A. (2009). Optimal cost-effective designs of phase II proof of concept trials and associated go-no go decisions. *Journal of Biopharmaceutical Statistics, 19*(3), 424–436.

Chen, C., & Beckman, R. A. (2014). Maximizing return on socioeconomic investment in Phase 2 proof-of-concept trials. *Clinical Cancer Research, 20*(7), 1730–1734.

DiMasi, J. A., Grabowski, H. G., & Hansen, R. W. (2016). Innovation in the pharmaceutical industry: New estimates of R&D costs. *Journal of Health Economics, 47*, 20–33.

Götte, H., Schüler, A., Kirchner, M., & Kieser, M. (2015). Sample size planning for phase II trials based on success probabilities for phase III. *Pharmaceutical Statistics, 14*(6), 515–524.

ICH E1. (1994). The extent of population exposure to assess clinical safety for drugs intended for long-term treatment of non-life-threatening conditions.

Marchenko, O., Miller, J., Parke, T., et al. (2013). Improving oncology clinical programs by use of innovative designs and comparing them via simulations. *Therapeutic Innovation & Regulatory Science, 47*(5), 602–612.

Mehta, C. R., & Patel, N. R. (2006). Adaptive, group sequential and decision theoretic approaches to sample size determination. *Statistics in Medicine, 25*(19), 3250–3269.

Mussen, F., Salek, S., & Walker, S. (2007a). A quantitative approach to benefit-risk assessment of medicines—Part 1: The development of a new model using multi-criteria decision analysis. *Pharmacoepidemiology and Drug Safety, 16*(Suppl 1), S2–S15.

Mussen, F., Salek, S., & Walker, S. (2007b). A quantitative approach to benefit-risk assessment of medicines—Part 2: The practical application of a new model. *Pharmacoepidemiology and Drug Safety, 16*(Suppl 1), S16–S41.

Ouellet, D., Werth, J., Parekh, N., et al. (2009). The use of a clinical utility index to compare insomnia compounds: A quantitative basis for benefit-risk assessment. *Clinical Pharmacology & Therapeutics, 85*(3), 277–282.

Patel, N. R., & Ankolekar, S. (2007). A Bayesian approach for incorporating economic factors in sample size design for clinical trials of individual drugs and portfolios of drugs. *Statistics in Medicine, 26*(27), 4976–4988.

Patel, N., Bolognese, J., Chuang-Stein, C., et al. (2012). Designing phase 2 trials based on program-level considerations: A case study for neuropathic pain. *Drug Information Journal, 46*(4), 439–454.

Pinheiro, J., Sax, F., Antonijevic, Z., et al. (2010). Adaptive and model-based dose-ranging trials: Quantitative evaluation and recommendations. *Statistics in Biopharmaceutical Research, 2*(4), 435–454.

Robertson, T., Wright, F. T., & Dykstra, R. L. (1988). *Order restricted statistical inference.* John Wiley & Sons.

Stallard, N., Whitehead, J., & Cleall, S. (2005). Decision-making in a phase II clinical trial: A new approach combining Bayesian and frequentist concepts. *Pharmaceutical Statistics, 4*(2), 119–128.

Chapter 12
Discounting Prior Results to Account for Selection Bias

> *...it is the peculiar and perpetual error of the human understanding to be more moved and excited by affirmatives than by negatives.*
> —Francis Bacon

12.1 Introduction

In Chap. 5, we described how information from completed trials could be incorporated in future trial planning. In that chapter, we ignored the possibility of any bias in the way that the completed trials were selected for use. In this chapter, we consider possible selection bias that can occur due to the fact that a Phase 2 trial is usually selected for use in future trial planning only when it has produced a positive response.

We first illustrate the phenomenon of selection bias and relate it to the general concept of regression to the mean.

We next consider the methods for correcting for selection bias introduced by Wang et al. (2006) and Kirby et al. (2012). The correction is needed so that trialists do not plan Phase 3 trials thinking their treatment candidates to be more efficacious than they actually are. Both sets of authors take the simplified situation of using results from a single Phase 2 trial that compared a single-dose arm versus control to plan a Phase 3 trial. We first consider their results for when there are no differences between the Phase 2 and Phase 3 trials in terms of endpoint, population or any other factor. For this simple scenario, it is shown by using simulation results that we may need to discount the Phase 2 result for planned power to match actual power or for estimated assurance to match so-called theoretical assurance. In the succeeding subsection, we consider their results for when the population and/or endpoint differ between Phase 2 and Phase 3 but other factors are held constant. To extend the results given by Kirby et al., we introduce a dose-response study between the Phase 2 POC study and the Phase 3 study. In doing this, we require the POC study result to be positive and the combined result from POC and dose-response studies also to be positive. We show

C. Chuang-Stein and S. Kirby, *Quantitative Decisions in Drug Development*, Springer Series in Pharmaceutical Statistics, https://doi.org/10.1007/978-3-030-79731-7_12

that the incorporation of additional Phase 2 information can lessen the amount of discounting required to be able to match estimated and theoretical assurance.

A different, empirical approach to examining the amount of discounting required due to bias in the selection of positive Phase 2 studies is to compare the estimated treatment effect for the Phase 2 trial data alone with the estimate obtained from a posterior distribution when the Phase 2 data are combined with an appropriate prior distribution.

Finally, we consider estimating selection bias using the maximum likelihood method and three further bias correction methods introduced in Kirby et al. (2020).

In Sect. 12.6, we describe a comparison for the seven bias correction methods described in this chapter and one additional method proposed by De Martini (2011).

We include the results of an empirical study by Kirby et al. (2012) on the amount of discounting required in Sect. 12.7 and offer additional comments on selection bias in drug development in Sect. 12.8.

12.2   Selection Bias

To illustrate selection bias, we take a simple example. We suppose that the true treatment effect for a treatment versus a comparator is 1 unit for a certain measurement. We further suppose that the variability between subjects in this measurement can be characterized by a Normal distribution with a variance of $2^2 = 4$. We now suppose that a parallel group study is to be run with 100 subjects randomly assigned with equal proportions to a new treatment or a placebo. The distribution for the difference in sample means is $N\left(1; \frac{2 \times 2^2}{50}\right)$. A result is to be declared positive if the difference in sample means is greater than a target value of 1.2. It is immediately obvious in this case that a result greater than 1.2 gives a biased estimate of the true treatment effect. What may be less obvious is that if the target value were say 0.8 then we would still get a biased estimate of the true treatment effect. We can see this by looking at the estimated mean effect calculated only from samples where the effect exceeds the target value of 0.8. For 10,000 random samples using a particular seed, we obtain an estimated treatment effect of 1.20. The bias in the estimation of the true treatment effect comes about because part of the sampling distribution for the difference in means, that part below the target value of 0.8, is ignored.

One way to display a similar result pictorially for a Phase 2 study with a confirmatory Phase 3 follow-up study is shown in Fig. 12.1. We assume that a Phase 2 study is run as described above and that a follow-on Phase 3 study with 400 subjects randomly allocated to the new treatment or a placebo may be run. Figure 12.1 displays 50 random Phase 2 observed effects (differences in the sample mean responses between the two groups) without any selection of results in the top panel together with linked results for a Phase 3 follow-on trial which is assumed to take place irrespective of the Phase 2 result. Even though a Phase 3 trial is linked to a Phase 2 trial, it was generated independently of the Phase 2 trial. The bottom panel displays results of

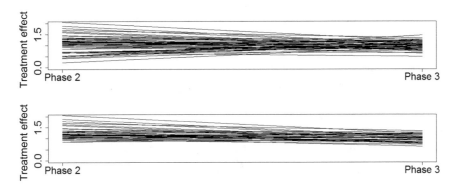

Fig. 12.1 Illustration of the effect of selecting a Phase 2 study when the observed treatment effect exceeds a target value of 0.8—the top panel shows simulated paired Phase 2 and 3 results without selection, and the bottom panel shows simulated paired Phase 2 and 3 results when the observed Phase 2 result needs to exceed 0.8 for the Phase 3 study to be launched

Phase 2 trials that have an observed effect greater than 0.8 and their linked Phase 3 trials among the same 50 simulated pairs of trials. We can see that there is no particular tendency for the lines to go up or down in the top panel but in the bottom panel there is a tendency for the lines to go down. The narrower range of values for Phase 3 trials is due to the larger sample size of these trials (i.e., 400 vs. 100).

The biased estimate of the treatment effect means that if we repeat the Phase 2 study and estimate the treatment effect without any requirement on the magnitude of the effect then we are most likely to obtain a treatment effect estimate that is less than our initial estimate. We can study this further by examining the average of the estimated Phase 2 treatment effect among trials (out of 10,000 randomly generated trials) with an observed effect greater than a target value. The target value may be the value needed to launch the subsequent Phase 3 trials. Figure 12.2 shows the average

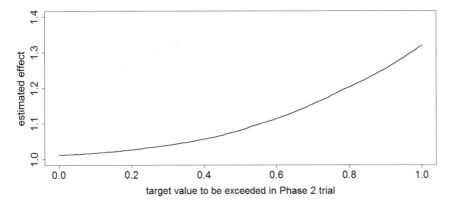

Fig. 12.2 Plot of the average of the estimated Phase 2 treatment effects among trials with an observed treatment effect exceeding a target value versus the target value

described above plotted against the target value with the target value ranging from 0 to 1. We can see that the average of the estimated treatment effect among Phase 2 trials meeting the target value requirement increases sharply as the target value increases. It should be noted that as the target value increases, the number of trials out of the 10,000 randomly generated trials meeting the target value requirement decreases steadily.

The selection bias illustrated above is a particular instance of the general situation that if a phenomenon is extreme on its first measurement then it will tend to be closer to the average on the second measurement. This phenomenon is known as regression to the mean (Chuang-Stein & Kirby, 2014).

12.3   The Wang, Hung and O'Neill and Kirby et al. Methods for Discounting Phase 2 Results

In this section, we describe the methods for discounting Phase 2 results introduced by Wang et al. (2006) and Kirby et al. (2012).

Both sets of authors considered the effect of using the result from a single Phase 2 study to plan a Phase 3 study. They assumed that the endpoint of interest has a Normal distribution with standard deviation equal to 1 and that both Phase 2 and Phase 3 trials are parallel group trials comparing a new treatment versus a comparator.

Wang et al. introduced the idea of a launch threshold, represented by Δ_{0L}. This is the value that the estimated treatment effect in the Phase 2 study needs to exceed for planning to continue with the design of a Phase 3 trial. They applied Δ_{0L} to three statistics: the observed treatment effect $(\widehat{\Delta})$, the observed treatment effect minus one standard error $(L_1 = \widehat{\Delta} - 1 \times s.e.)$ and the observed treatment effect minus 1.96 standard errors $(L_2 = \widehat{\Delta} - 1.96 \times s.e.)$. In other words, the Phase 3 study would be launched if $\widehat{\Delta}$, L_1 or L_2 exceeded Δ_{0L}. For simplicity, $\widehat{\Delta}$ is taken to be $\overline{X}_T - \overline{X}_C$ in this chapter where $\overline{X}_T$ and $\overline{X}_C$ are the observed mean responses on the primary endpoint in the treatment and the control group, respectively.

To decide how much discounting of the observed Phase 2 effect was necessary, Wang et al. looked at equating planned and actual power for the Phase 3 study. In each case, the planned power for the Phase 3 trial was 80%, and a one-sided 2.5% significance level was used in the sample size calculation given by

$$\frac{(Z_{0.025} + Z_{0.2})^2 2}{\tilde{\Delta}^2} \tag{12.1}$$

where $\tilde{\Delta}$ is $\widehat{\Delta}$, L_1 or L_2 and Z_{γ} is the upper $(100 \times \gamma)\%$ percentile of the standard Normal distribution. The actual power was defined as statistical power in the Phase 3 trial that was launched. The actual power was estimated by Wang et al. using simulation.

Wang et al. simulated 100,000 Phase 2 trials for each combination of sample size and launch threshold. For each simulation, they first generated an estimated Phase 2 treatment effect and assessed whether a Phase 3 trial was to be launched for each of the three statistics (i.e., $\widehat{\Delta}$, L_1 or L_2) and a given launch threshold. If the Phase 3 trial were to be launched for a statistic, then the sample size for the Phase 3 trial was determined using (12.1) with a treatment effect given by the statistic. They then generated a test statistic for the Phase 3 trial under an assumed treatment effect for the Phase 3 trial. If the test statistic was greater than the critical value, then the Phase 3 trial was regarded as providing evidence of superiority to the comparator.

Instead of seeking to equate planned and actual power, Kirby et al. looked to equate the estimated assurance probability for a statistically significant result in the Phase 3 trial with what they termed theoretical assurance. They defined theoretical assurance as assurance calculated using the true standard deviation and Phase 3 treatment effect. Estimated and theoretical assurance were obtained using the following general expression (O'Hagan et al., 2005)

$$1 - \Phi\left(\frac{1.96\sqrt{\tau} - \Delta}{\sqrt{\tau + \upsilon}}\right)$$

which was also discussed in Chap. 5 (see 5.5).

For estimated assurance, Δ was set equal to $\widehat{\Delta}$, L_1 or L_2, τ equal to $\frac{2\widehat{\sigma}^2}{n}$, υ equal to $\frac{2\widehat{\sigma}^2}{m}$ where n is the sample size per group for the Phase 3 trial, m is the sample size per group in the Phase 2 study, $\widehat{\sigma}$ is estimated from the Phase 2 data, and Φ is the cumulative distribution of the standard Normal distribution. For theoretical assurance, Δ was set equal to the true Phase 3 effect, and σ was set equal to the true standard deviation. It should be noted that the estimation of σ differs from the setting of σ equal to a known value in earlier chapters. It is expected, however, that there is little difference between these two approaches for the sample sizes considered.

Kirby et al. also looked at three further possible launch criteria. These criteria are as follows:

1. $M_f > \Delta_{0L}$
2. $L_{0.10} > \text{MAV}$ and $U_{0.25} > \text{TV}$
3. $L_{f,0.10} > \text{MAV}$ and $U_{f,0.25} > \text{TV}$.

In the first launch criterion above, $M_f = \widehat{\Delta} \times f$, and f is the fraction of the treatment effect to be retained and will be referred to as a retention factor. For example, a value of 0.9 for f means retaining 90% of the initial estimate for the treatment effect, or equivalently, discounting the initial estimate by 10%.

In the second launch criterion, $L_{0.10}$ is the lower one-sided 90% confidence interval limit for the treatment effect, and $U_{0.25}$ is the upper one-sided 75% confidence interval limit for the treatment effect. As introduced in Chap. 7, MAV represents a minimum acceptable value for the treatment effect, and TV is a target value for the treatment effect. The second launch criterion requires the lower one-sided 90% confidence

Table 12.1 Three additional launch criteria used by Kirby et al. and associated effects used to calculate the Phase 3 sample size

Launch criterion	$\tilde{\Delta}$ Used in Sample Size Calculation in (12.1)
$M_f > \Delta_{0L}$	M_f
$L_{0.10} > \text{MAV}$ and $U_{0.25} > \text{TV}$	$\hat{\Delta}$
$L_{f,0.10} > \text{MAV}$ and $U_{f,0.25} > \text{TV}$	M_f

interval limit ($L_{0.10}$) for the treatment effect to exceed the MAV and the upper one-sided 75% confidence interval limit ($U_{0.25}$) to exceed TV. This criterion is similar to the LPDAT approach described in Chap. 7 (see Sect. 7.2.3).

In the third launch criterion, $L_{f,0.10}$ and $U_{f,0.25}$ represent the same one-sided confidence interval limits, but M_f is used as the estimated treatment effect rather than $\hat{\Delta}$.

Kirby et al. calculated the required sample size for the Phase 3 study for the three additional launch criteria by setting $\tilde{\Delta}$ in (12.1) to different values as shown in Table 12.1.

Kirby et al. simulated 100,000 Phase 2 trials for each combination of threshold and Phase 2 sample size.

We consider the scenarios used by Wang et al. (2006) and also by Kirby et al. (2012).

12.3.1 Results When There is No Difference Between Phase 2 and 3 Populations and Endpoints or Any Other Factors

In this section, we assume that the Phase 2 and 3 studies do not differ in terms of population, endpoint or any other factor.

Scenario 1

$$\Delta_{02} = 0.3, \ \Delta_0 = 0.3, \ m = 50, 100, 200, \ \Delta_{0L} = 0.2, 0.15, 0.1$$

In the above description, Δ_{02} represents the true Phase 2 treatment effect, and Δ_0 represents the true Phase 3 treatment effect.

Selected results obtained by Wang et al. for the actual power are shown in Table 12.2 where $L_1 = \hat{\Delta} - 1 \times \text{s.e.}$, $L_2 = \hat{\Delta} - 1.96 \times \text{s.e.}$ and s.e. represents the standard error of $\hat{\Delta}$. The columns with headings $\hat{\Delta}$, L_1 and L_2 in Table 12.2 contain the estimated actual powers when applying the launch threshold to these three statistics. For convenience, we use "estimated powers" to mean "estimated actual powers".

Table 12.2 Estimated powers for Phase 3 trials run when a launch threshold is exceeded by each of the three statistics $\hat{\Delta}$, L_1 and L_2 under Scenario 1

Δ_{0L}	m	$\hat{\Delta}$	L_1	L_2
0.2	50	0.61	0.74	0.82
0.2	100	0.68	0.80	0.86
0.2	200	0.73	0.84	0.90
0.1	50	0.68	0.84	0.92
0.1	100	0.73	0.88	0.95
0.1	200	0.77	0.90	0.97

It can be seen from the table that to require estimated power to equal or exceed planned power for all sample sizes and the launch thresholds included in Table 12.2, we would need to use L_2, i.e., requiring that L_2 exceed a given launch threshold. Since the power for the Phase 3 study is set at 80%, L_1 is almost as good as L_2 except for the case when m is small and the launch threshold is high.

The difficulty with L_2 is the low probability of initiating Phase 3 trials associated with this choice. We include in Table 12.3 approximate proportions of Phase 3 studies launched when $\hat{\Delta}$, L_1 and L_2 are required to exceed a given launch threshold. The proportions are approximate because they were obtained by visual inspection of Fig. 1 in the paper of Wang et al.

It can be seen from Table 12.3 that the probability of launching Phase 3 trials under the criterion that $L_2 > \Delta_{0L}$ is low for all Phase 2 sample sizes. When the Phase 2 sample size is 200 per group, use of just the observed treatment effect and a launch threshold of 0.1 gives an estimated power of 0.77 (Table 12.2) while keeping the proportion of trials not launched fairly low at about 0.1 (result not shown in Table 12.2).

Table 12.4 includes a selection of the results obtained by Kirby et al. Only results for launch criterion (1) (i.e., $M_f > \Delta_{0L}$) are shown because Kirby et al. considered the other two launch criteria using MAV and TV as not demonstrating much additional value.

Table 12.4 shows results for a launch threshold of 0.1. It can be seen that M_f with $f = 0.8, 0.9$ or 1.0 causes estimated assurance to be closest to the corresponding theoretical assurance when the Phase 2 sample size per arm is 50, 100 or 200. For the larger Phase 2 sample sizes (100 or more patients per group), the probability

Table 12.3 Estimated proportion of Phase 3 trials launched when each of the three statistics $\hat{\Delta}$, L_1 and L_2 is required to exceed a launch threshold under Scenario 1

Δ_{0L}	m	$\hat{\Delta}$	L_1	L_2
0.15	50	0.75	0.4	0.1
0.15	100	0.85	0.5	0.2
0.15	200	0.9	0.7	0.3

Table 12.4 Estimated assurance, theoretical assurance and probability of launching a Phase 3 trial for Scenario 1 (m denotes Phase 2 sample size per treatment arm)

Launch criterion	$m = 50$			$m = 100$			$m = 200$		
	Est. Ass	Theo. Ass	P(launch)	Est. Ass	Theo. Ass	P(launch)	Est. Ass	Theo. Ass	P(launch)
$\hat{\Delta} > 0.1$	0.67	0.59	0.84	0.69	0.66	0.92	0.73	0.72	0.98
$L_1 > 0.1$	0.63	0.70	0.50	0.66	0.78	0.66	0.70	0.84	0.84
$L_2 > 0.1$	0.61	0.76	0.16	0.64	0.85	0.28	0.67	0.91	0.50
$M_{0.9} > 0.1$	0.66	0.63	0.83	0.68	0.70	0.91	0.72	0.77	0.97
$M_{0.8} > 0.1$	0.65	0.66	0.81	0.67	0.74	0.89	0.71	0.82	0.96

of launching a Phase 3 trial is estimated to be 0.89 or greater. Thus, for a launch threshold of 0.1, no discounting when sample size is 200 or more per group or a small amount of discounting (e.g., 10%) of the observed Phase 2 treatment effect approximately equates estimated and theoretical assurance without greatly affecting the probability of launching a Phase 3 trial.

Although not reproduced here a launch threshold of 0.15 also gives discounting factors of 0.8, 0.9 and 1.0 as those approximately equating estimated and theoretical assurance. For a launch threshold of 0.2, results in Kirby et al. show that the discounting factors are 0.6, 0.8 and 0.9 for Phase 2 sample sizes of 50, 100 and 200 per arm. For both the 0.15 threshold and the 0.2 threshold, the probability of launching a Phase 3 trial is reduced, but it is still greater than that associated with criteria using the L_1 and L_2 statistics.

The Phase 3 launch probability is higher under the M_f launch criterion compared with the criteria involving L_1 and L_2. This is also true under the null case when there is no Phase 2 or Phase 3 treatment effect. Kirby et al. found that provided the Phase 2 sample size was reasonable and a higher launch threshold was used then the probability of launching a Phase 3 trial in the null case was reasonably small. For example, if the sample size per group in the Phase 2 study is 200 and the launch threshold is 0.15, then the launch probability is estimated to be 0.047 for the $M_{0.90}$ criterion when the new treatment has no effect.

12.3.2 Results for Different Phase 2 Endpoint and/or Population Compared to Phase 3 (Other Factors Assumed the Same)

To examine the effect of having a different endpoint and/or population in the Phase 2 and 3 trials while other factors are held constant, Wang et al. and Kirby et al. looked at three other scenarios. They are as follows:

Scenario 2

$$\Delta_{02} = 0.3, \ \Delta_0 = 0.2, \ m = 50, 100, 200, \ \Delta_{0L} = 0.2$$

Scenario 3

$$\Delta_{02} = 0.3, \ \Delta_0 = 0.2, \ m = 50, 100, 200, \ \Delta_{0L} = 0.1$$

Scenario 4

$$\Delta_{02} = 0.4, \ \Delta_0 = 0.2, \ m = 50, 100, 200, \ \Delta_{0L} = 0.2, 0.15, 0.1$$

Table 12.5 Estimated powers for Phase 3 trials run when a launch threshold is exceeded for each combination of launch threshold, Phase 2 sample size and the use of $\widehat{\Delta}$, L_1 and L_2 for Scenarios 2 and 3 ($\Delta_0 = 0.2$, $\Delta_{02} = 0.3$)

Scenario	Δ_{0L}	m	$\widehat{\Delta}$	L_1	L_2
2	0.2	50	0.36	0.46	0.53
2	0.2	100	0.40	0.51	0.58
2	0.2	200	0.44	0.55	0.62
3	0.1	50	0.46	0.65	0.77
3	0.1	100	0.50	0.69	0.82
3	0.1	200	0.51	0.70	0.84

We present the results for Scenarios 2 and 3 because they represent a less severe diminution of the true treatment effect from Phase 2 to Phase 3. We first present the results obtained by Wang et al. in Table 12.5 for these two scenarios.

We recall that the planned power was 80%. Table 12.5 suggests that only the L_2 launch criterion ever gives an estimated power of 80% or more for any combination of threshold and sample size. As can be expected, the estimated probability of launching Phase 3 trials for the 0.2 threshold becomes even lower than that observed for the 0.15 threshold shown in Table 12.3 (see also Fig. 2 in Wang et al.).

We again present selected results from Kirby et al. for the same scenarios for the approach of finding the amount of discounting of the observed Phase 2 treatment effect required to equate estimated and theoretical assurance.

Table 12.6 suggests that there is rather little chance of launching a Phase 3 trial for values of f that approximately equate estimated and theoretical assurance when a launch threshold of 0.2 is used. By comparison, there is a far greater chance of launching a Phase 3 trial if the threshold is set at 0.1. The retention factors that give approximate equality of estimated and theoretical assurance when the launch threshold is set at 0.1 are 0.5, 0.6 and 0.6 for the Phase 2 sample sizes of 50, 100 and 200 per arm. It can be seen that these are roughly two thirds of the retention factors that equate estimated and theoretical assurance for Scenario 1, as one might expect given that the true Phase 3 effect is two thirds of the true Phase 2 effect.

12.3.3 Planning a Phase 3 Trial Using the Results of a Phase 2 POC Study and a Phase 2 Dose-Response Study

In this section, we extend the results obtained in Sects. 12.3.1 and 12.3.2 for the bias correction method described by Kirby et al. by assuming that after a successful POC study at the maximum tolerated dose, a dose-response study is conducted. We assume that the dose-response study includes three doses plus a placebo and that the highest dose is the maximum tolerated dose. The result from the dose-response study

Table 12.6 Estimated assurance, theoretical assurance and probability of launching a Phase 3 trial for Scenarios 2 and 3 (m denotes Phase 2 sample size per treatment arm)

Launch criterion	$m = 50$			$m = 100$			$m = 200$		
	Est. Ass	Theo. Ass	P(launch)	Est. Ass	Theo. Ass	P(launch)	Est. Ass	Theo. Ass	P(launch)
Scenario 2									
$\hat{\Delta} > 0.2$	0.68	0.39	0.69	0.71	0.42	0.76	0.74	0.44	0.84
$L_1 > 0.2$	0.66	0.46	0.31	0.69	0.49	0.38	0.72	0.52	0.50
$L_2 > 0.2$	0.65	0.49	0.07	0.68	0.53	0.10	0.71	0.57	0.16
$M_{0.3} > 0.2$	0.62	0.58	0.03	0.66	0.62	0.01	0.69	0.67	0.00
$M_{0.2} > 0.2$	0.62	0.60	0.00	NA	NA	0.00	NA	NA	0.00
Scenario 3									
$\hat{\Delta} > 0.1$	0.67	0.44	0.84	0.69	0.47	0.92	0.73	0.49	0.98
$L_1 > 0.1$	0.63	0.54	0.50	0.66	0.59	0.66	0.70	0.63	0.84
$L_2 > 0.1$	0.61	0.60	0.16	0.64	0.67	0.28	0.67	0.73	0.50
$M_{0.6} > 0.1$	0.62	0.57	0.75	0.65	0.64	0.83	0.68	0.71	0.91
$M_{0.5} > 0.1$	0.61	0.61	0.69	0.63	0.68	0.76	0.66	0.76	0.84

is combined with that from the POC study for the common dose (i.e., the maximum tolerated dose) by using the Normal approximation to the sampling distribution of the observed mean from the POC study as a prior distribution to be combined with the approximate Normal likelihood for the highest dose from the dose-response study. If the combined estimate also exceeds a threshold, then a Phase 3 study will be launched.

We consider the following extended scenarios which apply to the dose-response study as well as the POC study.

Scenario 1b

$$\Delta_{02POC} = 0.3, \ \Delta_{02DR} = (0, 0.1, 0.2, 0.3), \ \Delta_0 = 0.3,$$
$$m = 50, 100, 200, \ \Delta_{0L} = 0.2, 0.15, 0.1$$

Scenario 2b

$$\Delta_{02POC} = 0.3, \ \Delta_{02DR} = (0, 0.1, 0.2, 0.3), \ \Delta_0 = 0.2,$$
$$m = 50, 100, 200, \ \Delta_{0L} = 0.2$$

Scenario 3b

$$\Delta_{02POC} = 0.3, \ \Delta_{02DR} = (0, 0.1, 0.2, 0.3), \ \Delta_0 = 0.2,$$
$$m = 50, 100, 200, \ \Delta_{0L} = 0.1$$

Scenario 4b

$$\Delta_{02POC} = 0.4, \ \Delta_{02DR} = (0, 0.133, 0.267, 0.4), \ \Delta_0 = 0.2,$$
$$m = 50, 100, 200, \ \Delta_{0L} = 0.2, 0.15, 0.1$$

The total sample size for the dose-response study was 200 if the sample size per arm of the POC study was 50 or 100, and 400 if the sample size per arm of the POC study was 200. The total sample size in the Phase 2 dose-response study was split equally among the four groups. For convenience, we assume that the true dose-response is linear up to the maximum tolerated dose. Such a scenario could correspond to the linear part of an Emax dose-response model.

We assume that for the dose-response study to be launched a launch threshold must be exceeded by an estimate of the treatment effect, denoted by $\bar{d}_{POC}$, in the POC study. For the analysis of the dose-response study, we assume that a Normal prior distribution with mean equal to $\bar{d}_{POC}$ and variance equal to the estimated variance of $\bar{d}_{POC}$ is used. Furthermore, we assume that the sampling distribution of the treatment effect estimate at the maximum dose in the dose-response study, denoted by $\bar{d}_{DR}$, is Normal. Here, $\bar{d}_{DR}$ represents the predicted mean effect for the maximum dose from the linear regression of outcome on dose. Then, the posterior mean of the predicted mean response at the maximum dose is given by

Table 12.7 Retention factors f that approximately equate estimated and theoretical assurance when just a POC study is run (top scenario in each row) before Phase 3 and when both a POC study and a dose-response study (bottom scenario in each row) are run before Phase 3

Scenario (launch thresholds in brackets)	$n = 50$ per arm for POC study and 50 per arm for dose-response study	$n = 100$ per arm for POC study and 50 per arm for dose-response study	$n = 200$ per arm for POC study and 100 per arm for dose-response study
1 (0.1, 0.15, 0.2)	0.8, 0.8, 0.6	0.9, 0.9, 0.8	1.0, 1.0, 0.9
1b (0.1, 0.15, 0.2)	0.9, 0.8, 0.7	0.9, 0.9, 0.8	1.0, 1.0, 0.9
2 (0.2)	0.2	0.3[a]	0.3[a]
2b (0.2)	0.3[a]	0.3[a]	0.4[a]
3 (0.1)	0.5	0.6	0.6
3b (0.1)	0.6	0.6	0.6
4 (0.1, 0.15, 0.2)	0.4, 0.3, 0.2	0.5, 0.4, 0.2	0.5, 0.5, 0.3[a]
4b (0.1, 0.15, 0.2)	0.5, 0.4, 0.3[a]	0.5, 0.4, 0.3[a]	0.5, 0.5, 0.3[a]

[a]No result obtained using a smaller value for f because the proportion of Phase 3 trials estimated to be launched was zero in these cases

$$\overline{d}_{com} = \left(\frac{w_1 \overline{d}_{POC} + w_2 \overline{d}_{DR}}{w_1 + w_2} \right)$$

where w_1 is the inverse of the estimated variance for $\overline{d}_{POC}$, and w_2 is the inverse of the estimated variance for $\overline{d}_{DR}$. The Phase 3 study is launched provided the launch threshold is exceeded by a chosen function of the combined estimate $\overline{d}_{com}$ (e.g., 90% of $\overline{d}_{com}$).

Estimated assurance was calculated in the same way as before except that a pooled estimate of the variance was obtained by combining the estimates from the POC and dose-response studies. Results for 10,000 POC studies were simulated for each launch threshold and sample size.

In Table 12.7, we show the retention factor f for the launch criterion M_f that approximately equates estimated and theoretical assurance for the four scenarios when just a POC study is run and when both a POC study and a dose-response study are run.

It can be seen that for a number of combinations of launch threshold and sample size the discounting factor (i.e., $1 - f$) required to equate estimated and theoretical assurance is generally less when a dose-response study is run after the POC study and before considering launching a Phase 3 trial. This seems intuitively reasonable as more information is obtained before making the decision to launch a Phase 3 trial. The additional information dilutes the selection bias, especially in the case of a small but very positive POC trial.

12.4   Estimation of the Regression to the Mean Effect Caused by Phase 2 Trial Selection Using a Prior Distribution

Zhang (2013) presented an approach of assessing the regression to the mean effect caused by selection of a Phase 2 study result because it was positive. Zhang compared the observed Phase 2 effect with the expected effect obtained using a posterior distribution where the posterior distribution was calculated using the Phase 2 data and an appropriate prior distribution. He attributed the difference between the observed Phase 2 effect and the posterior mean to the effect of regression to the mean.

To illustrate Zhang's approach, we return to the example considered in Sect. 5.7. In that example, we considered a mixture distribution for a prior distribution for the treatment effect on TOTPAR6, total pain relief in the first six hours post-surgery, in a dental pain study. A lump of 20% of the prior distribution was placed at 0, and the remaining 80% of the distribution was taken to be a Normal distribution centered at 2.5 with a standard deviation of 0.8.

As in Sect. 5.7, we assume that the Phase 2 study randomized 200 patients equally to the new treatment and a comparator in a parallel group design. Similarly, we assume that the TOTPAR6 endpoint is Normally distributed with standard deviation equal to 7.

For each possible observed effect in the Phase 2 study, we can calculate the posterior distribution obtained by combining the Phase 2 study result with the prior distribution described above. Here, we do this by evaluating both the prior and the likelihood over a fine grid and approximating the likelihood for the Phase 2 result by a Normal likelihood. Using the posterior distribution, we can obtain the expected effect (i.e., posterior mean) that can be plotted against the observed effect to see the amount of regression to the mean. We show such a plot in Fig. 12.3 for observed treatment effects that would lead to rejection of the null hypothesis of no treatment difference using a Z-test with a one-sided 2.5% significance level. It can be shown that with 100 patients per group, an observed treatment effect greater than 1.94 on the TOTPAR6 scale would lead to rejection of the null hypothesis since $\sqrt{\frac{2*7^2}{100}} * 1.96 = 1.94$.

The shaded area between the 45-degree line and the curved line represents the regression to the mean effect, i.e., the difference between the observed Phase 2 effect and the posterior expected value. We can see that this difference becomes larger as the observed effect becomes large above where the line and the curve cross.

It is interesting to note that the posterior mean is higher than the observed effect estimate in the Phase 2 trial when the latter is <2.5. This is because 80% of the mass of the prior distribution follows a $N(2.5; 0.8^2)$ distribution which devotes 68% of its own mass to the range (1.7, 3.3). This represents a strong prior probability for a non-zero effect. Thus, when the observed treatment effect is low, the prior helps lift up the observed treatment effect so that the posterior expected value is higher than the observed effect.

Fig. 12.3 Observed Phase 2 effect (*x*-axis) versus posterior expected effect for prior distribution and clinical trial described in the text

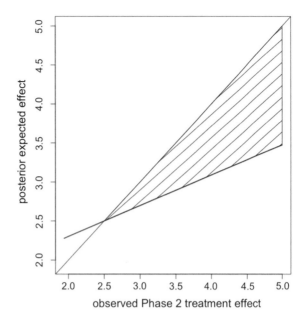

We can plot the difference between the observed Phase 2 effect and the posterior expected value as a percentage of the observed effect against the observed effect to examine the effect due to the regression to the mean. Such a plot is shown in Fig. 12.4. In Fig. 12.4, we only include observed Phase 2 effects that are greater than or equal

Fig. 12.4 Observed Phase 2 effect minus posterior expected effect plotted as a percentage of the observed Phase 2 effect versus observed Phase 2 effect

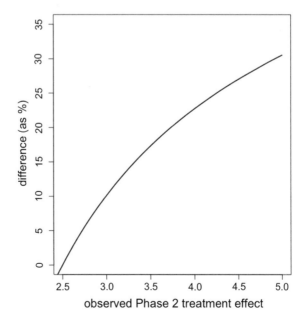

to the corresponding posterior expected values (i.e., when the observed effect in the Phase 2 trial is 2.5 or above).

From Fig. 12.4, it can be seen that the percentage increases up to around 30% when the observed Phase 2 effect is 5.0. Thus, an observed effect of 5.0 would be discounted down to a value of approximately 3.5. This approach differs from that of Kirby et al. by allowing a variable percentage discounting of the observed Phase 2 effect depending upon the value of the observed effect. It offers a theoretical justification for the level of discounting. Both the precision of the Phase 2 result and the prior distribution can have a substantial influence on the level of discounting under this approach.

To illustrate the effect of a larger POC study, we consider a POC study with twice the number of subjects per arm, i.e., with 200 subjects per arm. We obtain the graph shown in Fig. 12.5 for the regression to the mean effect with this sample size.

Figure 12.5 shows that the regression to the mean effect is now smaller. As before, we can plot the regression to the mean effect as a percentage of the observed Phase 2 effect versus the observed Phase 2 effect. This plot is shown in Fig. 12.6.

We can see from Fig. 12.6 that the discounting percentage for an observed Phase 2 effect of 5.0 has been reduced to approximately 22% compared with roughly 30% for the smaller POC trial.

We next illustrate the effect of the prior distribution on the regression to the mean effect. For this, we assume that instead of the mixture prior for the treatment effect we have just a Normal prior centered as before at 2.5 but now with a standard deviation of 2 instead of 0.8. Using this prior we obtain the regression to the mean effect shown in Fig. 12.7.

Fig. 12.5 Observed Phase 2 effect (*x*-axis) versus posterior expected effect for prior distribution and POC trial described in the text with POC sample size per arm increased to 200

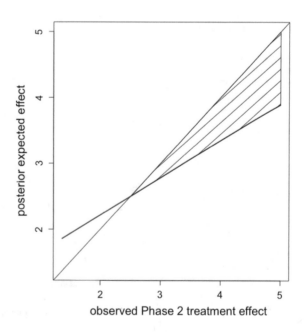

Fig. 12.6 Observed Phase 2 effect minus posterior expected effect plotted as a percentage of the observed Phase 2 effect versus observed Phase 2 effect for the POC trial described in the text with the larger sample size of 200 subjects per arm

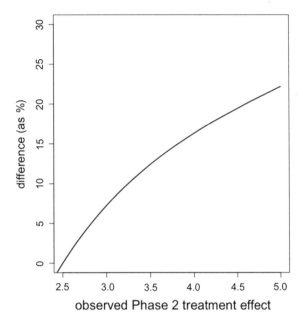

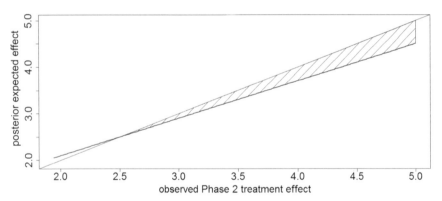

Fig. 12.7 Regression to the mean effect for the POC trial described in the text with 100 subjects per treatment arm and the prior $N(2.5; 2^2)$

It can immediately be seen from Fig. 12.7 that the regression to the mean effect is much smaller for the new prior distribution. The percentage by which the observed effect needs to be discounted when it is equal to 5.0 is now approximately just 10%. Compared to the mixture prior distribution, the Normal prior assigns a higher probability to larger treatment effects. For example, the mixture prior distribution assigns 42% probability to a treatment effect greater than 2.44, while the Normal prior assigns 51%. As a result, the posterior predicted value is higher under the Normal prior for large observed Phase 2 treatment effects.

It should also be noted that the regression to the mean will be affected by the location of the prior distribution. Thus, in the example above if the prior distribution had a mean of 3.0 instead of 2.5 then there would be less regression to the mean for observed values above 3.0.

Thus, provided an appropriate prior is available and acceptable, the expected value of the posterior distribution obtained from combining the prior with the Phase 2 data gives a theoretical basis for discounting a very promising observed Phase 2 effect.

12.5 The Maximum Likelihood Method and Three Other Methods for Estimating the Bias in a Phase 2 Result

As in Sect. 12.3, we assume that the endpoint of interest has a Normal distribution with a known variance and that we consider a parallel group trial comparing a new treatment versus a comparator. Further, we assume that the result for the Phase 2 trial is considered positive if the estimated treatment effect is bigger than some threshold value Δ_{PD} where the subscript PD stands for positive decision. This threshold serves a similar role as Δ_{OL} introduced in Sect. 12.3 even though Δ_{OL} may imply a greater commitment on a sponsor's part. Because we do not consider results corresponding to estimated treatment effects below the threshold, the sampling distribution for the estimated treatment effect is a truncated Normal distribution as depicted in Fig. 12.1.

Maximum likelihood estimation for a truncated Normal distribution is a much-studied problem (see, e.g., Johnson & Kotz, 1970; Barr & Sherrill, 1999). The maximum likelihood estimator of the treatment effect Δ is obtained by solving the following expression for Δ

$$\frac{\partial l_c\left(\Delta, \widehat{\Delta}\right)}{\partial \Delta} = \frac{\widehat{\Delta} - \Delta}{\frac{2\sigma^2}{m}} - \frac{-\varphi\left(\frac{\Delta_{PD}-\Delta}{\sqrt{\frac{2\sigma^2}{m}}}\right)\left(-\frac{1}{\sqrt{\frac{2\sigma^2}{m}}}\right)}{1 - \Phi\left(\frac{\Delta_{PD}-\Delta}{\sqrt{\frac{2\sigma^2}{m}}}\right)} = 0 \qquad (12.2)$$

In (12.2), m is the sample size per group of the Phase 2 trial, $\varphi(\bullet)$ is the density function of the standard Normal distribution, and $\Phi(\bullet)$ is the cumulative distribution function of the standard Normal distribution. In (12.2), $l_c(\Delta, \widehat{\Delta})$ is the log likelihood for the truncated Normal distribution based on the conditional probability density function of $(\widehat{\Delta}|\widehat{\Delta} > \Delta_{PD})$ which is

$$\frac{\left(\frac{1}{\sqrt{\frac{2\sigma^2}{m}}}\right)\varphi\left(\frac{\widehat{\Delta}-\Delta}{\sqrt{\frac{2\sigma^2}{m}}}\right)}{1 - \phi\left(\frac{\Delta_{PD}-\Delta}{\sqrt{\frac{2\sigma^2}{m}}}\right)} \qquad (12.3)$$

for $\widehat{\Delta} > \Delta_{PD}$ and 0 otherwise.

Equation (12.2) can be solved using numerical methods such as the uniroot method in R (R Core Team, 2020). The resulting estimate for Δ will be referred to as the maximum conditional likelihood estimate (MCLE) in this chapter.

We have illustrated via Fig. 12.1 that using $\widehat{\Delta}$ under the condition that $\widehat{\Delta} > \Delta_{PD}$ could result in a bias in estimation. The bias is given by the expression in (12.4)

$$b\left(\widehat{\Delta}|\widehat{\Delta} > \Delta_{PD}\right) = E\left(\widehat{\Delta}|\widehat{\Delta} > \Delta_{PD}\right) - \Delta \tag{12.4}$$

In the case of a Normally distributed endpoint, $\widehat{\Delta}$ has a Normal distribution with mean Δ and a standard deviation of $\left(\sqrt{2/m}\sigma\right)$. The bias in (12.4) can be found in the following closed form for a given Δ.

$$\sqrt{\frac{2\sigma^2}{m}} \, \frac{\varphi\left(\frac{\Delta_{PD}-\Delta}{\sqrt{\frac{2\sigma^2}{m}}}\right)}{1 - \Phi\left(\frac{\Delta_{PD}-\Delta}{\sqrt{\frac{2\sigma^2}{m}}}\right)} \tag{12.5}$$

Kirby et al. (2020) introduced three other bias correction methods. They referred to their first method as the "likelihood weighted bias" method. This method calculates the average bias by weighting the bias at a true treatment effect in (12.4) by its likelihood as in (12.6) below.

$$\text{abias} = \int_{-\infty}^{+\infty} b(\widehat{\Delta}|\widehat{\Delta} > \Delta_{PD}) L(\Delta, \widehat{\Delta}) \, d\Delta \, / \int_{-\infty}^{+\infty} L(\Delta, \widehat{\Delta}) d\Delta \tag{12.6}$$

In (12.6), $L(\Delta, \widehat{\Delta})$ is the likelihood of Δ for a given observed $\widehat{\Delta}$. Since the denominator on the right hand side of the equation in (12.6) is equal to 1 and $L(\Delta, \widehat{\Delta})$ is given by

$$L\left(\Delta, \widehat{\Delta}\right) = \frac{1}{\sqrt{2\pi}\sqrt{\frac{2\sigma^2}{m}}} \exp\left\{ -\frac{1}{2}\left(\frac{\widehat{\Delta} - \Delta}{\sqrt{\frac{2\sigma^2}{m}}}\right)^2 \right\}$$

the average bias in (12.6) can be simplified to

$$E\left(\sqrt{\frac{2\sigma^2}{m}} \, \frac{\varphi\left(\frac{\Delta_{PD}-\widehat{\Delta}}{\sqrt{\frac{2\sigma^2}{m}}} - X\right)}{1 - \Phi\left(\frac{\Delta_{PD}-\widehat{\Delta}}{\sqrt{\frac{2\sigma^2}{m}}} - X\right)}\right)$$

where X has a standard Normal distribution.

The "likelihood weighted bias" method subtracts the average bias from $\widehat{\Delta}$ to give a bias-corrected estimate.

Kirby et al.'s second method uses a Bayesian approach with a vague uniform prior for the treatment effect. The posterior distribution is calculated, and the bias corresponding to the 20th percentile of this posterior distribution for the treatment effect obtained. Kirby et al. subtracted this quantity from $\widehat{\Delta}$ and obtained another bias-corrected estimate. Kirby et al. referred to this method as the "percentile bias" method.

Kirby et al.'s third method subtracted the estimator of bias given in (12.7) below from $\widehat{\Delta}$.

$$\text{bias} = \int_{-\infty}^{+\infty} b(\widehat{\Delta}|\widehat{\Delta} > \Delta_{\text{PD}}) L_c(\Delta, \widehat{\Delta}) d\Delta \Big/ \int_{-\infty}^{+\infty} L_c(\Delta, \widehat{\Delta}) d\Delta \qquad (12.7)$$

In (12.7), $L_c(\Delta, \widehat{\Delta})$ is the likelihood based on the conditional probability density function for $\widehat{\Delta}|\widehat{\Delta} > \Delta_{\text{PD}}$ given in (12.3). Kirby et al. referred to this method as the "conditional likelihood weighted bias" method.

12.6 A Comparison of the Seven Bias Correction Methods and One Further Bias Correction Method

Kirby et al. (2020) compared the seven bias correction methods described so far in this chapter with respect to the (remaining) bias and the probability of incorrect decisions. They included the uncorrected estimate in the comparisons as a reference.

For the Wang, Hung and O'Neill bias correction method, Kirby et al. just used the option of subtracting one standard error from the estimated treatment effect and labeled it as the "one s.e." method. Only this option was used because Wang, Hung and O'Neill (Wang et al., 2006) concluded that this option did best in approximately equating planned and actual power across a range of scenarios. For the Kirby et al. (2012) bias correction method, Kirby et al. (2020) just used multiplication of the observed treatment effect by 0.9 and referred to this as the "0.9 multiplication" method. They only chose this option because they felt it performed best in equating estimated and theoretical assurance when the treatment effect remains the same between Phase 2 and Phase 3 trials. Kirby et al. (2020) referred to Zhang's informative prior method as the "posterior mean (informative prior)" method. The informative prior used by Kirby et al. (2020) was the mixture prior shown in (12.8)

$$p(\Delta) = (0.5)(3.3) \exp(-3.3\Delta), \ \Delta > 0$$
$$p(0) = 0.5, \ \Delta = 0 \qquad\qquad\qquad\qquad (12.8)$$

Kirby et al. (2020) started by considering two examples. In the first example, they assumed a proof-of-concept (POC) parallel group trial comparing a new treatment with a control with 50 subjects randomly allocated to each group, The endpoint X was assumed to be Normally distributed with mean μ_T for the new treatment and mean μ_C for the control with a known common variance equal to 1 for the two groups. Higher values of X are taken to indicate a better result, and the trial is declared a success if

$$Z = \frac{(\overline{X}_T - \overline{X}_C)}{\sqrt{\frac{2\sigma^2}{m}}} > Z_{0.05} \qquad (12.9)$$

The decision criterion in (12.9) corresponds to a threshold Δ_{PD} for the observed treatment effect of 0.33.

For the second example, the trial design and endpoint were kept the same, but the trial was declared a success if the observed treatment effect was greater than 0.5. In this example, Δ_{PD} is set at 0.5.

Kirby et al. (2020) calculated the bias of the bias-corrected estimators for the two examples for the range of true treatment effects from 0 to 1 and plotted the bias for the observed treatment effect $\widehat{\Delta}$ as well as the 7 bias-corrected estimators against the true treatment effect as shown in Fig. 12.8.

It can be seen from the figure that when the true treatment effect is small the bias is smallest for the MCLE, one s.e. and percentile bias methods. When the true treatment effect is large, the smallest magnitude of bias is for the likelihood weighted bias, conditional likelihood weighted bias and MCLE methods.

Kirby et al. considered the broader set of scenarios given by all combinations of $m = 50, 100, 200, 500$ and $\Delta_{PD} = 0.1, 0.2, 0.3, 0.4, 0.5$. The qualitative findings were generally the same as those shown in Fig. 12.8.

Kirby et al. also looked at the probability of making an incorrect decision using the bias-corrected estimators of treatment effect. For $\Delta < \Delta_{PD}$, they defined an incorrect decision as $\widehat{\Delta}_{corr} > \Delta_{PD}$, and for $\Delta > \Delta_{PD}$, they defined it as $\widehat{\Delta}_{corr} \leq \Delta_{PD}$. Here, $\widehat{\Delta}_{corr}$ refers to any of the bias-corrected estimators of treatment effect. The probabilities of these two incorrect decisions are shown in Fig. 12.9 for Examples 1 and 2. It can be seen that the different bias-corrected estimators perform well in different situations. Thus, if the main concern is with not making a wrong decision when $\Delta < \Delta_{PD}$ then the one s.e., posterior mean (informative prior), MCLE or percentile method would likely be preferred. If the main concern is with not making a wrong decision when $\Delta > \Delta_{PD}$, then the 0.9 multiplication method might be preferred. To balance the risk of the two errors, a method such as the likelihood weighted bias or conditional likelihood weighted bias could be used. Again, Kirby et al. (2020) found generally similar qualitative results for the other scenarios listed above.

Finally, Kirby et al. (2020) looked at the average power for a Phase 3 trial sample sized using the bias-corrected estimate when the launch threshold is also exceeded by the bias-corrected estimate under different methods. The launch threshold used

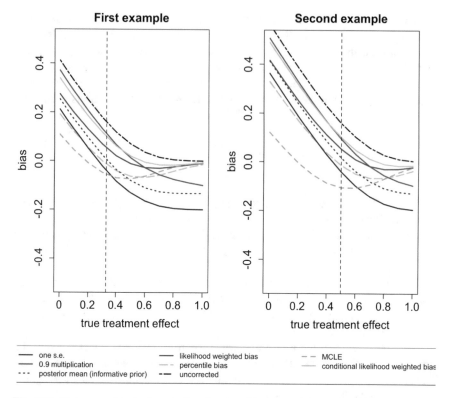

Fig. 12.8 Bias versus true treatment effect for seven bias correction methods and the unadjusted treatment effect for Examples 1 and 2

was the same as that used to declare a positive result for the observed Phase 2 effect, i.e., Δ_{PD}.

Kirby et al. (2020) included one additional method in this evaluation. The new addition is the calibrated optimal γ conservative strategy (COS) introduced by De Martini (2011) in the comparison of average power among different methods. The COS strategy consists of using the γ-lower bound for the effect size, the one-directional confidence interval with coverage probability γ in order to estimate the sample size for Phase 3. De Martini proposed selecting γ using the concept of overall power, which is the probability of launching a Phase 3 trial times the average power of the Phase 3 trial, given that a launch threshold has been exceeded by the observed Phase 2 effect. De Martini found that the COS strategy was better on average in achieving overall power than six other classical and Bayesian strategies with which it was compared. Kirby et al. (2020) adopted the COS strategy but required that the γ-lower bound exceeds the launch threshold rather than just the observed effect. They did so because all the other methods require that the bias-corrected estimate exceeds the launch threshold. Besides, the γ-lower bound may be regarded as a better

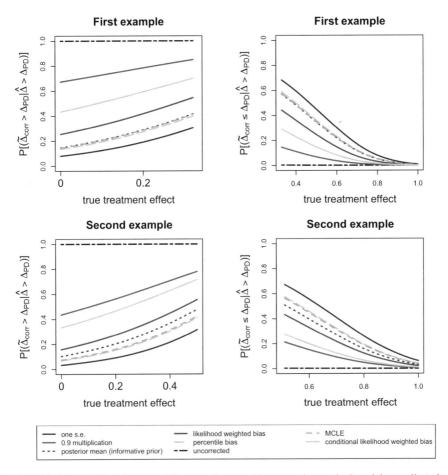

Fig. 12.9 Probabilities of two possible errors for seven bias correction methods and the unadjusted treatment effect for Examples 1 and 2

estimator of the true treatment effect in view of the existing bias. Kirby et al. chose to compare the average power instead of the overall power in their evaluation.

The average power for the seven methods, the COS method and the unadjusted observed treatment effect is plotted against true treatment effect for Examples 1 and 2 in Fig. 12.10. It can be seen from the figure that the conditional likelihood weighted bias method has the largest average power before it first reaches 80% power. The one s.e., posterior mean (informative prior) and 0.9 multiplication methods achieve 80% power as the true treatment effect is further increased but then proceed to overpower as the treatment gets even larger. A similar finding that the conditional likelihood weighted bias method tended to perform best was generally found for the other scenarios.

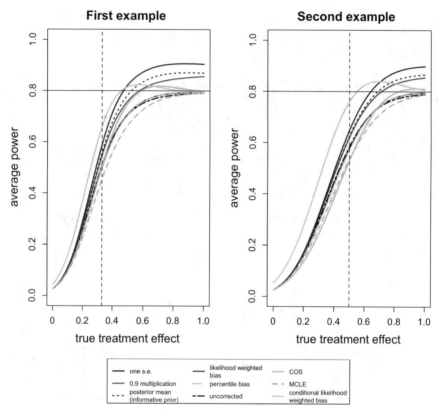

Fig. 12.10 Average power versus true treatment effect for eight bias correction methods (including COS method) and the unadjusted treatment effect for Examples 1 and 2

12.7 An Empirical Assessment of the Amount of Discounting Required for Observed Phase 2 Effects

Kirby et al. (2012) investigated empirically the amount of discounting required for observed Phase 2 results by looking at Pfizer development projects with completed Phase 2 and Phase 3 studies between 1998 and 2009. To evaluate the amount of discounting required, they compared average estimated assurance with the observed Phase 3 success probability. To do this, they excluded projects without comparative Phase 2 trials but did allow the time point of evaluation to differ between Phase 2 and Phase 3. They found 11 drug projects satisfying these selection criteria. The drug projects spanned the disease areas of osteoporosis, obesity, hypertension, pain, overactive bladder, atrial fibrillation, smoking cessation, migraine and arthritis.

Generally, the Phase 3 trials were initiated in 2005 or earlier when recruitment was concentrated heavily in the West and for the most part had similar inclusion/exclusion criteria to their Phase 2 counterparts. The empirical assessment exercise was thus to focus on selection bias alone rather than selection bias in combination with changed population or endpoint.

To calculate the estimated average assurance and compare it with the Phase 3 success probability, it was necessary to match the Phase 3 trials with the Phase 2 trials that would have been used to plan the Phase 3 trials. This proved very challenging because of multiple Phase 2 studies and not being able to consult with individuals who would have made programme-level decisions. Consequently, Kirby et al. formed all possible pairs of Phase 2 and Phase 3 studies under each programme. When multiple doses were included in either the Phase 2 or Phase 3 studies, the doses that provided the best match were chosen.

Kirby et al. found that the above matching led to some failed Phase 2 studies being linked with Phase 3 trials. As a result, they decided to exclude all matches that gave an estimated assurance of less than 0.1 as being unlikely for the Phase 2 trial to have led to the launching of the Phase 3 trial. This gave them 104 matches from 11 drug projects with 32 distinct Phase 2 studies and 54 distinct Phase 3 studies.

For continuous endpoints, Kirby et al. calculated estimated assurance using a Normal prior distribution with mean equal to the Phase 2 estimated treatment effect and standard deviation equal to the corresponding standard error. For binary endpoints, they used beta distributions as priors for each treatment group with means equal to the Phase 2 estimated proportions and standard deviation equal to the corresponding estimated binomial standard deviation.

Kirby et al. found that averaging the estimated assurance from the 104 matched pairs of trials gave a value of 0.801. Most of the estimated assurances were found to be large so it is possible the Phase 3 trials were powered using a minimum clinically important difference rather than the observed Phase 2 effect. Additionally, most of the trials appeared to show robust efficacy results. Among the 104 matched pairs of studies, a proportion 0.779 of the Phase 3 trials produced statistically significant results. The average planned power by comparison for the 104 pairs was 0.858. Thus, the average estimated assurance was closer to the proportion of statistically significant results than the average planned power.

To see if the average estimated assurance could be brought even closer to the proportion of statistically significant results, Kirby et al. multiplied each of the observed Phase 2 effects by 0.9. This gave an average estimated assurance of 0.777 which is very close to the proportion of statistically significant results.

Kirby et al. did caution, however, against over interpretation of this result for a number of reasons. First, the proportion of statistically significant results among distinct Phase 3 trials (54 in total) was 81% which is much greater than the 50–60% figure that has generally been reported for the Phase 3 success rate. Kirby et al. conjectured that the higher success rate might be attributable to the multiple Phase 2 trials that were run. Second, it seems that at least some of the Phase 3 trials were sized using the concept of a minimum clinically important difference. This affects the estimated assurance and the success probability. Finally, it is not clear how decisions were made to move development to Phase 3 in the period 1998–2005 which predated a Pfizer initiative to make the decision-making process more quantitative and transparent.

12.8 Discussion

In this chapter, we looked at the bias that could be produced by the direct use of Phase 2 results as estimates for the treatment effect when the results were selected because of a favorable outcome. We then looked at eight proposals for how to discount the observed Phase 2 results when needed.

Wang et al. recommend that subtracting one standard error from the observed Phase 2 effect might be reasonable. We have seen, however, that this level of discounting may not be necessary and that it can lead to a relatively low probability of launching a Phase 3 trial. By comparison, Kirby et al. recommend that multiplying the observed Phase 2 effect by 0.9 might be sufficient when there are no differences between Phase 2 and Phase 3 trials in terms of the treatment effect and the launch threshold is sufficiently low (e.g., 1/3 of the true treatment effect). Their recommendation is backed up by a limited and possibly selective amount of empirical data. Zhang proposed discounting an observed Phase 2 effect by combining it with a prior distribution and using the expected effect from the posterior distribution as the discounted estimate for future planning. We review four additional methods including maximum likelihood estimation of the treatment effect for a truncated Normal distribution and three new methods introduced by Kirby et al. (2020). A final method is the COS method which is applied to obtain an estimate to sample size a Phase 3 trial. Kirby et al. (2020) found that these different estimators have different properties, and so their possible use will depend on the situation under consideration.

The topic of this chapter is important because Pereira et al. (2012) concluded that most large effect sizes were observed in small studies and the observed effect sizes became typically much smaller when additional trials were performed. In addition to the potential change in patient populations and endpoints, the effect of regression to the mean offers another explanation for the disappearing or shrinking effect.

Previously, in Chaps. 4 and 5, we have seen how the idea of an average replication probability and the calculation of an assurance probability give a more realistic assessment of probability of a successful study (POSS) in a succeeding trial than using the initial point estimate alone. In this chapter, we have learned that it may also be necessary to adjust the assurance calculation because of the possibility of a selection bias.

The bias identified in this chapter for Phase 2 results could also be manifested in moving between Phase 3 and Phase 4 because there may be a selection effect in only considering Phase 3 trials that are successful. Given the usual size of Phase 3 studies, however, one can expect that this selection bias is much smaller (and may even be negligible) than that which can occur between Phase 2 and Phase 3.

Another message from this chapter is the importance of obtaining sufficient information in Phase 2. The results obtained in Sect. 12.3 show that when the Phase 2 and 3 true effects are the same and just a POC study is run, then no or little discounting is required provided a bigger Phase 2 sample size is used together with not too high a launch threshold. Including a dose-response study in this scenario lessens the discounting required when the POC study is small. One can expect a similar result of no or little discounting needed for an observed Phase 2 effect under the Zhang method and the other methods when the Phase 2 result is based on sufficient information and the prior distribution before the start of Phase 2 is not informative.

References

Barr, D. R., & Sherrill, E. T. (1999). Mean and variance of truncated normal distributions. *The American Statistician, 53*(4), 357–361.

Chuang-Stein, C., & Kirby, S. (2014). The shrinking or disappearing observed treatment effect. *Pharmaceutical Statistics, 13*(5), 277–280.

De Martini, D. (2011). Adapting by calibration the sample size of a phase III trial on the basis of phase II data. *Pharmaceutical Statistics, 10*, 89–95.

Johnson, N. L., & Kotz, S. (1970). *Continuous univariate distributions – 1*. Wiley. Chapter 13.

Kirby, S., Burke, J., Chuang-Stein, C., & Sin, C. (2012). Discounting phase 2 results when planning phase 3 clinical trials. *Pharmaceutical Statistics, 11*(5), 373–385.

Kirby, S., Li, J., & Chuang-Stein, C. (2020). Selection bias for treatments with positive phase 2 results. *Pharmaceutical Statistics, 19*(5), 679–691.

O'Hagan, A., Stevens, J. W., & Campbell, M. J. (2005). Assurance in clinical trial design. *Pharmaceutical Statistics, 4*(3), 187–201.

Pereira, T. V., Horwitz, R. I., & Ioannidis, J. P. A. (2012). Empirical evaluation of very large treatment effects of medical intervention. *Journal of the American Medical Association, 308*(16), 1676–1684.

R Core Team. (2020). *A language and environment for statistical computing*. R Foundation for Statistical Computing. https://www.R-project.org/

Wang, S. J., Hung, H. M. J., & O'Neill, R. T. (2006). Adapting the sample size planning of a phase III trial based on phase II data. *Pharmaceutical Statistics, 5*(2), 85–97.

Zhang, J. (2013). Evaluating regression to the mean of treatment effect from phase II to phase III. https://www.amstat.org/meetings/jsm/2013/onlineprogram/AbstractDetails.cfm?abstractid=309685. Accessed 11 Mar 2021.

Chapter 13
Adaptive Designs

The Measure of intelligence is the ability to change.
—Albert Einstein.

13.1 Introduction

The FDA guidance *Adaptive Designs for Clinical Trials of Drugs and Biologics* (FDA, 2019) defines an adaptive design as "a clinical trial design that allows for prospectively planned modifications to one or more aspects of the design based on accumulating data from subjects in the trial." As such, this broad definition allows for many different types of design including those which allow early stopping for success or futility, those which allow the sample size to be re-estimated and those which allow treatment arms to be dropped. We describe a fuller classification based on the FDA guidance in the following section. The EMA Reflection Paper on *Methodological Issues in Confirmatory Clinical Trials Planned With An Adaptive Design* (EMA, 2007) has a similar definition of an adaptive design, but given its focus on confirmatory trials emphasizes that for those trials there must be full control of the Type I error. The definition in the EMA document is that a study design is adaptive "if statistical methodology allows the modification of a design element (e.g., sample size, randomization ratio, number of treatment arms) at an interim analysis with full control of the Type I error." Although not mentioned in this definition the EMA Reflection Paper concurs with the FDA guidance that modifications should be prospectively planned and pre-specified in the protocols.

Adaptive designs can potentially help with quantitative decision making by allowing designs to be amended so that better decisions can be made in the light of emerging data. Thus, rather than rigidly adhering to a fixed design which is based on assumptions which may not be supported by the emerging data, an adaptive design allows adjustments to certain aspects of the trial. A key part of an evaluation of an

C. Chuang-Stein and S. Kirby, *Quantitative Decisions in Drug Development*, Springer Series in Pharmaceutical Statistics, https://doi.org/10.1007/978-3-030-79731-7_13

adaptive design thus becomes how well the design can adapt to emerging data and in particular whether it can perform better than a fixed design.

In Sect. 13.2, we consider some principles for adaptive designs before reviewing the many types of adaptive design in Sect. 13.3. In Sects. 13.4–13.7, we look at examples of each of four particular types of adaptive design. In Sect. 13.4, we look at a group sequential design with an interim analysis for futility. In Sect. 13.5, we look at a Phase 2 dose-ranging study where doses can be dropped or added. In Sect. 13.6, we look at an example of a Phase 2/3 enrichment design where the trial could be enriched by focusing on the correct patient population. Then, in Sect. 13.7, we look at a confirmatory trial where the adaptation is to decide on two doses before accumulating confirmatory evidence on these doses.

We conclude with some general comments on adaptive designs in Sect. 13.8.

13.2   Adaptive Designs—Principles

The FDA guidance describes four key principles that should be satisfied in the design, conduct and analysis of an adaptive clinical trial. These four key principles are as follows: The chance of erroneous conclusions should be adequately controlled, estimation of treatment effects should be sufficiently reliable, details of the design should be completely pre-specified, and finally, trial integrity should be maintained. The guidance advocates following these principles even in early development to lessen the risk of adversely affecting a drug development program.

A number of situations can lead to the chance of erroneous conclusions not being controlled such as, for example, when multiple hypothesis tests are conducted each at a significance level α so that the overall Type I error rate is greater than α. Other adaptive design features may similarly lead to Type I error rate inflation. Adaptive design proposals with tests of null hypotheses should therefore address control of the overall Type I error rate.

Estimation of treatment effects needs to be sufficiently reliable so that benefit–risk can be properly assessed and new drugs appropriately labeled. Some adaptive designs can lead to statistical bias in the estimation of treatment effects, so this may need to be addressed. For some designs, there are known methods for adjusting estimates, but for other designs, there may not be any available methods. In either case, the extent of any bias should be evaluated, and the results should be presented with stated cautions if the potential bias is found via simulation to be large.

An important point is that all details of an adaptive design are prospectively specified. Pre-specification is important for at least three reasons. First, for many adaptive designs, it may not be possible to control the Type I error rate and obtain reliable estimates if all details are not pre-planned. Second, pre-specification gives confidence that decisions to adapt the design were not done in an unplanned manner. Third, pre-specification can help motivate careful planning at the design stage. Having said all these, there may be occasions when a DMC advises, for good reasons, departures from the pre-specified design. Ideally these circumstances should be anticipated and suitably robust methods proposed. But if something totally unexpected happens, a good approach is for the sponsor to discuss the situation with the regulators, especially if the trial is designed to be a confirmatory trial.

It is vital that trial integrity is maintained because knowledge of accumulating data can affect the course and conduct of a trial. As such, it is strongly recommended that access to accumulating data be strictly limited to those who need to know and are independent of the conduct and management of an adaptive trial.

By construction, possible changes are built into the design of an adaptive trial. It is important to know how likely these changes will take place and how well they are able to achieve the goals of the adaptations. These properties are referred to as the operating characteristics of an adaptive design. Understanding these characteristics is an integral and critical part of designing an adaptive trial. Simulations are usually needed to conduct the assessment. Depending on the nature of the adaptations and the statistical methods required to analyze the trial data, the required simulations could be extensive.

13.3　Types of Adaptive Design

The FDA guidance identifies seven distinct types of adaptive design. These are as follows:

i.   Group sequential designs
ii.   Adaptations to the sample size
iii. Adaptations to the patient population (e.g., adaptive enrichment)
iv.   Adaptations to treatment arm selection
v.   Adaptations to patient allocation
vi.   Adaptations to endpoint selection
vii. Adaptations to multiple design features.

13.3.1　Group Sequential Designs

Group sequential designs allow one or more prospectively planned interim analyses with pre-specified criteria for stopping a trial (Jennison & Turnbull, 2000; Wassmer & Brannath, 2016). They can be useful for reducing the expected sample size and duration of a trial so can have ethical and efficiency advantages.

The stopping rules for efficacy and/or futility can be implemented using a variety of methods for controlling the Type I error rate. A popular approach is the one proposed by O'Brien and Fleming (1979) which requires very persuasive results to stop a trial early for efficacy. This approach requires the pre-specification of the number and timings of the interim analyses. An alternative that offers more flexibility is the alpha spending approach due to Lan and DeMets (1983). The Lan and DeMets approach specifies a function for how Type I error rate is to be spent during a trial and hence allows for flexibility in number and timing of interim analyses. It is possible, however, if analysis times are chosen based on accumulating results, that the Type I error rate could be inflated. Consequently, it is recommended that a schedule for number and approximate timing of analyses is included.

There are a number of further considerations for group sequential designs. One is that the trial should only be terminated for efficacy if the stopping criteria are met. A second is that any binding futility boundaries must be respected for the Type I error rate to be controlled if the strategy to control the Type I error rate assumes a binding futility rule. Third, a trial stopped early for efficacy will have less data for secondary endpoints and safety data. Therefore, early stopping should only be undertaken when there is a big treatment effect and strong evidence in its favor. Lastly, the usual estimates of treatment effect for fixed designs tend to be biased, so adjustments for the stopping rules are needed (Jennison & Turnbull, 2000; Wassmer & Brannath, 2016).

13.3.2   Adaptations to the Sample Size

A popular adaptation is to allow the sample size for a trial to be changed based on interim results. There are two key types of sample size adaptation. The first type uses blinded data to estimate nuisance parameters. This type of sample size adaptation usually has no effect or miniscule effect on the Type I error rate (Friede & Kieser, 2006).

The second type of sample size adaptation uses information on comparative interim results. This is often referred to as unblinded sample size re-estimation. Its value is that the desired statistical power can be maintained even when a treatment effect is less than expected. Just as special methods are required to control the Type I error rate in group sequential designs, so similarly special methods are required to control the Type I error rate for unblinded sample size re-estimation. A number of approaches have been proposed for hypothesis testing based on combining test statistics or p-values from different stages of a trial or preservation of conditional Type I error probability (Bauer & Köhne, 1994; Cui et al., 1999; Müller & Schäfer, 2001).

Pre-specification of the rule including when to adapt the sample size is important. A subtle caveat to this is that not too much information on the sample size re-estimation should be widely available in case individuals other than those who strictly need to know are able to back-calculate an interim estimate of treatment effect.

13.3.3   Adaptations to the Patient Population

Sometimes it is expected that the treatment effect will be greater or may only exist in a subset of the trial population. This subpopulation could be defined in a number of ways, e.g., by a genetic marker that is related to the drug's mechanism of action. For such a setting, an adaptive design could be considered that allows selection of the patient population based on interim trial results. Such a design is often referred to as an adaptive enrichment design. Compared to a fixed design, an adaptive enrichment design could provide advantages in terms of increased statistical power for detecting a treatment effect in the selected subpopulation and reducing drug exposure in the de-selected subpopulation.

Modification of the population and the multiple hypothesis tests involved can be accommodated by combining test statistics from the different stages of the trial in a pre-planned method and using appropriate multiple testing procedures (Wassmer & Brannath, 2016).

An important point to make about an adaptive enrichment design is that the design should be motivated by results from previous trials or some strong biologic plausibility. In addition, a threshold (or a rule to select the threshold) will have to be set if the characteristic defining the subpopulation is continuous and an in vitro diagnostic procedure is needed to diagnose the subpopulation.

We illustrate the use of an adaptive enrichment design by describing the TAPPAS trial in Sect. 13.6.

13.3.4   Adaptations to Treatment Arm Selection

Another adaptive design pertains to the treatment arms. This could be adding or dropping treatment arms or indeed doing both of these things. This sort of design often occurs in early development dose-ranging trials. We describe such an example in Sect. 13.5. Adaptive treatment arm selection can also occur, however, in confirmatory trials. In the latter case, methods for control of the Type I error rate must be used. These could be group sequential designs with a multiple testing approach if no other adaptations are considered. Alternatively, if there are other adaptations, the approach indicated above for population enrichment can be used.

A special case of this design is the platform design (see Sect. 1.4.2 in Chap. 1) where potentially many treatments are compared with a control to select promising treatments. Because these trials may involve multiple sponsors, carry on for an unstated length of time and involve complex adaptations, it is recommended that they are discussed with regulators at the planning stage.

In Sect. 13.7, we describe the INHANCE trial which selected treatment arms in a confirmatory trial.

13.3.5   Adaptations to Patient Allocation

Covariate-adaptive treatment assignment seeks to achieve balance between treatment groups on baseline groups and is one type of adaptive patient allocation. A popular method for this type of adaptation is minimization proposed by Pocock and Simon (Pocock & Simon, 1975). These methods do not increase the Type I error rate if analyzed appropriately.

A second type of adaptive patient allocation is response-adaptive randomization in which the randomization ratio for different arms changes based on accumulating data on treatment response. In some circumstances, these designs can have statistical advantages produced by minimizing the variance of the test statistic and can also lead to more subjects being allocated promising treatments. The designs are controversial, however, among some researchers who do not like the idea of using inconclusive interim results to change treatment allocation ratios. One strategy to address this concern is to require a minimum number of patients on all treatments before considering changing the randomization ratio. Similar to covariate-adaptive treatment methods, adaptive patient allocation does not usually increase the Type I error rate provided that appropriate analysis methods are used.

13.3.6   Adaptations to Endpoint Selection

Adaptive designs which choose among acceptable primary endpoints are possible. However, because of the clinical considerations involved in selecting an endpoint, it is recommended that such a design adaptation be discussed with regulators in advance.

13.3.7   Adaptations to Multiple Design Features

In principle, it is possible to have an adaptive design which contains many possible adaptations. In practice, such a design may be hard to pre-specify, hence, control of the Type I error rate may become problematic, and it may also be difficult to estimate its operating characteristics. The regulators have tended to discourage such designs while still indicating their openness to discuss proposed adaptive designs.

13.4   A Group Sequential Design with an Interim Analysis for Futility

A group sequential design with an interim analysis for futility can be regarded as a simple adaptive design. We take as our example the parallel group design in Sect. 5.5. We recall that the study uses a parallel group design with a total of 200 subjects randomized equally to a new drug, SC-75416 or ibuprofen and the endpoint TOTPAR6 (total pain relief over the first 6 h after dental surgery) was assumed to be Normally distributed with a standard deviation of 7. Further, a prior distribution for the difference in means between SC-75416 and ibuprofen is $N(3.27; 0.6^2)$. The sponsor would be interested in SC-75416 if the true difference in means is at least three points on the TOTPAR6 scale.

We suppose that an interim analysis is to be conducted when TOTPAR6 is available in half of the subjects and the study will be stopped early unless the predictive power calculated using the interim TOTPAR6 data is greater than 0.20. The calculation of the predictive power is the same as that of probability of study success, but done at the interim analysis (Grieve, 1991; Jennison & Turnbull, 2000). Using an improper prior $p(\Delta) = 1$ for Δ (the difference in means), the posterior distribution for Δ given the data at the interim is $N(\bar{x}_{1,SC} - \bar{x}_{1,IBU}; 2\sigma^2/n_1)$ where n_1 is the sample size per treatment group at the interim, and $\bar{x}_{1,SC}$ and $\bar{x}_{1,IBU}$ are the sample means at the interim in the SC-75416 and ibuprofen group, respectively. In the SC-75416 example, n_1 is 50. The predictive power is then given by (Grieve, 1991)

$$1 - \Phi\left(z_\alpha - \frac{\bar{x}_{1,SC} - \bar{x}_{1,IBU}}{\sqrt{\frac{\sigma^2}{n_1}}}\right) \tag{13.1}$$

where $\Phi(.)$ is the cumulative distribution of the standard Normal distribution and z_α is the upper $100\alpha\%$ percentile of the standard Normal distribution to be used as the critical value for the one-sided test at the end of the trial. We use $\alpha = 0.025$ for the one-sided test of the null hypothesis $H_0 : \Delta \leq 0$ versus the alternative hypothesis $H_A : \Delta > 0$ at the end of the study. An alternative to the assumption of the improper prior would be to use the prior distribution for the treatment effect. The use of the improper prior gives, however, an interim analysis robust to the specification of the prior for the treatment effect.

We show in Table 13.1 the results from 10,000 simulated trials where we treat trials stopped for futility at the interim analysis as negative trials (i.e., do not reject H_0) and group them with trials that completed but had negative results. The pooled sample variance is used for σ^2 in calculating the predictive power at interim in (13.1).

The probabilities in Table 13.1 are quite similar to those in Table 5.2. The probability of rejecting H_0 is slightly lower when the design has a futility interim analysis (85% vs. 88%). This is due to a small chance of stopping the trial early even though

Table 13.1 Estimated probabilities for combinations of truth and hypothesis test decision from 10,000 simulated trials

		Truth		Total
		$\Delta < 3$	$\Delta \geq 3$	
Decision	Do Not Reject H_0	0.10	0.06	0.16
	Reject H_0	0.23	0.62	0.85
	Total	0.33	0.68	

[*] probabilities do not sum to 1.00 due to rounding

Table 13.2 Estimated probabilities for combinations of truth and decision to stop or continue at interim analysis from 10,000 simulated trials

		Truth		Total
		$\Delta < 3$	$\Delta \geq 3$	
Decision at Interim Analysis	Stop	0.05	0.03	0.08
	Continue	0.28	0.64	0.92
	Total	0.33	0.67	

$\Delta \geq 3$. The PPV of the design with an interim futility analysis is 73% (=0.62/0.85) which is slightly higher than the 72% reported when the study does not include any interim futility analysis (see Sect. 5.5).

One may be also interested in other properties such as the percentage of trials that will be stopped at the interim analysis. We include the estimated percentage in Table 13.2.

It can be seen that a relatively small proportion of trials (estimated to be around 8%) will be stopped after the interim analysis. Of these an estimated 62.5% (=0.05/0.08) would be stopped correctly. Table 13.2 also shows that there is an estimated 3% chance that the trial will be terminated early and the effect is at least 3. An interesting statistic from Table 13.2 is the probability that $\Delta \geq 3$ given that the trial is allowed to continue. This probability is 70% (=0.64/0.92), which is higher than the prior probability of 67% that $\Delta \geq 3$, but less than the PPV of 73% at the end of the trial.

13.5   An Example of an Adaptive Dose-Ranging Study

We consider an adaptive dose-ranging study for an oral factor Xa inhibitor PD 0348292 (an anticoagulant candidate by Pfizer) for thromboprophylaxis after total knee replacement surgery. Much of the material related to this example came from Cohen et al. (2013) supplemented by our working knowledge about the project while working at Pfizer.

Developing an anticoagulant is difficult and expensive. In the case of PD 0348292, the sponsor hoped to find a dose expected to be similar to a standard anticoagulant (enoxaparin 30 mg, given twice a day) for preventing venous thromboembolic events (VTE) after total knee replacement while minimizing the risk of bleeding.

In preparing for the trial, the sponsor extracted results on VTE and bleeding from past trials on anticoagulants. The sponsor also obtained key in vitro biomarker data on inhibition of thrombin generation (TG) of these anticoagulants. Assuming relative potency for clinical response (VTE and bleeding) is a function of the relative potency for inhibition of TG, the sponsor used results from past trials to build models linking the biomarker to VTE and bleeding, respectively. These models, together with the known effect of PD 0348292 on the biomarker, offered a predicted range of PD 0348292 doses necessary to achieve the goal on VTE and bleeding.

There were two options in building the models. One option assumed that PD 0348292 behaved more like other anticoagulants with an FXa mechanism. Under this option, the modelers used only data pertaining to FXa drugs in building the models. A second option was to make no assumption and use all anticoagulants to build the models. The FXa-only drug models suggested a narrower dose range ($1\times$ to $20\times$), while the all-drug models suggested that a wider range (up to $100\times$ dose range) should be explored.

Since there was uncertainty concerning which option was closer to the truth and the therapeutic index was likely to be narrow, the sponsor decided to explore a sufficient number of doses and use an adaptive design to explore a 100-fold dose range with enoxaparin 30 mg bid as the active comparator. The doses considered were 0.1, 0.3, 0.5, 1.0, 2.5, 4.0 and 10 mg to be given once a day. The plan was to start with a set of lower doses and add or drop doses as more data were accumulated in the trial in an adaptive manner.

At the start of the trial, subjects were randomized to one of the five lowest doses (0.1, 0.3, 0.5, 1.0 or 2.5 mg) of PD 0348292 or subcutaneous enoxaparin 30 mg in a 1:1:1:1:1:2 ratio. The primary efficacy endpoint was VTE, and the primary safety endpoint was the incidence of total bleeding (TB, including major or minor bleeding in accordance with the International Society on Thrombosis and Haemostasis definition described in Schulman and Kearon 2005). A total of four dose decision interim analyses were planned, each being conducted after every 147 additional subjects were randomized and treated. The study targeted a total of 735 evaluable subjects. To be evaluable, an individual needed to have an evaluable bilateral venogram to allow a VTE assessment or have symptomatic VTE that was objectively confirmed.

At each dose decision analysis, the lowest dose was to be dropped if the one-sided 90% lower confidence interval bound of the estimated odds ratio for VTE (vs. enoxaparin) was >1.5. Any dose arm would also be discontinued if the one-sided lower confidence bound of estimated major bleeding (MB) incidence was $>5\%$. A higher dose would be added if the predicted odds ratio for VTE at that dose did not meet the above criterion on VTE and the predicted incidence of major bleeding was acceptable. The predictions were based on fitted models for VTE and MB at the most recent interim analysis. The higher doses available were 4 and 10 mg. These pre-specified dose decision analyses were assessed by an independent Data Monitoring Committee.

Efficacy was modeled using the logistic regression model in (13.2). For simplicity, indicator variables that reflect different treatment groups are not used in (13.2).

$$\log[p/(1-p] = E_0 + \alpha(\text{Enoxaparin}) + \beta \log(\text{Dose}_{292}) + \lambda(\text{region}) \quad (13.2)$$

In (13.2), p is the probability of a VTE, E_0 is the intercept, α is the treatment effect of enoxaparin 30 mg, Dose_{292} is the dose of PD 0348292, and λ is the effect of region (North America vs outside of the North America). The dose of PD 0348292 equivalent to 30 mg enoxaparin in VTE reduction was estimated to be

$$\text{Deq}_{292} = \exp\left(\hat{\alpha}/\hat{\beta}\right) \tag{13.3}$$

where $\hat{\alpha}$ and $\hat{\beta}$ are parameter estimates.

Total and major bleeding incidence was both modeled by the same logistic equation except that Dose_{292} was used rather than $\log(\text{Dose}_{292})$.

The trial ran to completion, and all seven available doses of PD 0348292 were used, i.e., higher doses were added after dose decision analyses. The dose of PD 0348292 equivalent to enoxaparin 30 mg for VTE prevention was estimated to be 1.16 mg (95% confidence interval, 0.56 to 2.41mg). Both drugs were considered to be well tolerated, and it was concluded that the characterization of the dose-response relationship for VTE and bleeding using an adaptive Phase 2 study design provided a strong quantitative basis for Phase 3 dose selection. The estimated dose-response relationship for VTE was found to be very similar to the FXa-only drug model developed from the literature at the trial planning stage.

To illustrate the assessment of an adaptive dose-ranging design, we use the final data from the trial described above to reconstruct the two scenarios considered possible at the design stage. The final data for VTE and total bleeding (TB) are given in Tables 13.3 and 13.4. TB was used in our illustration because the number of MB in the actual trials was too low to allow good estimation of the dose-response relationship for MB.

The numbers of subjects in each dose group differ between Tables 13.3 and 13.4. This is due to the requirement that to be included in the VTE assessment, an individual needed to have either a bilateral venogram that allowed for a VTE assessment or have symptomatic VTE that was objectively confirmed. Seven hundred and forty-nine (749) subjects met this requirement. As for the assessment of safety on TB, an individual just needed to receive at least one dose of the study drug to be included in the analysis. There are 1,389 subjects in the safety assessment.

Table 13.3 Final VTE data for PD 0348292 dose-ranging study (Cohen et al., 2013)

PD 0348292

	0.1 mg	0.3 mg	0.5 mg	1 mg	2.5 mg	4 mg	10 mg	Enoxaparin 30 mg
N	35	89	104	120	112	74	27	188
VTE n (%)	13 (37.1)	33 (37.1)	30 (28.8)	23 (19.2)	16 (14.3)	1 (1.4)	3 (11.1)	34 (18.1)

Table 13.4 Final total bleeds data for PD 0348292 dose-ranging study (Cohen et al., 2013)

PD 0348292

	0.1 mg	0.3 mg	0.5 mg	1 mg	2.5 mg	4 mg	10 mg	Enoxaparin 30 mg
N	61	141	183	202	200	140	65	397
TB n (%)	3 (4.9)	8 (5.7)	19 (10.4)	16 (7.9)	16 (8.0)	15 (10.7)	9 (13.8)	25 (6.3)

For the first scenario, we estimate the following two logistic regression models using the data given above,

$$\log\left(\frac{p_{\text{VTE}}}{1 - p_{\text{VTE}}}\right) = \mu + \alpha(\text{Enoxaparin}) + \beta\log(\text{Dose}_{292}) \qquad (13.4)$$

and

$$\log\left(\frac{p_{\text{TB}}}{1 - p_{\text{TB}}}\right) = \mu + \alpha(\text{Enoxaparin}) + \beta(\text{Dose}_{292}) \qquad (13.5)$$

Equations (13.4) and (13.5) are the same as those estimated for VTE and TB in the study except that the term for the region effect is omitted here as no data for this are given in Cohen et al. (2013).

To obtain the second scenario, we perturb the estimated value for μ (and correspondingly perturb the estimated value for α) for both equations such that the estimated dose required to give the same effect on VTE as enoxaparin is likely to be outside the range of the initial doses and the dose-response relationship for TB gives a lower incidence of TB for any particular dose. This scenario mimics the all-drug models developed by the sponsor's modelers initially.

The transformed estimated dose-response for VTE and TB together with transformed 99.9% pointwise confidence interval (covariance matrix assumed unchanged for perturbed fit) for the corresponding linear predictors is plotted in Figs. 13.1 and 13.2.

We consider a simplified adaptive dose-ranging design with just one interim analysis and assume a total possible sample size of 740 evaluable patients with 210 patients randomized to enoxaparin and a maximum of 106 patients randomized to each dose of PD 0348292. The initial doses of PD 0348292 are the same as those initially used in the actual trial, these being 0.1, 0.3, 0.5, 1 and 2.5 mg. At the interim analysis, a maximum of two doses can be dropped or added such that a maximum of five doses of PD 0348292 are used in the remainder of the trial. The lowest dose (0.1 mg) is dropped if the lower 90% confidence interval for the odds ratio for VTE compared to enoxaparin is greater than 1.5. When this happens, the 4 mg dose will be added, provided that the predicted TB for 4 mg is less than 12%. If the second lowest dose (0.3 mg) also has a lower 90% confidence interval for the odds ratio for VTE compared to enoxaparin greater than 1.5, it is also dropped and replaced by the 10 mg dose provided that the predicted TB for 10 mg is less than 12%. Doses with an estimated TB risk greater than 12% will also be dropped.

We use simulation to assess the operating characteristics of the simplified dose-ranging adaptive design. Data are generated in the following fashion. First, random samples for parameters in (13.4) and (13.5) are drawn from the prior distributions that are multivariate Normal with mean vector equal to estimated or perturbed parameter values and with covariance matrix given by the estimated covariance matrix. The generated parameters create new dose-response relationships on VTE and TB, which act as the true dose-response relationship for that particular run. In our assessment,

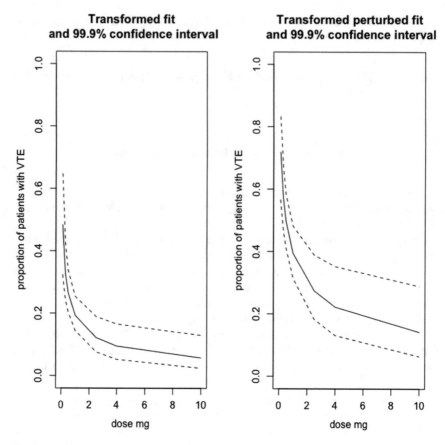

Fig. 13.1 Estimated and perturbed fit for (13.4) for final PD 0348292 VTE data

10,000 true dose-response curves were generated for VTE and TB. Next, incidence rates of VTE and TB for a dose under the new true dose-response relationships are used to create counts of VTE and TB at that dose (the trial data). This process is repeated for each scenario. If the slope for the VTE dose-response relationship was estimated to be greater than 0 at the interim analysis, the term $\beta \log(\text{Dose}_{292})$ was dropped from (13.4). This was done because β in (13.4) is not expected to be positive. Similarly, if the slope for the TB dose-response relationship was estimated to be less than 0 at the interim analysis, the term $\beta(\text{Dose}_{292})$ was dropped from (13.5). This was done because β in (13.5) is not expected to be negative.

As in the actual trial, the dose estimated to be equivalent to enoxaparin 30 mg bid is calculated using (13.3). The dose closest to the estimated dose among the seven investigated doses is then taken to be the selected dose. The selected dose is considered correct if the ratio of the true VTE incidence to that for enoxaparin is <1.3 and the ratio of true TB incidence to that for enoxaparin is <1.5. The true incidences are given by (13.4) and (13.5) using the generated true parameter values.

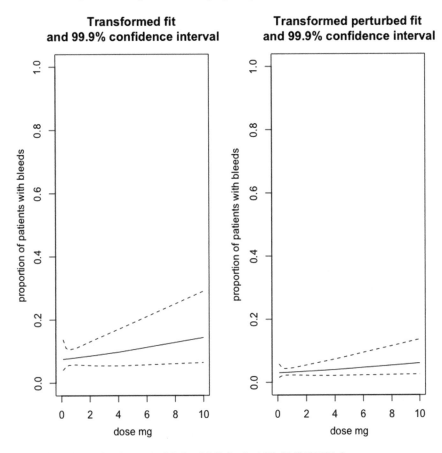

Fig. 13.2 Estimated and perturbed fit for (13.5) for final PD 0348292 TB data

We consider a number of metrics of interest. These are as follows: the proportion of times a correct dose is selected using the criteria described above, the doses chosen and the reasons for a selected dose failing to be correct.

We take as a comparator for the adaptive design the fixed design given by just using the initial set of doses.

We consider first the fixed design for the two scenarios and obtain, for 10,000 simulations, the results shown in Table 13.5 for the proportion of times a correct dose is selected.

Table 13.5 Proportion of times a correct dose is selected using the fixed design with PD 0348292 doses 0.1, 0.3, 0.5, 1 and 2.5 mg

	Scenario 1	Scenario 2
Proportion of times a correct dose selected	0.6602	0.2230

Table 13.6 Proportion of times a selected dose is incorrect for a given reason under the fixed design

	Scenario 1	Scenario 2
VTE ratio > 1.3	0.1002	0.777
TB ratio > 1.5	0.2596	0.0
VTE ratio > 1.3 and TB ratio > 1.5	0.0200	0.0

The reasons for incorrect dose selection are given in Table 13.6.

It can be seen from Table 13.5 that the estimated probability of correctly selecting a dose using the fixed design differs greatly between Scenario 1 and Scenario 2. This is to be expected given the likely higher dose required for Scenario 2. The reason for failure for Scenario 2 is estimated to be exclusively due to the ratio of true VTE relative to enoxaparin being too high. The enoxaparin true rate is estimated to be 0.063 under Scenario 2, so the true rate of VTE for a dose needs to be $< 0.063 * 1.5 = 0.0945$ for the dose to have an acceptable rate of VTE. Looking at Fig. 13.1, it can be seen that such a true rate is extremely unlikely even for the top dose of 2.5 mg.

We now consider the performance of the adaptive dose-ranging design described above. The proportion of times a dose is correctly selected for each of the two scenarios is given in Table 13.7.

As before, we also tabulate in Table 13.8 the proportion of times a dose was incorrectly selected for differing reasons.

Table 13.7 shows that the proportion of times a correct dose is selected for Scenario 1 is estimated to slightly decrease under the adaptive design compared with the fixed design but the probability of correctly selecting a dose for Scenario 2 is estimated to increase greatly. Recall that for the fixed design, the main reason for incorrectly selecting a dose is true TB ratio too high for Scenario 1 and true VTE ratio too high for Scenario 2.

It is of interest to look in more detail at how the adaptive design obtains these results. Consequently, we look at another metric which is the proportion of times a

Table 13.7 Proportion of times a correct dose is selected using the adaptive dose-ranging design with available PD 0348292 doses 0.1, 0.3, 0.5, 1, 2.5, 4 and 10 mg

	Scenario 1	Scenario 2
Proportion of times a correct dose selected	0.6447	0.7971

Table 13.8 Proportion of times a selected dose was incorrect for a given reason under the adaptive design

	Scenario 1	Scenario 2
VTE ratio > 1.3	0.1003	0.1574
TB ratio > 1.5	0.2754	0.0498
VTE ratio > 1.3 and TB ratio > 1.5	0.0204	0.0043

Table 13.9 Proportion of times different doses are selected under the fixed design

Dose (mg)	Proportion of times selected	
	Scenario 1	Scenario 2
0.1	0.0002	0.0
0.3	0.0128	0.0
0.5	0.1630	0.0
1.0	0.5454	0.0057
2.5	0.2786	0.9943

Table 13.10 Proportion of times different doses are selected under the adaptive design

Dose (mg)	Proportion of times selected	
	Scenario 1	Scenario 2
0.1	0.0004	0.0
0.3	0.0176	0.0
0.5	0.1609	0.0
1.0	0.5393	0.0052
2.5	0.2217	0.1327
4.0	0.0459	0.3730
10.0	0.0142	0.4891

particular dose is selected. We look at this metric for both the fixed and the adaptive design to compare the two designs. The metric is tabulated in Tables 13.9 and 13.10.

It can be seen from Table 13.9 that the fixed design almost always selects the highest possible dose for Scenario 2 but this dose usually does not satisfy the requirement for the ratio of VTE relative to enoxaparin. By comparison, the adaptive design mostly selects the two doses not initially used. A consequence of the extra flexibility of the adaptive design is that it may sometimes select doses higher than necessary as evidenced for Scenario 1.

For this example, the performance of the adaptive dose-ranging design as measured by its probability of selecting a correct dose is close to that of the fixed design for Scenario 1 and much better than the fixed design for Scenario 2. Consequently, it would likely be favored in a choice between the two designs, especially when there is uncertainty concerning the choice of doses to investigate. Some researchers have criticized the dose range chosen for most dose-ranging studies as being too narrow (Thomas et al., 2014), resulting in a repeat of some form of a dose-ranging study. In our experience, adaptive dose-ranging studies that allow the addition or dropping of doses offer a good alternative to a fixed design with minimum compromise during this critical phase of drug development.

To understand the operating characteristics such as those described above requires extensive simulations. This is especially so in the case of the PD 0348292 trial with four planned interim dose decision analyses and the need to quantitatively balance between the benefit (VTE) and the risk (TB). Nevertheless, for the expense of conducting a large outcome trial to decide on a critical dose like the PD 0348292 trial, running simulations represented a more efficient alternative to the possibility of needing to run a second trial with a different dose range.

13.6   An Example of a Phase 3 Adaptive Population Enrichment Design with Sample Size Re-estimation

We consider the example of the TAPPAS (TRC105 And Pazopanib versus Pazopanib alone in patients with advanced AngioSarcoma) trial. This trial was designed as an adaptive design incorporating population enrichment and sample size re-estimation. Nearly all of the materials in this subsection come from Jones et al. (2019) and Mehta et al. (2019a, b).

A Phase 3 adaptive design was chosen because of the ultra-orphan status of the disease (about 2000 cases per year in the United States and Europe) and the lack of reliable data on progression free survival (PFS) and overall survival (OS). Population enrichment was included as an option because there was some indication of greater tumor sensitivity in the subgroup with cutaneous lesions.

The primary objective of the TAPPAS trial was to demonstrate superior PFS of the combination treatment (TRC105 plus pazopanib) versus pazopanib alone in patients with angiosarcoma (AS). Patients were stratified by AS sub-type (cutaneous versus non-cutaneous) and the number of lines of previous therapy for AS (none, 1 or 2) and randomized in a 1: 1 ratio to the two treatment groups. Efficacy was assessed by RECIST (Response Evaluation Criteria In Solid Tumours, Eisenhauer et al., 2009) every 6 weeks following randomization.

The adaptive strategy for the trial was to have one interim analysis at which the Data Monitoring Committee (DMC) could recommend one of three options: continue as planned with the full population, continue with the full population with an increase in sample size or continue with just the cutaneous subgroup with a target number of PFS events for the subgroup.

A number of design parameters had to be set for this trial, and, as described by Mehta et al. (2019b), these were determined by a combination of theory, graphical display and simulation. We review the design parameters finally used and the corresponding operating characteristics for a comparison of the adaptive design with a fixed design.

The initial specification of the number of patients required was obtained by first determining that 95 events had 83% power to detect a hazard ratio of 0.55 for a one-sided $\alpha = 0.025$ test using the equation

$$Number\ of\ PFS\ Events = 4 \left[\frac{Z_\alpha + Z_\beta}{\ln(HR)} \right]^2$$

(see, e.g., Schoenfeld, 1983). The ratio of 0.55 is based on the assumptions that the median PFS for pazopanib alone is 4.0 months (from past experience) and a conjectured median PFS for the combination therapy is 7.27 months (based on single-arm experience). These assumptions lead to a HR of 0.55 (=4.0/7.27) on the exponential scale.

Mehta et al. (2019b) used the methods proposed by Kim and Tsiatis (1990) that assumed piecewise linear enrollment and piecewise exponential time to progression to estimate the number of patients needed in order to observe 95 events within a reasonable period of time. A blinded review 16 months after study initiation suggested that the enrollment averaged 1 patient per month for the first 5 months, 4 patients per month for the next 11 months and 9 patients per month thereafter. The hazard rate for dropouts was estimated to be 0.1. This information together with the assumed median PFS times for the two groups led Mehta et al. (2019b) to decide that a sample size of 190 patients was needed to obtain 95 events within three years. It should be mentioned that the blinded review of enrollment and dropout rates resulted in a larger target number of patients than originally anticipated. This experience led Mehta et al. (2019b) to recommend blinded reviews be conducted routinely in future adaptive trials.

A key consideration for the statistical validity of making adaptive changes based on an unblinded interim analysis is to keep the data used for the interim analysis independent of the data that results from the adaptive change. This is a challenge for outcome-based trials like TAPPAS because patients who have not experienced the event of interest before the interim analysis will continue to contribute efficacy data after the interim analysis. To this end, the study adopted the approach suggested by Jenkins et al. (2010) of splitting the study population into two cohorts whose initial size and PFS events are pre-specified. At an interim analysis, which occurs while Cohort 1 is being enrolled, the data are unblinded to an independent DMC which makes a decision about any adaptations. The adaptations apply only to Cohort 2. Patients in Cohort 1 continue to proceed until the pre-specified events have been observed.

For TAPPAS, it was decided that an interim analysis after 40 PFS events was a reasonable compromise between too late an interim analysis when data from Cohort 2 patients already recruited could not be used in the final analysis and too early an interim analysis when there might be insufficient PFS events to make decisions about sample size re-assessment or enrichment. Ultimately, the decision was made to recruit 120 patients to Cohort 1 and 70 patients to Cohort 2 to achieve a reasonable balance between the two cohorts. Cohort 1 would be followed for 60 PFS events, while Cohort 2 followed for 35 events.

The decision rules for whether to increase sample size and if so, by how much and whether to enrich the population, were obtained by extensive simulations by Mehta et al. (2019a; b) and are set out in Table 13.11. The decision rules are based on conditional power (CP) which is defined as the probability that, conditional on the current value of the test statistic, the test statistic will achieve statistical significance at the final analysis. For TAPPAS, the interim estimate for the hazard ratio is used as the true hazard ratio assumed for the remaining (yet to be observed) data in calculating

Table 13.11 Recommended actions determined by values of conditional power

Zone and corresponding conditional power requirement for full (CP_F) and/or cutaneous subpopulation (CP_S)	Recommended action
Unfavorable zone: $CP_F < 0.3$ and $CP_S < 0.5$	No Change: Continue the trial as planned Test treatment effect in the full population at the final analysis
Enrichment zone: $CP_F < 0.3$ and $CP_S > = 0.5$	Enrichment: Enroll 160 patients from the cutaneous subpopulation only in Cohort 2. Follow these patients until 110 events have been observed in the cutaneous subgroup in Cohort 1 and Cohort 2 combined Only test treatment effect in the cutaneous subgroup in the final analysis
Promising zone: $0.3 < = CP_F < = 0.95$	Sample size increase: Enroll 220 patients from the full population in Cohort 2. Follow these patients until 110 events have been observed in Cohort 2 Test treatment effect in the full population
Favorable zone: $CP_F > 0.95$	No change Enroll 70 patients from the full population in Cohort 2. Follow these patients until 35 events have been observed in Cohort 2 Test treatment effect in the full population
In all cases	Continue follow-up of patients in Cohort 1 until 60 events have been observed from Cohort 1

the CP. Conditional power is calculated for both the full population (CP_F) and the cutaneous subpopulation (CP_S).

The terminology unfavorable zone, promising zone and favorable zone come from a paper by Mehta and Pocock (2011) in which they showed that, without other adaptations, a promising zone can be constructed using conditional power which allows a sample size increase without any effect on the Type I error rate. As the name suggests, promising zone indicates that a positive result may be obtained if the sample size is increased. The enrichment zone is similarly constructed where sample size can be increased to try to achieve a positive result in the enriched population. Enrichment is considered only if the conditional power for the full population falls in the unfavorable zone and the interim data provide some evidence for a positive treatment effect in the cutaneous subpopulation.

To control the Type I error rate, the closed testing principle (Marcus et al., 1976) was used to account for the multiplicity due to selecting either the full population or the subpopulation. The inverse normal method (Wassmer & Brannath, 2016) was used to combine p-values from the two cohorts. We describe the methodology below.

Let H_o^F denote the null hypothesis for the full population, H_0^S denote the null hypothesis for the cutaneous subgroup and $H_0^{FS} = H_0^F \cap H_0^S$ denote the global null hypothesis. Closed testing ensures that the overall Type I error rate is strongly controlled under any configuration of the null hypotheses provided that two requirements are met. First, each of the hypotheses in the closed family is tested at level α. Second, significance is claimed for H_0^F only if both tests for H_0^F and H_0^{FS} are significant at level α. Similarly, significance is claimed for H_0^S only if both tests for H_0^S and H_0^{FS} are significant at level α.

One-sided p-values for full population and cutaneous subpopulation were obtained using logrank tests and denoted by p_1^F and p_1^S for Cohort 1 and by p_2^F and p_2^S for Cohort 2. The p-value for the test of the global null hypothesis for the first cohort was obtained by the Simes method (Wassmer & Brannath, 2016) and computed as

$$p_1^{FS} = min\left[2min\{p_1^F, p_1^S\}, max\{p_1^F, p_1^S\}\right]$$

Similarly, the p-value for the test of the global null hypothesis for the second cohort in the case of no enrichment was obtained as

$$p_2^{FS} = min\left[2min\{p_2^F, p_2^S\}, max\{p_2^F, p_2^S\}\right]$$

Finally, the inverse normal method was used to combine p-values for the two cohorts. If the trial is not enriched after the interim, then the p-value combination for testing the global null hypothesis is given by

$$p^{FS} = 1 - \Phi\left\{w_1\Phi^{-1}\left(1 - p_1^{FS}\right) + w_2\Phi^{-1}\left(1 - p_2^{FS}\right)\right\}$$

and the p-value combination for testing H_o^F is given by

$$p^F = 1 - \Phi\left\{w_1\Phi^{-1}\left(1 - p_1^F\right) + w_2\Phi^{-1}\left(1 - p_2^F\right)\right\}$$

Significance is claimed for the full population if both one-sided p-values are less than 0.025.

If the trial is enriched, then correspondingly, we have

$$p^{FS} = 1 - \Phi\left\{w_1\Phi^{-1}\left(1 - p_1^{FS}\right) + w_2\Phi^{-1}\left(1 - p_2^S\right)\right\}$$

and

$$p^S = 1 - \Phi\left\{w_1\Phi^{-1}\left(1 - p_1^S\right) + w_2\Phi^{-1}\left(1 - p_2^S\right)\right\}$$

and significance is claimed for the cutaneous subgroup if both one-sided p-values are less than 0.025. The weights w_1 and w_2 are pre-specified to be $\sqrt{60/95}$ and $\sqrt{35/95}$, reflecting the split of the initial target event number between the two cohorts.

Mehta et al. (2019a) compared the adaptive design with the fixed design of the same planned sample size. We include in Table 13.12 some of the simulation results

Table 13.12 Operating characteristics of adaptive and fixed sample designs based on 10,000 simulations

HR cutaneous/non-cutaneous		Zone	Prob of zone	Power		Average study duration (months)		Average PFS events		Average sample size (number of patients)	
				Adap	Fixed	Adap	Fixed	Adap	Fixed	Adap	Fixed
0.55	0.65	Enrich	0.09	0.80		56		139		275	
		Unfav	0.19	0.24		39		95		190	
		Prom	0.40	0.89		50		170		338	
		Fav	0.32	0.88		39		95		190	
		Total	1.00	0.76	0.83	45	40	129	129	257	257
0.55	0.75	Enrich	0.14	0.81		57		139		275	
		Unfav	0.22	0.18		38		95		190	
		Prom	0.40	0.84		50		170		338	
		Fav	0.24	0.86		38		95		190	
		Total	1.00	0.70	0.71	45	40	131	131	261	261
0.55	0.85	Enrich	0.19	0.79		57		138		274	
		Unfav	0.24	0.15		37		95		190	
		Prom	0.38	0.79		49		170		336	
		Fav	0.19	0.80		38		95		190	
		Total	1.00	0.64	0.58	45	40	131	131	261	261

provided in Mehta et al. (2019a). Table 13.12 shows the power, average study duration, average PFS events and average sample size from 10,000 simulations for the
case where the hazard ratio for the cutaneous subgroup is 0.55 and that for the
non-cutaneous subgroup is 0.65, 0.75 or 0.85. Simulation results for the scenarios
presented here can be obtained using the East statistical software (East 6, 2020).

Two general features of this table are apparent. First, the fixed design has a higher
overall power when the hazard ratios are similar between the cutaneous and the non-
cutaneous subgroups, but a lower overall power as the ratios become very dissimilar.
Second, the fixed design has a shorter average study duration across all scenarios.

As noted by Mehta et al. (2019a) the real benefit of the adaptive design arises,
however, from its learning and consequent improvements in power in certain situations. For example, for the case of a 0.55 HR for the cutaneous subgroup and a
0.75 HR for the non-cutaneous subgroup, we can see that although the overall
power is approximately the same, the power for the enrichment zone is increased
to 0.81, and the power for the promising zone is increased to 0.84. The greater
the heterogeneity in the two subgroups the greater is this benefit for the adaptive
design. Instead of having to conduct a second study to confirm a possible benefit
of the combination therapy in the cutaneous subpopulation, the proposed adaptive
trial provides the opportunity to enrich the study population and obtain a definitive
answer for this question in the same trial.

Unfortunately, the TAPPAS study was discontinued at the interim for futility.
Even though futility was not formally part of the TAPPAS design, the DMC had the
flexibility to use its clinical judgment to recommend terminating the trial for futility.

13.7 An Example of an Adaptive Confirmatory Study with Dose Selection

We take as an example of an adaptive two-stage confirmatory study (INHANCE)
(Barnes et al., 2010; Donohue et al., 2010; Lawrence et al., 2014) of indicaterol
for the treatment of chronic obstructive pulmonary disease (COPD). Indicaterol is a
beta-2 adrenergic agonist bronchodilator. The characteristics of indicaterol powder
changed on scaling up for Phase 3 supplies. This meant that the Phase 2 dose-ranging
studies already done could no longer be regarded as applicable. To avoid delay, it
was decided to combine dose-ranging and confirmation of efficacy for selected doses
into a single two-stage adaptive trial.

The first stage of the study explored several doses (given once a day, o.d.) and
selected two doses based on 14 days of treatment. The second stage evaluated the
safety and efficacy of the two chosen doses during 26 weeks of treatment. This study
is perhaps one of the first well-documented and much-discussed seamless Phase 2/3
trials. Most of the materials pertaining to this example come from Lawrence et al.
(2014). The study design is shown in Fig. 13.3.

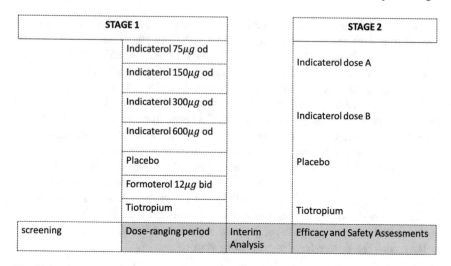

Fig. 13.3 Study design

The doses selected for the second stage are labeled as Indicaterol dose A and Indicaterol dose B.

The primary objective of the study was to demonstrate superiority of at least one dose of indicaterol selected in stage 1 versus placebo with respect to 24 h post-dose trough FEV_1 (forced expiratory volume during the first second of the forced breath) after 12 weeks of treatment in patients with COPD. The important secondary objective was to demonstrate non-inferiority of at least one of the selected indacaterol doses to tiotropium in trough FEV_1 after 12 weeks of treatment.

At stage 1, patients were randomly assigned in 1: 1: 1: 1: 1: 1: 1 ratio to receive open label tiotropium or one of the six double-blind, double dummy treatments as shown in Fig. 13.3. The primary aim of this stage of the trial was to allow a risk–benefit analysis of the four indicaterol doses in order to select two doses to carry forward to stage 2. A Data Monitoring Committee independent of the study conduct was tasked to perform this and provided with a set of dose-selection guidelines. Randomization was paused when interim results were being evaluated for dose selections.

The interim analysis was planned for when 770 evaluable patients had each completed two weeks of treatment. This sample size was calculated to ensure that at least one of the selected doses would be efficacious with a probability of at least 75%. Interim data were used to obtain adjusted (least squares) means for the four doses in a predefined mixed-effects model. The model contains treatment as a fixed effect and the baseline FEV_1 as a covariate. The model also includes smoking status (current/ex-smoker) and country as fixed effects with center nested within country as a random effect.

Because the trial is designed as a confirmatory trial, control of the Type I error rate is essential. To achieve this, a Bonferroni adjustment with a significance level of $\alpha/4$ was used for comparing each of the two selected doses against placebo in the final analysis. The choice of $\alpha/4$ is because the study started with four indicaterol doses. The significance level α is what would have been used for a single comparison. The primary, key and important study objectives were tested sequentially at level $\alpha/4$ in a pre-specified hierarchy for each of the doses separately.

The dose-selection guidelines were complicated by the need to take account of risk as well as benefit. The efficacy guidelines are described below and are included in the DMC charter. It was understood that the DMC had the discretion to deviate from the guidelines as necessary. In addition, a communication plan was put in place in case the DMC experienced unanticipated complexities and needed to reach out to the sponsor.

The dose-selection guidelines focused on comparing placebo-adjusted means for indacaterol doses from the mixed-effects model against two thresholds. The first dose to be selected was to be the lowest dose that exceeded both thresholds, and the second dose was to be the next highest dose unless the highest dose was selected first in which case the next highest dose was also to be selected.

The two thresholds were as follows:

X (for trough FEV_1 after two weeks of treatment)—the maximum of

i.   Minimum clinically important difference (MCID) pre-specified as 120 ml
ii.   Adjusted mean effect of formoterol versus placebo
iii. Adjusted mean effect of tiotropium versus placebo.

Y (for the area under the curve of FEV_1 for 1 to 4 h after two weeks of treatment)—the maximum of

i.   Adjusted mean effect of formoterol versus placebo
ii.   Adjusted mean effect of tiotropium versus placebo.

Pre-specified dose-selection guidelines are given in Table 13.13.

Interim safety data were also presented to the DMC for the committee to carry out risk–benefit deliberations.

At the interim analysis, the 150 μg dose of indicaterol was found to be the lowest dose exceeding both of the thresholds defined above. Because the DMC did not find any safety concerns with this dose and the next higher dose (i.e., 300 mg), they selected these two doses to move forward to stage 2 of the trial. Patients who were randomized to the discontinued indacaterol doses or formoterol continued their treatment until a completion visit could be scheduled. After the completion visit, they were prescribed therapy deemed necessary to treat their COPD. Patients who were randomized to 150 μg, 300 μg, placebo and tiotropium in stage 1 continued with their treatment for a total of 26 weeks treatment.

In stage 2, an additional 285 patients were randomized to each of the four treatment groups until the total number of patients per group reached 400 patients. This number of patients was judged to be necessary to have at least 85% power for the key secondary objective of non-inferiority of at least one indacaterol dose versus tiotropium in trough FEV_1.

For the two selected indacaterol doses, placebo and tiotropium, data from both stages were used in the final analysis. As stated above, one-sided Bonferroni adjusted

Table 13.13 Possible outcomes of interim analysis and corresponding recommended dose-selection decisions

Possible outcome	Decision
More than one dose beats X and Y	Select lowest dose that beats X and Y and the next higher dose
One dose beats X and Y	Select this dose and the next higher dose
More than one dose beats X but not Y	Select the dose that beats X and is closest to Y and the next higher dose
One dose beats X but not Y	Select this dose and the next higher dose
More than one dose beats Y but not X	Select the dose that beats Y and is closest to X and the next higher dose
One dose beats Y but not X	Select this dose and the next higher dose
One dose beats X but not Y and one dose beats Y but not X	Select the dose that beats X and the next higher dose
No dose beats X or Y	Select the dose that is closest to X and the next higher dose

significance level of 0.00625 (=0.025/4) was used for comparing each of the two indacaterol doses with the placebo. More powerful approaches using, for example, p-value combination functions or conditional error rates could have been applied, but were not chosen for INHANCE because of the complexity of the trial design and a desire to test for both primary and some key secondary endpoints.

Both of the selected doses were found to be superior to placebo in trough FEV_1. The estimated differences were 180 ml for both doses. This difference was bigger than the estimated difference versus placebo for tiotropium.

The regulatory outcome from the use of this adaptive design is interesting. INHANCE was completed during the 3rd quarter of 2008. A new drug application for 150 μg and 300 μg was submitted in late 2008. In 2009, the European Union approved indacaterol for 150 μg and 300 μg. The FDA, on the other hand, requested the sponsor to explore lower doses of indacaterol. The sponsor conducted two 12-week studies to compare 75 mg versus placebo. The FDA eventually approved indacaterol in July 2011 for the 75 μg dose.

This adaptive design therefore successfully speeded up regulatory approval by the EU but not by the FDA. The trial was carefully designed and brilliantly executed. The example illustrates the potential advantages and possible risks in decision making from using a seamless Phase 2/3 design. The design saved time and number of patients compared with following all four dose arms throughout the study. But the quality of the decision making about dose selection was not uniformly regarded as optimal by all of the regulators.

In our opinion, the inability to thoroughly explore the risk–benefit profiles of different doses and seek regulatory input on dose selection before moving into the confirmatory stage is perhaps the biggest drawback of a seamless Phase 2/3 design.

13.8 Discussion

Adaptive designs offer the opportunity to change a clinical trial design in response to emerging data. This can be increasing sample size to maintain power, stopping a study early for efficacy or futility, changing treatment arms, selecting the patient population or other possibilities. This ability to change a clinical trial design can speed up development and be more efficient in some aspects. It does, however, come at a cost. The cost is that an adaptive design needs to be planned in detail and thoroughly evaluated. There can also be increased risk as exemplified by the INHANCE trial described in this chapter. The selection of doses in the INHANCE trial was acceptable to the EU regulators but not to the FDA.

When Cui et al. (1999) first proposed a weighted statistic to combine test statistics from data before and after an unblinded interim analysis to re-estimate the sample size of a study, researchers were quick to comment on the inefficiency of the proposed methodology. (The weighted statistic is a special case of the inverse normal combination statistic described in Sect. 13.6.) For example, Tsiatis and Mehta (2003) demonstrated that for any adaptive design with the sample size modification using the weighted statistic, they could construct a group sequential design utilizing the usual sufficient statistic that would stop the trial earlier with a higher probability of rejecting the null hypothesis if the new treatment was effective and also stop the trial earlier with a higher probability of accepting the null hypothesis if the treatment had no effect. Jennison and Turnbull (2003) demonstrated a similar result. Over time, Mehta and Pocock (2011) realized that the conditions that resulted in appreciable efficiency gains from an ideal group sequential design, such as no trial overruns, a large number of interim analyses and a large up-front sample size commitment and aggressive early stopping boundaries, were not always possible in the real world of drug development. They observed that many developers prefer investing limited resources initially and increasing commitment only after seeing interim results that were promising. In fact, the latter may be a necessity for developers who are being financially supported by venture capital groups. The financial model, plus the real challenge of conducting many interim analyses with aggressive stopping boundaries, has led many developers to see the value of an adaptive design with a built-in unblinded sample size re-estimation during the past 10 years.

After an initial period when some viewed adaptive designs as likely to radically change drug development, there now seems to be a consensus that adaptive designs should be selectively used in situations in which they can be carefully justified. They are simply one additional tool for our design toolkit. At the same time, regulators have gradually evolved their opinions about when and how adaptive designs might be used and the potential risks involved. Along with the experience with adaptive designs came a greater understanding of when adaptive designs may have their greatest value in drug development. Readers who would like to learn more about adaptive designs are recommended to read the texts by Chang (2014), Menon and Zink (2015) and Wassmer and Brannath (2016).

It is not the strongest of the species that survives, nor the most intelligent that survives. It is the one that is most adaptable to change.

Charles Darwin

References

Barnes, P. J., Pocock, S. J., Magnussen, H., et al. (2010). Integrating indacaterol dose selection in a clinical study in COPD using an adaptive seamless design. *Pulmonary Pharmacology & Therapeutics, 23*, 165–171.

Bauer, P., & Köhne, K. (1994). Evaluation of experiments with adaptive interim analyses. *Biometrics, 50*(4), 1029–1041 (Correction in 1996 *Biometrics*, 52, 380).

Chang, M. (2014). *Adaptive design theory and implementation using SAS and R* (2nd ed.). Chapman and Hall.

Cohen, A. T., Boyd, R. A., Mandema, J. W., et al. (2013). An adaptive-design dose-ranging study of PD 0348292, an oral factor Xa inhibitor, for thromboprophylaxis after total knee replacement surgery. *Journal of Thrombosis and Haemostasis, 11*, 1503–1510.

Cui, L., Hung, H. M. J., & Wang, S.-J. (1999). Modification of sample size in group sequential clinical trials. *Biometrics, 55*, 853–857.

Donohue, J. F., Fogarty, C., Lotvall, J., et al. (2010). Once-daily bronchodilators for chronic obstructive pulmonary disease: Indacaterol versus tiotropium. *Ann. J. Respir. Crit. Care Med., 182*, 155–162.

East 6. (2020). *Statistical software for the design, simulation and monitoring clinical trials.* Cytel Inc.

Eisenhauer, E. A., Therasse, P., Bogaerts, J., et al. (2009). New response evaluation criteria in solid tumours: Revised RECIST guideline (version 1.1). *European Journal of Cancer, 45*, 228–247.

EMA. (2007). *Reflection Paper on Methodological issues in confirmatory clinical trials planned with an adaptive design.*

Friede, T., & Kieser, M. (2006). Sample size recalculation in internal pilot study designs: A review. *Biometrical Journal, 48*(4), 537–555.

Grieve, A. (1991). Predictive probability in clinical trials. *Biometrics, 47*(1), 323–329.

Jenkins, M., Stone, A., & Jennison, C. J. (2010). An adaptive seamless phase II/III design for oncology trials with subpopulation selection using correlated survival endpoints. *Pharmaceutical Statistics, 4*, 347–356.

Jennison, C., & Turnbull, B. W. (2000). *Group Sequential methods with applications to clinical trials.* Chapman & Hall/CRC Press.

Jennison, C., & Turnbull, B. W. (2003). Mid-course sample size modification in clinical trials based on the observed treatment effect. *Statistics in Medicine, 22*, 971–993.

Jones, R. L., Ravi, V., Brohl, A. S., et al. (2019). Results of the TAPPAS trial: An adaptive enrichment phase III trial of TRC105 and pazopanib (P) versus pazopanib alone in patients with advanced angiosarcoma (AS). *Annals of Oncology, 30* (Supplement 5), v683–v709. https://doi.org/10.1093/annonc/mdz283

Kim, K., & Tsiatis, A. A. (1990). Study duration for clinical trials with survival response and early stopping rule. *Biometrics, 46*, 81–92.

Lan, K. K. G., & DeMets, D. L. (1983). Discrete sequential boundaries for clinical trials. *Biometrika, 70*(3), 659–663.

Lawrence, D., Bretz, F., & Pocock, S. (2014). INHANCE: An adaptive confirmatory study with dose selection at interim. In A. Trifilieff (Ed.), *Indicaterol, Milestones in Drug Therapy.* Springer. https://doi.org/10.1007/978-3-0348-0709-8_2.

Marcus, R., Peritz, E., & Gabriel, K. R. (1976). On closed testing procedures with special reference to ordered analysis of variance. *Biometrika, 63,* 655–660.

Mehta, C. R., Liu, L., & Theuer, C. (2019a). An adaptive population enrichment phase III trial of TRC105 and pazopanib versus pazopanib alone in patients with advanced angiosarcoma (TAPPAS trial). *Annals of Oncology, 30,* 103–108.

Mehta, C. R., Liu, L., & Theuer, C. (2019b). Supplementary material for An adaptive population enrichment phase III trial of TRC105 and pazopanib versus pazopanib alone in patients with advanced angiosarcoma (TAPPAS trial). *Annals of Oncology, 30,* 103–108.

Mehta, C., & Pocock, S. (2011). Adaptive increase in sample size when interim results are promising: A practical guide with examples. *Statistics in Medicine, 30*(28), 3267–3284.

Menon, S., & Zink, R. (2015). *Modern approaches to clinical trials using SAS®: Classical, adaptive, and Bayesian methods.* SAS Institute.

Müller, H. H., & Schäfer, H. (2001). Adaptive group sequential designs for clinical trials: Combining the advantages of adaptive and of classical group sequential approaches. *Biometrics, 57,* 886–891.

O'Brien, P. C., & Fleming, T. R. (1979). A multiple testing procedure for clinical trials. *Biometrics, 35,* 549–556.

Pocock, S. J., & Simon, R. (1975). Sequential treatment assignment with balancing for prognostic factors in the controlled clinical trial. *Biometrics, 31*(1), 103–115.

Schoenfeld, D. (1983). Sample-size formulae for the proportional-hazards regression model. *Biometrics, 39*(2), 499–503.

Schulman, S., Kearon, C; on behalf of the subcommittee on control of anticoagulation of the scientific and standardization committee of the International Society on Thrombosis and Haemostasis. (2005). Definition of major bleeding in clinical investigations of antihemostatic medicinal products in non-surgical patients. *Journal of Thrombosis and Haemostasis, 3,* 692–694.

Thomas, N., Sweeney, K., & Somayaji, V. (2014). Meta-analysis of clinical dose response in a large drug development portfolio. *Statistics in Biopharmaceutical Research, 6*(4), 302–317.

Tsiatis, A., & Mehta, C. (2003). On the inefficiency of the adaptive design for monitoring clinical trials. *Biometrika, 90,* 367–378.

U.S. Food and Drug Administration. (2019). *Adaptive designs for clinical trials of drugs and biologics.*

Wassmer, G., & Brannath, W. (2016). *Group sequential and confirmatory adaptive designs in clinical trials.* Springer.

Chapter 14
Additional Topics

It always seems impossible until it's done.
—Nelson Mandela.

14.1 Probability of Program Success Further Examined

In Sect. 6.5.1, we estimated the success probability of a confirmatory program. For convenience, we assumed that the confirmatory program consists of two Phase 3 trials of similar design. As such, the effect of a new investigational drug, while unknown, is assumed to be the same in the two Phase 3 trials.

There are diseases whose management is typically composed of two distinct phases. An example is ulcerative colitis (UC) which is an inflammatory bowel disease affecting the colon. Patients with UC experience recurrent flares of abdominal pain and bloody diarrhea. A successful treatment for UC needs to induce remission and maintain remission once a remission is achieved. Dose or the administration frequency used during the induction phase is often higher than that used during the maintenance phase. A Phase 2 development program typically includes trials that investigate the induction and the maintenance effect. For a confirmatory program to be successful, the new treatment needs to demonstrate effect for both induction and maintenance.

Induction trials follow a standard design. They are randomized trials of a short duration such as 6–8 weeks. The primary endpoint is the remission rate at the end of the short treatment period based on the Mayo score. A Mayo score consists of four parts: stool frequency, rectal bleeding, endoscopic findings and physician's global assessment. Each part has a score ranging from 0 to 3, resulting in a total score between 0 and 12. One definition of remission is a complete Mayo score ≤ 2 with no individual subscore > 1 and rectal bleeding subscore of 0. Variations of this definition have also been used.

C. Chuang-Stein and S. Kirby, *Quantitative Decisions in Drug Development*, Springer Series in Pharmaceutical Statistics,
https://doi.org/10.1007/978-3-030-79731-7_14

Trials to investigate maintenance effect generally follow two strategies. One is to conduct a long-term trial (e.g., 52 weeks) and evaluate the remission rate at the end of the 52-week treatment in addition to that at the end of week 8. This strategy was used for Humira® (adalimumab) and Remicade® (infliximab). Another strategy is to use a randomized withdrawal design by selecting patients with an initial clinical response to an investigational treatment and randomizing them to a placebo or the investigational treatment. The primary endpoint is remission rate at, for example, week 52. It is not unusual to include two doses or two administration schedules in a randomized withdrawal design because a lower dose or a less frequent administration may be capable of achieving a long-term remission. A clinical response used in the selection criteria, while less than a full remission, signals a meaningful response to the new treatment during the initial treatment period. A clinical response could be a reduction in the total Mayo score of ≥ 3 points and $\geq 30\%$ from baseline with an accompanying reduction in rectal bleeding subscore of ≥ 1 point or absolute rectal bleeding subscore ≤ 1 point. This is the strategy used for Entyvio® (vedolizumab), Stelara® (ustekinumab) and Xeljanz XR® (tofacitinib).

Because a randomized withdrawal maintenance trial was enriched with early clinical responders, the long-term remission rate in a randomized withdrawal trial is likely to be higher than their counterpart in a long-term maintenance trial without the upfront enrichment.

In the above situation, it is reasonable to expect the effect in induction trials to be related to that in the maintenance trials. This relationship could be actively modeled and utilized when estimating the probability of a successful Phase 3 program. One such approach was proposed by Mukhopadhyay (2019) who used a Bayesian latent relationship modeling (BLRM) framework to describe the relationship. We will apply a simple version of the framework in the remainder of Sect. 14.1.

We assume that the Phase 2 program of a new drug for the UC indication includes an induction trial of 8 weeks and a randomized withdrawal maintenance trial of 30 weeks. Based on past experience, the sponsor believes that the maintenance effect observed at week 30 could reasonably predict the effect at the end of week 52. The primary endpoint is clinical remission, and the comparison is against a placebo in both trials.

The confirmatory program calls for conducting two identical induction trials of 8-week duration and a randomized withdrawal trial of 52 weeks. All trials will randomize an equal number of participants to the investigational drug or a placebo. Each induction trial will enroll 260 subjects (130 per group) while the maintenance trial will enroll 300 subjects (150 per group). The sponsor is interested in estimating the probability that all three trials show a statistically significant effect at the one-sided 2.5% level.

We can break down the assessment of the Phase 3 program success into six parts as described below:

A. Find a prior distribution for the remission rate for the placebo group in an induction trial.

Table 14.1 Observed placebo remission rates in seven confirmatory induction trials and the Phase 2 induction trial of the new investigational drug

Induction trials	Observed remission rate (%)	Sample size (N)
Adalimumab UC-I	9.2	130
Adalimumab UC-II	9.3	246
Infliximab UC-I	15	121
Infliximab UC-II	6	123
Vedolizumab UC-I	5	149
Tofacitinib XR UC-I	8	122
Tofacitinib XR UC-II	4	112
Phase 2 Trial of the New Drug	10	50

B.   Find a prior distribution for the remission rate for the placebo group in a randomized withdrawal trial.

C.   Find a prior distribution for the effect of the new investigational drug on the remission rate during the induction phase.

D.   Find a prior distribution for the effect of the new investigational drug on the remission rate during the maintenance phase.

E.   Find the correlation (e.g., Pearson's correlation coefficient) between the effect during the induction phase and that in the maintenance phase.

F.   Estimate the probability of success through simulations utilizing the information above.

Part A

To find a prior for the remission rate for placebo in an induction trial, we examined remission data from confirmatory trials involving adalimumab, infliximab, vedolizumab, tofacitinib and the completed Phase 2 trial of the new drug. These data are given in Table 14.1. We have decided not to include results from trials of ustekinumab because ustekinumab adopted a remission definition that did not include the total Mayo score as one of the requirements. Except for the Phase 2 trials of the new drug, all results in Tables 14.1, 14.2 and 14.3 come from the labels of these drugs. The labels are downloadable from the US FDA site (www.fda.gov).

Table 14.2 Observed placebo remission rates in two confirmatory randomized withdrawal trials and the Phase 2 maintenance trial of a new investigational drug

Randomized withdrawal trials	Observed remission rate (%)	Sample size (N)
Adalimumab UC-I	11	198
Adalimumab UC-II	16	126
Phase 2 Trial of the New Drug	13	50

Table 14.3 Observed treatment effects in the pivotal trials for vedolizumab and tofacitinib as well as those observed in the Phase 2 trials of a new drug

Product	Observed effect in the induction phase[a] (%)	Observed effect in the maintenance phase[a] (%)
Vedolizumab	11.5	23
Tofacitinib	12	26
New Drug	14	27

[a]The observed effects for the new drug in the Phase 2 trials were discounted to account for possible selection bias

Using sample size as weight, the weighted average of the observed remission rates was found to be 8.3%. The weighted average of the squared differences between the remission rates in Table 14.1 and 8.3% is $(0.031)^2$. Based on these results, we choose Beta(6.3, 70.3) as the prior for the remission rate in the placebo group in an induction trial. This beta prior has a mean of 0.083 and standard deviation of 0.031.

Part B

To construct a prior for the placebo remission rate in a randomized withdrawal trial, we use results from two pivotal randomized withdrawal trials and the completed Phase 2 trial of the new drug displayed in Table 14.2.

Using sample size as weight, a weighted average of the observed remission rates was found to be 13.0%. The weighted average of the squared differences between the remission rates in Table 14.2 and 13.0% is $(0.023)^2$. Based on these results, we choose Beta(28.2, 189.8) as the prior for the remission rate in the placebo group in a randomized withdrawal trial. This beta prior has a mean of 0.130 and standard deviation of 0.023.

Part C

For the drug chosen to be further tested in the induction trials in Phase 3, the Phase 2 induction trial suggested a remission effect around 14% (over placebo) after employing some discounting strategies as discussed in Chap. 12. With 10% as the placebo remission rate, this translates to a discounted remission rate of 24% for the new drug. With 50 subjects per group in the Phase 2 trial, this yields a sampling distribution for the estimated effect of $N(0.14; (0.074)^2)$.

Part D

For the drug chosen to be further tested in a confirmatory maintenance trial (randomized withdrawal trial), the Phase 2 maintenance trial suggested an effect around 27% (over placebo), again after considering some form of discounting. With 13% as the placebo remission rate, this means a discounted remission rate of 40% for the new drug. With 50 subjects per group, this translates to a sampling distribution for the estimated effect of $N(0.27; (0.084)^2)$.

Part E

In Table 14.3, we include the reported treatment effects for vedolizumab and tofacitinib in their confirmatory program. We also include the effects reported in Part C and Part D for the new drug. There are two pivotal induction trials for tofacitinib. We averaged the treatment effects reported for these two trials in the product label. Two doses were included in the maintenance trial of tofacitinib. We included the effect reported for the lower dose since it is the recommended starting dose for the maintenance phase according to tofacitinib's product label.

Pearson's correlation coefficient between the observed induction and maintenance effects is 0.817.

Part F

The assessment on the success probability of the Phase 3 program could be conducted by following steps 1–5 below:

1. Draw a random value $p_{C,I}$ from Beta(6.3,70.3) and a random value $p_{C,M}$ from Beta(28.2,189.8). These two values will serve as the remission rates for placebo in the induction and the maintenance trials, respectively.
2. Draw a random pair (μ_I, μ_M) from a bivariate normal distribution with marginal distributions of $N(0.14;(0.074)^2)$ and $N(0.27;(0.084)^2)$ and a correlation coefficient of 0.817 between the two components.
3. Set $p_{N,I} = p_{C,I} + \mu_I$ and $p_{N,M} = p_{C,M} + \mu_M$. $p_{N,I}$ and $p_{N,M}$ will serve as the remission rates for the new drug in the induction and maintenance trials, respectively. If either rate is negative, replace it by 0. If either rate is greater than 1, replace it by 1.
4. Generate 3 pairs of independent binomial random variables to represent outcomes in the three studies. Two pairs will be generated from $b(130;p_{C,I})$ and $b(130;p_{N,I})$ (induction trials), and the third pair will be generated from $b(150;p_{C,M})$ and $b(150;p_{N,M})$ (maintenance trial). Compare the binomial outcomes within each study and denote the resulting three one-sided P-values by p_1, p_2 and p_3.
5. Repeat the above steps 100,000 times and calculate the percentage of times when all three P-values are ≤ 0.025.

For the UC example, the probability of success was estimated to be 66.0%. This estimation incorporates the correlation between the observed induction effect and maintenance effect. If we ignore this relationship and assess the success probability for the induction trials and the maintenance trial separately, the estimated success probably is 64.6%.

Incorporating a correlation coefficient of 0.817 did not increase the probability of program success by much. An interesting question is whether the increase may be more noticeable if the correlation coefficient is higher, for example, 0.90. Using 0.90 as the correlation coefficient in the codes provided in the Appendix, we found the success probability to be 66.6%, a mere 2% increase over the success probability that ignores the correlation altogether.

So, while the correlation coefficient could affect the success probability, it is not an important factor. The dominating factor continues to be the prior mean, and to some degree, the prior variance of the treatment effect of interest.

14.2   Joint Analysis of an Efficacy and a Safety Endpoint

So far, we have focused primarily on the analysis of efficacy endpoints. It may be the case, however, that a joint analysis of a safety and an efficacy endpoint is of interest. An example is the development of new oral anticoagulants. The efficacy endpoint could be the prevention of venous thromboembolism. At the same time, it is desired that the number of bleeding events be kept at an acceptable level.

Thall et al. (2006) described a Bayesian outcome-adaptive procedure that used both efficacy and toxicity to choose doses for an experimental agent for successive cohorts of patients in an early-phase clinical trial. For simplicity, they considered the bivariate binary case. Their approach has three basic components. The first one is a Bayesian model for the joint probabilities of efficacy and toxicity as functions of dose. The second component is to decide which doses are acceptable. A dose is considered acceptable if, given the current data, the posterior probability that the chance of efficacy at the dose being greater than a fixed lower limit $\underline{\pi}_E$ exceeds a pre-specified value p_E and the posterior probability that the chance of toxicity at the same dose being less than a fixed upper limit $\overline{\pi}_T$ exceeds a pre-specified value p_T. Values $\underline{\pi}_E$, p_E, $\overline{\pi}_T$, and p_T are design parameters. The third component is to construct a family of efficacy-toxicity trade-off contours in the region $[0, 1] \times [0, 1]$ of probability of efficacy and probability of toxicity, based on elicited probability pairs that are considered to be equally desirable targets. Thall et al. (2006) used three target probability pairs to determine the shape of the contours. The point $(1,0)$ in the $[0, 1] \times [0, 1]$ region represents the ideal state of guaranteed efficacy and absence of toxicity. Contours closer to the ideal state are considered more desirable than contours further away from $(1,0)$.

One can design a trial by choosing a total sample size, a cohort size, models linking probability of efficacy and probability of toxicity to doses, $\underline{\pi}_E$, p_E, $\overline{\pi}_T$, p_T, prior means for the probability of efficacy and toxicity at each dose, and three equally desirable target probability pairs to construct the shape of efficacy-toxicity trade-off contours.

A study proceeds by allocating the first cohort a starting dose decided by the physician. The data will be used to update the model and determine the acceptability of the doses. At any interim point in the trial, there is either no acceptable dose or at least one acceptable dose. In the former case, the trial is stopped, while in the latter case the next cohort is treated with the dose having the maximum acceptability. No untried dose may be skipped as long as the dose meets the selection criteria. If the trial is not stopped early for futility, then at the end of the trial, the most desirable acceptable dose is selected to be the optimal dose.

The operating characteristics of the design can be evaluated for plausible scenarios using simulation. Scenarios can be defined by $\underline{\pi}_E$, p_E, $\overline{\pi}_T$, p_T, and the treatment effect. Thall et al. suggested that metrics of interest included the probabilities that a dose was selected and the average sample sizes at each dose, and the probabilities of stopping the trial early.

Tao et al. (2015) considered a method for jointly modeling a continuous efficacy and a safety endpoint in Phase 2 studies. They recommended fitting a bivariate Normal nonlinear model to estimate the dose response for both endpoints simultaneously. The nonlinear function used for the efficacy endpoint can differ from that used for the safety endpoint. The joint modeling is used to estimate both the minimum effective dose (MED) and the maximum safe dose (MSD). Following Bretz et al. (2005), they estimated the MED as the lowest dose to have an effect that exceeded the clinically meaningful minimum difference and for which simultaneously the lower confidence limit for the predicted mean value, for some chosen confidence level, also exceeded this minimum difference. The MSD is estimated as the maximum dose for which the upper confidence limit, for some chosen confidence level, is less than the largest clinically acceptable safety response.

Before the joint modeling, Tao et al. described a first stage of testing whether proof of concept (POC) existed for efficacy and safety using the MCP-Mod approach of Bretz et al. (see Sect. 6.3.2 for a description of MCP-Mod.) POC for safety here means evidence of a dose response relationship for the safety endpoint. If POC is established for efficacy using typically a Type I error rate of 0.05 and one of the doses is estimated as the MED, Tao et al. suggested testing POC for safety using a different Type I error rate such as 0.20. If POC for both efficacy and safety are established and the estimated MSD is greater than or equal to the estimated MED, then joint modeling of efficacy and safety responses will proceed.

Tao et al. discussed two strategies for fitting a joint model. The first strategy starts with the most significant models obtained from fitting efficacy and safety models separately. The most significant models are then fitted jointly by generalized least squares with an assumed variance–covariance structure for the efficacy and safety endpoints. The MED and MSD are estimated from the jointly fitted models.

The second strategy keeps all the significant models obtained from fitting efficacy and safety models separately at the first stage to establish the POC. Joint model fitting is then undertaken for all possible combinations of these significant efficacy and safety models. The best combination is chosen based on the lowest Akaike Information Criterion (Akaike, 1973) defined as

$$AIC = 2k - 2\ln(L) \qquad (14.1)$$

where k is the number of parameters to be estimated in the pair of (efficacy, safety) models and $\ln(L)$ is the log of the maximum value of the likelihood function for the pair. The best combination is then used to estimate the MED and MSD. Tao et al. found that the second strategy appeared to be the better of the two.

The performance of this joint modeling approach can be assessed by simulation under plausible scenarios.

14.3   Use of a Sampling Distribution as a Prior Distribution

At various points throughout the book, a sampling distribution or a Normal approximation to a sampling distribution has been used as a prior distribution. One justification for doing this is that, on some occasions, the sampling distribution is the same as the posterior distribution that would have been obtained from a Bayesian analysis with a given appropriate prior, albeit the interpretation of the distribution differs (Cox & Hinkley, 1974). For example, for the case of a Normal distribution with unknown mean and known variance, the posterior distribution for the mean is the same as the sampling distribution for the mean if the improper prior $p(\Delta) = 1$ (for all Δ) is used.

A possible justification for using a Normal approximation to a sampling distribution as a prior is that when a flat prior is used the maximum likelihood estimate will coincide with the maximum a posteriori probability estimate from the Bayesian analysis, and subject to regularity conditions the posterior distribution will converge, as sample size increases, to a Normal distribution with mean given by the maximum likelihood estimate and posterior variance given by the variance of the maximum likelihood estimate (Gelman et al., 2004). We should point out that care is needed for this interpretation as convergence may require large sample sizes particularly for multi-parameter problems.

Alternatively, as described in Sect. 5.11, a sampling distribution or a Normal approximation to a sampling distribution is simply a convenient and objective way to describe our current knowledge about the parameters of interest.

It is important to remember, as discussed in Chap. 12, that discounting may be needed when the sampling distribution of the treatment effect estimate from a small and positive POC trial is used to help plan future trials.

14.4   Using Prior Information at the Pre-clinical Stage

So far, we have focused on the clinical phase of drug development. Before clinical testing of a new drug can begin, the drug has to be evaluated first in animal studies. Traditionally, pre-clinical animal studies have not received as much statistical support as clinical studies. There are several reasons for this. In our opinion, the most important two are probably the comparatively less statistical resource dedicated to pre-clinical activities and the generally cookie-cutter designs of repeat animal studies. As a result, many pre-clinical biologists analyze the studies themselves, using automated statistical packages that employ bar charts, t-tests and the analysis of variance technique.

However, repeat animal studies are particularly suited for utilizing knowledge from past studies and offering information to future studies. As Walley et al. (2016) pointed out, animals in these studies are typically from the same strain, and approximately the same age and within the same range of body weights. The same equipment and room is often used for each study. Some studies include an extra control group (besides the standard control group) that receives no challenge and serves as a check on the consistency of results with previous studies. The uniformity and similarity in design and animals make it highly feasible to borrow information from previous studies, especially with respect to the standard control group that is typically treated in the same way across studies.

Walley et al. (2016) described their experience in introducing a Bayesian meta-analytic predictive approach to repeat animal studies. They focused on the standard control group with an objective to reduce the number of animals in this group. Their approach leads to either an informative prior for the standard control group as part of a full Bayesian analysis or a predictive distribution that could be used to replace the standard control group completely in the next study.

14.5 Data Sources

14.5.1 Pre-clinical Data

Except for a few conditions (most notably bacterial infections), pre-clinical efficacy models seldom exist that could be used to predict treatment effect in humans directly. On the other hand, pre-clinical insights on a drug's mechanism could help a sponsor better understand the potential use and side effects of the drug. For example, DiSantostefano et al. (2016) used Factor Xa and thrombin inhibitors as an example. They stated that emerging pre-clinical data for this class of molecular entities suggested that these entities might have benefits in reducing progression of atherosclerosis and atrial fibrillation as a consequence of their effects on inflammation, vascular remodeling, and fibrosis. In addition, their potential for direct vascular effects may increase the risk of bleeding in patients susceptible to microvascular bleeds.

In general, pre-clinical data offer qualitative information on what may be worthwhile exploring in humans, but any quantification of a suggested relationship will likely come from clinical trials.

14.5.2 Information from Observational Studies

Chapter 5 described how information from previous trials could be incorporated into future trial planning. The discussion focuses on comparisons within randomized trials. If there are no randomized trials comparing two treatments head to head and a network meta-analysis as described in Chap. 10 is not possible, it may be possible to derive a prior distribution for the comparative effect between two treatments by resorting to observational studies (Rosenbaum, 2010).

The interest in observational studies has intensified since the turn of the century, partly because of the increasing availability of large-scale healthcare databases and improvements in informatics to access them. Large-scale healthcare databases include administrative claims databases and electronic health records. Besides, it is cheaper and faster to conduct observational studies than randomized clinical trials. In some cases, randomized clinical trials are just not possible.

Observational studies could help a sponsor better understand a target patient population and the effectiveness of marketed drugs in the real-world setting. These studies range from population-based cohort studies with prospective data collection to targeted patient registries to retrospective case–control studies. Many potential biases and sources of variability threaten the validity of such studies and a substantial literature documents these concerns (Ioannidis, 2008).

Compared to randomized clinical trials, the most notable challenge of observational studies is the lack of randomization, which can result in different groups of patients receiving different treatments. Another challenge of observational studies is that patients in the studies may be drastically different from the average patient population. For example, the US Medicare database pertains primarily to people who are 65 years or older while claims databases of private insurance companies include predominantly younger people. Because older people tend to have more co-morbidity and receive more medications, it may be difficult to generalize findings from the Medicare database to the average patient population.

Furthermore, observational studies of healthcare databases represent a secondary use of the data. Consequently, the studies are often limited by what is available in these databases. For example, healthcare databases typically do not contain pain relief scores or responses on the Hamilton Depression Rating scale. They often do not include laboratory results in a consistent fashion either. Because of these limitations, observational studies are generally more suited for studies involving clinical events.

There are methods that have been proposed to handle potential bias due to treatment selection. One such approach is to calculate a propensity score (Austin, 2011). We discuss the construction of propensity scores in some detail in Sect. 5.10.1 in the context of using information from historical trials. Propensity scores can be used to compare treatments within strata defined by quintiles of the propensity score. When applying such an analysis, it is important that the propensity score is modeled using all appropriate covariates to avoid issues arising from unmeasured confounding variables. Austin suggests various diagnostics that can be used to check the validity of such an analysis.

14.5.3 General Principles on Handling Data from Different Sources

DiSantostefano et al. (2016) recommended a set of principles when using data from different sources to conduct benefit–risk assessment. Some of their recommendations are equally applicable when using data from different sources to evaluate a drug's efficacy and safety individually. We include relevant key points below.

- Consider all available data sources, their value and utility as well as their intended uses when extracting information from these data sources.
- When interpreting data across studies involving different data sources, it is important to be aware of the characteristics and limitations of the studies. In some cases, results from randomized clinical trials may be able to generalize to larger populations via standardization to the larger populations.
- Context, including how well an outcome of interest is captured and in whom, is important. Population, endpoint identification and analytical approach may all contribute to differences in results from different sources, limiting direct comparison of results across different sources.
- As a general rule, inferentially combining data from different sources is not recommended. Results from different sources should be used to assess if findings are similar and if not, explore why they are different. Existing research has shown that even studies within the same type of data source (e.g., observational studies) may yield different results.
- Phase 3 clinical trials generally have limited generalizability to the population with a medical condition of interest. Hence, there is a need to expand the evidence in the postmarketing setting. This is important to the planning of pragmatic trials, which have attracted a lot of attention in recent years.
- New study designs (e.g., pragmatic randomized trials, randomized studies using electronic health records) offer new opportunities. These designs blur the line between randomized clinical trials and observational studies, but also offer new opportunities to conduct robust efficacy and safety assessment of a new drug in a less controlled setting.
- Safety assessment and, increasingly, comparative effectiveness are major activities in the postmarketing setting. Because of the lack of randomization in observational studies, one needs to adjust for confounding and identify differences in populations relative to the clinical trial setting.

14.6 Changes Over Time

We mentioned in Sect. 9.8 the need to be aware of how missing data were handled in prior studies because the method to handle missing data affected the estimate for the treatment effect.

Methods to handle missing data are not the only change that occurred over the last several decades. The advent of "professional patients" who move from trial to trial or even participate in several trials simultaneously has created real challenges for trial sponsors (McCann et al., 2015). These professional patients often do not adhere to study medications and provide data that may be of limited value. This challenge is especially a problem for developing drugs to treat central nervous system disorders.

At the other end of the disease spectrum are conditions that, if left untreated, could lead to high mortality and serious morbidity. For ethical reasons, trials of such conditions typically use the standard of care as the comparator and mortality or clinically important morbidity as the primary endpoint. Due to the advances in modern medicines and patient support care, the event rate in the control group has decreased substantially in recent years. The assumption on the event rate in the control group based on historical information may not be valid and adjustment of the sample size in mid-trial may be necessary. While the latter could be planned as part of an adaptive design, this requires additional understanding and planning upfront.

Thanks to lifestyle improvement and medical advancements, people are living longer. This also means that today's seniors are taking more medications than their ancestors. The phenomenon of poly-pharmacy requires a sponsor to anticipate more drug–drug interactions and to optimize the dosing schedule (e.g., once a day instead of twice a day). This shift in the population could also impact how similar a past trial population is to today's population.

There has also been a societal shift toward preventive medicine. Vaccines and treatment guidelines have helped reduce the incidence of certain diseases. While this is something to celebrate as a society, the increasing use of vaccines or immuno-modulators could also have an impact on the human immune system in general.

The conduct of multi-regional clinical trials (MRCTs) to support simultaneous global drug development (Chen & Quan, 2016) has added another layer of complexity to modern-day trials. Rising interest in MRCTs has prompted the International Council for Harmonisation to convene an expert working group and publish a guideline document on the general principles for planning and design of MRCTs (ICH E17, 2017). An MRCT could have hundreds of sites all over the world. Chuang-Stein (2016) stated the risk of launching a confirmatory MRCT when there was little knowledge of how patients in most regions would respond to the new treatment. We shared the story of Dimebon in Sect. 6.6. Dimebon was a new drug intended to treat Alzheimer's Disease. Dimebon's failed global Phase 3 program was based on a single positive Phase 2 trial conducted in Russia.

A premise for this book is the need to take full advantage of prior information that is pertinent and translatable when planning a new trial. The requirement of translatability is critical. Using prior information blindly without checking this requirement could do more harm than good.

14.7   Further Extensions of the Concept of Success Probability

Although POSS (probability of study success), POPS (probability of program success) and POCS (probability of compound success) are of interest in their own right, they can be rolled up further with other considerations to determine a probability of technical success (PTS) and a probability of technical and regulatory success

(PTRS). The former is defined as the probability of a compound generating favorable data to support a filing to regulators. The latter is the probability of this occurring and the filing being successful. Additional factors affecting the PTS (beyond those included in POCS) include findings from animal studies (especially the 2-year rat and 6-month transgenic mouse carcinogenicity studies), emerging new mechanistic insights that may impact the safety profile, manufacturing issues related to scaling up the production and sourcing the active pharmaceutical ingredients at a reasonable price. Unlike the calculation of POCS, the assessment of these other factors is often done in a less quantitative manner and may even include a subjective component.

As for PTRS, it includes regulatory precedents in approving drugs for the same indication and how regulators view the benefit–risk profile of the new drug. Some regulators place a greater emphasis on the safety of a pharmaceutical product while others are more willing to accept a higher level of risk if the product can deliver a greater level of efficacy. In recent years, there has been a plethora of medical, statistical and decision-making literature dedicated to the subject of structured benefit–risk assessment methods to evaluate pharmaceutical products. Some of these methods are qualitative (e.g., Coplan et al., 2011) while others are quantitative (e.g., Mussen et al., 2009). A good overview of benefit–risk evaluation methods can be found in Quartey et al. (2016).

Health authorities have also shown interest in a more systematic and transparent way to conduct benefit–risk assessment. For example, the Center for Devices and Radiological Health at the US FDA (FDA-CDRH) issued two guidance documents related to benefit–risk determinations in medical device premarket approvals (FDA, 2018; 2019). In addition, there has been an increasing awareness among regulators, supported by patient advocacy groups, that patient preference needs to be incorporated in the assessment of pharmaceutical products. This awareness has led to the first national benefit–risk preference study conducted by the FDA-CDRH in collaboration with the Research Triangle Institute Health Solutions. The study surveyed 654 obese patients to assess how much risk they were willing to tolerate in order to lose weight. Insight from the study led to an FDA-CDRH proposal on the benefit–risk paradigm for clinical trial design of obesity devices (Talamini, 2013). In 2016, FDA-CDRH finalized a guidance on the voluntary submission of patient preference information and the role of such information on the decision and labeling of a premarket approval application of a device (FDA, 2016).

We can expect to see a greater outreach to patients during the entire process of a pharmaceutical product by both regulators and pharmaceutical sponsors. Patient engagement is not only important during the clinical testing phase of a product, but is also critical in the ultimate acceptance of the product by the patient community.

Because of the extra factors involved, PTRS will generally be lower than PTS, which in turn will be lower than POCS in most cases.

We would like to point out that even after a product has received marketing authorization in a country and is being looked upon favorably by the medical and patient communities in that country, the product's sponsor still needs to demonstrate that the product is cost-effective for the product to be covered under the national health plan if the country provides universal health care to its nationals. The decision on coverage is typically based on an economic assessment referred to as cost-effectiveness assessment (CEA) or health technology assessment (HTA). The primary objective of a CEA or a HTA is to identify those healthcare technologies that, if funded, would maximize total population health for the available healthcare budget. The optimization is achieved by estimating differences in costs and effects between technologies and choosing those with the lowest opportunity costs. The assessment may lead to a decision to cover the product only in a subgroup of the population for which the product is indicated (Paget et al., 2011).

The coverage decision needs to be made separately in each country with a HTA requirement and may be based on complex models comparing different treatments balancing treatment benefits and costs over a long period of time. Many HTA authorities have published method guidelines for health technology appraisals (e.g., National Institute for Health & Care Excellence, 2013). As a result, a sponsor has to interact with each authority and potentially conduct different analyses. This introduces another source of uncertainty and affects the overall chance of a product's becoming a commercially successful product. One can incorporate this additional uncertainty and calculate the probability that a product will be successful commercially. Understandably, this probability is likely to be lower than PTRS.

Readers who are interested in learning more about CEA or HTA are encouraged to read Briggs et al. (2006).

14.8 Wrapping Up

In this book, we show how clinical trials perform like a series of diagnostic tests and the condition to diagnose is whether a new drug has a clinically meaningful effect. The trials at the early stage serve as screening tests. As the need for more precision arises, subsequent trials will be designed with more sensitivity and specificity. Under this analogy, the positive predictive value (PPV) of a trial conveys useful information on the likelihood that the new drug has the desirable effect. This is conceivably one of the most relevant questions of concern to both the sponsor who develops the drug and regulators who need to decide if the drug is approvable.

The PPV of a diagnostic test may vary among subgroups of patients due to the intrinsic and extrinsic factors associated with patients in the subgroups. Similarly, intrinsic and extrinsic factors could affect a drug's effect in subgroups. Thus, the PPV of a drug may vary among different subgroups. For example, black people tend to receive less benefit from many antihypertensive drugs compared to other races.

We discuss the probability of success at the study, development stage and program level. We stress the importance to consider such probabilities in conjunction with statistical power when planning a trial or a series of trials. The distinction between the probability of success and statistical power is particularly pertinent for late stage development when we have accumulated a fair amount of information about a new drug's ability to induce a response. This knowledge should be incorporated into the planning of a future trial and the estimation of the likelihood of a positive outcome. We are glad to see the uptake of this concept in the statistical community. In our opinion, the concept of probability of success in general can help statisticians communicate with clinicians because many clinicians prefer thinking in terms of the chance of an outcome unconditionally instead of conditionally.

Product development is a continuum. As a general rule, a sponsor will progress only compounds that look promising to the next stage. This rule, while sensible and supported by the diagnostic analogy, creates a statistical challenge in estimating the true treatment effect. To understand this challenge, Chuang-Stein and Kirby (2014) drew a conceptual comparison between the Phase 2–3 development stages and interim analyses of a trial with a group sequential design. They considered the simple case when the target patient population stayed the same throughout Phase 2–3 and treatment effect was measured by the same endpoint at the same time point of interest. They compared Phase 2 and Phase 3 testing to a long-running clinical investigation structured by a group sequential design with a few pre-determined interim points labeled as end of POC, end of Phase 2b, and end of Phase 3. The design allows early stopping for efficacy and futility based on the observed treatment effect at these interim points. Zhang et al. (2012) discussed how overestimation could occur under a group sequential design if the efficacy boundary was crossed early in the trial and one used the observed treatment effect as an estimate for the true treatment effect. The same overestimation applies, for example, when we use the observed treatment effect to estimate the true treatment effect in a very positive proof-of-concept trial.

The overestimation mentioned above needs to be accounted for when we use results from a positive trial to plan a future trial. This is especially important if we hope to size the new study to detect an effect that is above the minimum clinically meaningful effect but considered plausible based on the results from a positive trial. We discussed in Chap. 12 several approaches that had been investigated to discount previous positive results. In our opinion, this is probably one area where awareness is not yet as widespread as we would like to see in the pharmaceutical industry. We hope this book will help increase this awareness as sponsors plan new trials.

Go/No-Go decisions are needed at the end of various development stages. It is useful to quantitatively assess the quality of the decisions by describing the risks associated with them. Simulation has become a regular tool to perform the assessment. In this book, we discuss metrics that are helpful to enable the decisions. We acknowledge the many possible metrics including those we have proposed and used ourselves. We want to emphasize that every situation is different and should be evaluated in its own right. Our goal of writing this book is to provide the setup for a general framework, well aware that customization is needed for specific applications.

Even though modeling can be conducted separately for efficacy and safety, dose decision and drug approval are ultimately based on the trade-off between benefits and risks of a new drug at the dose(s) submitted for regulatory approval. The emphasis on this trade-off has prompted some sponsors to consider ways to combine efficacy and safety into one endpoint. We included some of these efforts in Chap. 11 (see Sect. 11.5) and this chapter. We expect greater efforts to be devoted to this area in the future.

Some of our non-statistician colleagues are dismayed by the relatively low probability of success figures for Phase 3 studies obtained by the approaches discussed in this book, when comparing them to the statistical power (e.g., 90%) used to design the studies. A good way to help them understand the lower figures is to explain the need to calibrate our expectations concerning the outcome of these trials. The calibration takes into account what we have observed previously and how strong the existing evidence about the drug candidate is. As such, the probability of success figure for late stage trials is much more in line with the empirical success rate we have observed among these trials than the statistical power. Working on the probability of success scale can thus better prepare the research community for the phenomenon that a good portion of our late stage studies will fail.

We will end the book by sharing an interesting story that highlights a case of regulatory decisions on doses. Because all drugs have side effects and the incidences of drug-related adverse reactions typically increase with doses, regulators tend to favor lower doses if lower doses also meet the efficacy criterion set up in the confirmatory trials. This preference has led to the search for the minimum effective dose on many occasions. The minimum effective dose is usually defined as the lowest dose that yields a clinically meaningful therapeutic benefit to patients when compared to a placebo. Consequently, if multiple doses are submitted for approval and if a higher dose is considered to have much more unfavorable side effects than can be justified by its additional benefits, regulators often prefer not approving the high dose.

This is why the approval of the 150 and not the 110 mg of dabigatran was a surprise to many people. The FDA approved dabigatran for the reduction of the risk of stroke and systemic embolism in patients with non-valvular atrial fibrillation on October 19, 2010. As stated in Beasley et al. (2011), the approval was based on results from a multi-center, active-control trial, the Randomized Evaluation of Long-Term Anticoagulation Therapy (RE-LY). In RE-LY, patients were randomized in equal proportions to 150 mg of dabigatran, 110 mg of dabigatran or warfarin. The primary endpoint is a composite endpoint of stroke or systemic embolism. RE-LY is a non-inferiority trial. The non-inferiority margin for the primary efficacy endpoint (a dabigatran dose against warfarin) is 1.38. Both the 150 mg and 110 mg of dabigatran were shown to be non-inferior to warfarin on efficacy. In addition, the 150 mg was significantly superior to warfarin and the 110 mg on efficacy.

The main adverse drug reaction is major bleeding. For major bleeding, 110 mg dabigatran was superior to warfarin, while 150 mg was similar to warfarin. Looking at these results, it is clear that both 110 mg and 150 mg have some advantage over warfarin. For the 110 mg, it is the better bleeding profile without sacrificing the efficacy. For the 150 mg, it is the better efficacy profile without causing worse bleeding than warfarin. Beasley et al. (2011) acknowledged that either dose would have been considered safe and effective against warfarin (and therefore approvable) if studied alone in a trial.

There were 49 more stroke or systemic embolism events in the 110 mg group than in the 150 mg (183 versus 134). The number of additional stroke events in the 110 mg was also 49 (171 versus 122). On the other hand, the number of major bleeding episodes in the 150 mg group was 57 more than that in the 110 mg group (399 versus

342). The number of life-threatening bleeding episodes in the 150 mg group was 34 higher than that in the 110 mg group (193 versus 159). If stroke/systemic embolism and major bleeding were considered equally undesirable, 150 mg and 110 mg would have similar net benefit and risk. However, many consider the irreversible effects of stroke and systemic emboli to have greater clinical significance than non-fatal bleeding. From this perspective, 150 mg has an overall benefit–risk advantage over the 110 mg, based on the results in RE-LY.

As a side story, Beasley et al. (2011) described FDA's attempt to identify, within RE-LY, subgroups for whom the benefit–risk assessment of 110 mg could be more favorable than 150 mg since the 110 mg was associated with a lower bleeding risk. The FDA looked for patients with impaired renal function (since dabigatran is cleared primarily through the kidneys, impaired renal function implies a higher dabigatran blood level and a potentially higher chance for bleeding), patients who experienced hemorrhage previously (a pre-disposition for bleeding), and elderly patients (who tend to bleed more easily in general). The FDA was not able to find any subpopulation for whom 110 mg has a better benefit–risk profile.

In the end, Beasley et al. stated that the FDA felt that "playing it safe" (i.e., using 110 mg) for patients and by physicians represented an undesirable stimulus to using a less effective regimen and would lead to unnecessary strokes and disability. This consideration plus the inability to identify a subgroup for which 110 mg would be more favorable in terms of benefit and risk led the FDA to approve only the 150 mg dose for dabigatran.

Everybody is standing, but you must stand out.

Everybody is breaking grounds; but you must breakthrough!

Everybody scratching it; but you must scratch it hard!

Everybody is going, but you must keep going extra miles!

Dare to be exceptionally excellent and why not?

Israelmore Ayivor

References

Akaike, H. (1973). Information theory and an extension of the maximum likelihood principle. In B. N. Petrov, F. Csáki (Eds.), *2nd International Symposium on Information Theory* (pp. 267–281), Tsahkadsor, Armenia, USSR, September 2–8, 1971. Akadémiai Kiadó, Budapest.

Austin, P. C. (2011). An introduction to propensity score methods for reducing the effects of confounding in observational studies. *Multivariate Behavioural Research, 46*(3), 399–424.

Beasley, B. N., Unger, E. F., & Temple, R. (2011). Anticoagulant options—Why the FDA approved a higher but not a lower dose of dabigatran. *New England Journal of Medicine, 364*(19), 1788–1790.

Bretz, F., Pinheiro, J. C., & Branson, M. (2005). Combining multiple comparisons and modeling techniques in dose-response studies. *Biometrics, 61*(3), 738–748.

Briggs, A., Claxton, K., & Sculpher, M. (2006). *Decision modelling for health economic evaluation.* Oxford University Press.

Chen, J., & Quan, H. (2016). *Multiregional clinical trials for simultaneous global new drug development.* Chapman and Hall/CRC Press.

Chuang-Stein, C., & Kirby, S. (2014). The shrinking or disappearing observed treatment effect. *Pharmaceutical Statistics, 13*(5), 277–280.

Chuang-Stein, C. (2016). The journey to multiregional clinical trials in support of simultaneous global product development. In J. Chen, H. Quan (Eds.), *Multiregional Clinical Trials for Simultaneous Global New Drug Development*. Chapman and Hall/CRC Press.

Coplan, P. M., Noel, R. A., Levitan, B. S., et al. (2011). Development of a framework for enhancing the transparency, reproducibility and communication of the benefit–risk balance of medicines. *Clinical Pharmacology & Therapeutics, 89*(2), 312–315.

Cox, D. R., & Hinkley, D. V. (1974). *Theoretical statistics*. Chapman and Hall.

DiSantostefano, R., Berlin, J. A., Chuang-Stein, C., et al. (2016). Selecting and integrating data sources in benefit-risk assessment: Considerations and future directions. *Statistics in Biopharmaceutical Research, 8*(4), 394–403.

Gelman, A., Carlin, J. B., Stern, H. S., & Rubin, D. B. (2004). *Bayesian data analysis* (2nd ed.). Chapman and Hall/CRC Press.

International Council for Harmonisation E17. (2017). General principles for planning and design of multi-regional clinical trials.

Ioannidis, J. P. A. (2008). Why most discovered true associations are inflated? *Epidemiology, 19*(5), 640–648.

McCann, D. J., Petry, N. M., Bresell, A., et al. (2015). Medication nonadherence, "professional subjects", and apparent placebo responders: Overlapping challenges for medications development. *Journal of Clinical Psychopharmacology, 35*(5), 566–573.

Mukhopadhyay, S. (2019). *Predicting technical success of a Phase III program using Bayesian latent relationship model*. Presented at the Joint Statistical Meetings, Denver Colorado, July 30. Accessed 21 March 2021, from https://ww2.amstat.org/meetings/jsm/2019/onlineprogram/AbstractDetails.cfm?abstractid=304313.

Mussen, F., Salek, S., & Walker, S. (2009). *Benefit-risk appraisal of medicines: A systematic approach to decision-making*. Wiley.

National Institute for Health and Care Excellence. (2013). *Guide to the methods of technology appraisal*, UK, NHS. Available at: http://www.nice.org.uk/article/PMG9/chapter/Foreword. Accessed 21 March, 2021.

Paget, M.-A., Chuang-Stein, C., Fletcher, C., & Reid, C. (2011). Subgroup analyses of clinical effectiveness to support health technology assessments. *Pharmaceutical Statistics, 10*(6), 532–538.

Quartey, G., Ke, C., Chuang-Stein, C., et al. (2016). Overview of benefit-risk evaluation methods: A spectrum from qualitative to quantitative. In Q. Jiang, & W. He (Eds.), *Benefit-risk assessment methods in medicinal product development: Bridging qualitative and quantitative assessments*. Chapman and Hall/CRC Press.

Rosenbaum, P. R. (2010). *Design of observational studies*. Springer.

Talamini, M. A. (2013). Benefit-risk paradigm for clinical trial design of obesity devices: FDA proposal. *Surgical Endoscopy, 27*(3), 701.

Tao, A., Lin, Y., Pinheiro, J., & Shih, W. J. (2015). Dose finding method in joint modeling of efficacy and safety endpoints in phase II studies. *International Journal of Statistics and Probability, 4*(1), 33–45.

Thall, P. F., Cook, J. D., & Estey, E. H. (2006). Adaptive dose selection using efficacy-toxicity trade-offs: Illustrations and practical considerations. *Journal of Biopharmaceutical Statistics, 16*(5), 623–638.

U.S. Food and Drug Administration Guidance for industry, Food and Drug Administration Staff, and Other Stakeholders. (2016). *Patient preference information—Voluntary submission, review in premarket approval applications, humanitarian device exemption applications, and de novorequests, and inclusion in decision summaries and device labeling*.

U.S. Food and Drug Administration Guidance for Industry and Food and Drug Administration Staff. (2018). *Benefit-risk factors to consider when determining substantial equivalence in premarket notifications (510(k)) with different technological characteristics*.

U.S. Food and Drug Administration Guidance for Industry and Food and Drug Administration Staff. (2019). *Factors to consider when making benefit-risk determinations in medical device premarket approval and* de novo classifications.

Walley, R., Sherington, J., Rastrick, J., et al. (2016). Using Bayesian analysis in repeated preclinical *in vivo* studies for a more effective use of animals. *Pharmaceutical Statistics, 15*(3), 277–285.

Zhang, J. J., Blumenthal, G. M., He, K., et al. (2012). Overestimation of the effect size in group sequential trials. *Clinical Cancer Research, 18*(18), 4872–4876.

Appendix

In this appendix, we include selected R and WinBUGS programs that produced the results reported in the book. To make the programs easier to read functions have not been used but a competent R programmer could shorten at least some of the programs by making use of functions.

The R packages referred to in the text and used in some of the programs are available from https://cran.r-project.org/. The packages need to be installed and then loaded into R using the library() function.

The version of R used was version 4.0.2 and the version of WinBUGS used was WinBUGS 1.4.3. Please direct any question about codes to Simon Kirby at s.kirby1.kirby@btinternet.com.

Chapter 5, Table 5.2

```
#require statistical significance at one-sided 2.5% level


#set random number seed
set.seed(80835459)
#number of simulations
nsim<-10000
#required true treatment effect to be of interest
reqdelta<-3
#sample size per group
nsamp<-100
#true variance of the endpoint
var<-49
#correct positive decision counter
corrpos<-0
#incorrect positive decision counter
incorrpos<-0
```

```
#correct negative decision counter
corrneg<-0
#incorrect negative decision counter
incorrneg<-0


#begin the simulations
for (ss in 1:nsim){

    #sample true delta from a prior assumed to be a Normal
    #distribution with mean 3.27 and SD of 0.6
    delta<-rnorm(1,3.27,0.6)

    #sample difference in the observed means
    diff<-rnorm(1,delta,sqrt(2*var/nsamp))

    #construct the test statistic
    test<-diff/sqrt(2*var/nsamp)

    #correct positive decision
    if((test>=qnorm(0.975))&(delta>=reqdelta))
      corrpos<-corrpos+1

    #incorrect positive decision
    if((test>=qnorm(0.975))&(delta<reqdelta))
      incorrpos<-incorrpos+1

    #correct negative decision
    if((test<qnorm(0.975))&(delta<reqdelta))
      corrneg<-corrneg+1

    #incorrect negative decision
    if((test<qnorm(0.975))&(delta>=reqdelta))
      incorrneg<-incorrneg+1

}

#correct positive decision proportion
corrpos/nsim
#incorrect positive decision proportion
incorrpos/nsim
#correct negative decision proportion
corrneg/nsim
#incorrect negative decision proportion
incorrneg/nsim
```

Chapter 6, Table 6.3

```
#require statistical significance at one-sided 2.5% level
#and observed treatment effect ≥ 3 for a positive decision
#set random number seed
set.seed(58974595)
```

```
#number of simulations
nsim<-10000
#required true treatment effect to be of interest
reqdelta<-3
#sample size per group
nsamp<-225
#true variance of the endpoint
var<-49
#correct positive decision counter
corrpos<-0
#incorrect positive decision counter
incorrpos<-0
#correct negative decision counter
corrneg<-0
#incorrect negative decision counter
incorrneg<-0

#begin simulations
for (ss in 1:nsim){

              #sample true delta from a prior assumed to be a Normal
              #distribution with mean 3.27 and SD of 0.6
              delta<-rnorm(1,3.27,0.6)

              #sample difference in the observed means
              diff<-rnorm(1,delta,sqrt(2*var/nsamp))

              #construct the test statistic
              test<-diff/sqrt(2*var/nsamp)

              #correct positive decision
              if((test>=qnorm(0.975)&(diff>=3))&(delta>=reqdelta))
                corrpos<-corrpos+1

              #incorect positive decision
              if((test>=qnorm(0.975)&(diff>=3))&(delta<reqdelta))
                incorrpos<-incorrpos+1

              #correct negative decision
              if((test<qnorm(0.975)|(diff<3))&(delta<reqdelta))
                corrneg<-corrneg+1

              #incorrect negative decision
              if((test<qnorm(0.975)|(diff<3))&(delta>=reqdelta))
                incorrneg<-incorrneg+1
              }

#correct positive decision proportion
corrpos/nsim
#incorrect positive decision proportion
```

```
incorrpos/nsim
#correct negative decision proportion
corrneg/nsim
#incorrect negative decision proportion
incorrneg/nsim
```

Chapter 7, Figures 7.2 – 7.4

```
#first set of plot commands give Go probabilities
#second set of plot commands give Pause probabilities
#third set of plot commands give Stop probabilities

#minimum clinically important difference
MCID<-0.3
#target value
TV<-0.5
#assumed true standard deviation of the endpoint equal to 1
#vector of effect sizes with increment of 0.01
effectsize<-c(seq(0,1,0.01))

#sample size per group under Trad approach (one-sided 2.5%
#significance level and 80% power)
tradn<-ceiling(((qnorm(0.975)+qnorm(0.8))^2*2)/MCID^2)
tradn

#vectors to store Go and Stop probabilities for the Trad
#approach
tradgo<-NA
tradstop<-NA

#index for vectors to hold Trad results
index<-0

#calculate Trad Go and Stop probabilities for vector of
#effect sizes
for (ee in effectsize){


        index<-index+1
        tradgo[index]<-pnorm(sqrt(tradn*ee^2/2)-qnorm(0.975))
        tradstop[index]<-1-tradgo[index]
    }

#sample size per group for the ESOE approach
esoen<-ceiling(((qnorm(0.95)+qnorm(0.80))^2*2)/TV^2)

#vectors to store Go, Stop and Pause probabilities for ESOE
```

```
esoego<-NA
esoestop<-NA
esoepause<-NA

#index for vectors to hold results
index<-0

#calculate ESOE Go, Stop and Pause probabilities for vector
#of effect sizes
for (ee in effectsize){

     index<-index+1
     esoego[index]<-pnorm(sqrt(esoen*ee^2/2)-qnorm(0.95))
     esoestop[index]<-1-pnorm(sqrt(esoen*ee^2/2)-qnorm(0.80))
     esoepause[index]<-1-esoego[index]-esoestop[index]
  }

#number supplied from a separate sample size calculation for
#LPDAT
lpdatn<-135

#vectors to store Go, Stop and Pause probabilities for LPDAT
lpdatgo<-NA
lpdatstop<-NA
lpdatpause<-NA
#index for vectors to hold results
index<-0

#calculate LPDAT Go, Stop and Pause probabilities for vector
#of effect sizes
#NB Go probability can be calculated as below because
#requirement that lower confidence interval limit exceeds
#MCID dominates requirement that upper confidence interval
#limit exceeds TV for this example
for (ee in effectsize){

               index<-index+1
               lpdatgo[index]<-1-pnorm(MCID,ee-qnorm(0.80)*
               sqrt(2/lpdatn),sqrt(2/lpdatn))
               lpdatstop[index]<-pnorm(TV,ee+qnorm(0.95)*sqrt(2/lpdatn)
               ,sqrt(2/lpdatn))
               lpdatpause[index]<-1-lpdatgo[index]-lpdatstop[index]
            }

#sample size per group for TV
TVn<-ceiling(2*qnorm(0.95)^2/TV^2)
```

```
#vectors to store Go and Stop probabilities for TV
TVgo<-NA
TVstop<-NA
```

```
#index for vectors to hold results
index<-0
```

```
#calculate TV Go and Stop probabilities for vector of effect
#sizes
#NB Go probability can be calculated as below because
#precision requirement satisfied if observed
#effect >= TV
for (ee in effectsize){
```

```
            index<-index+1
            TVgo[index]<-(1-pnorm(TV,ee,sqrt(2/TVn)))
            TVstop[index]<-1-TVgo[index]
        }
```

```
#sample size per group for TVMCID
TVncomp<-ceiling(2*qnorm(0.95)^2/(TV-MCID)^2)
```

```
#vector to store Go and Stop probabilities for TVMCID
TVcompgo<-NA
TVcompstop<-NA
```

```
#index for vectors to hold results
#NB Go probability can be calculated as below because
#precision requirement is satisfied if observed effect >= TV
index<-0
```

```
#calculate Go and Stop probabilities for TVMCID
for (ee in effectsize){
```

```
            index<-index+1
            TVcompgo[index]<-(1-pnorm(TV,ee,sqrt(2/TVncomp)))
            TVcompstop[index]<-1-TVcompgo[index]
        }
```

```
#plot Go probabilities
plot(effectsize,tradgo,typ='l',lty=1,col='black',
ylab='probability',xlab='effect size',lwd=2,cex.axis=2,
cex.lab=2,xaxt='n')
lines(effectsize,esoego,lty=2,col='blue',lwd=2)
lines(effectsize,lpdatgo,lty=3,col='red',lwd=2)
lines(effectsize,TVgo,lty=4,col='brown',lwd=2)
```

```
lines(effectsize,TVcompgo,lty=5,col='brown',lwd=2)
legend(0.7,0.6,legend=c('Trad (n=175)','ESOE (n=50)',
'LPDAT (n=135)','TV (n=22)',expression(TV[MCID] ~"(n=136)"))
,lty=c(1,2,3,4,5),col=c('black','blue','red','brown','brown'),
lwd=2,cex=2)
axis(1,at=c(0.2,0.3,0.4,0.5,0.6,0.8),labels=c('0.2','MCID',
'0.4','TV','0.6','0.8'),cex.axis=2)

#plot Pause probabilities
plot(effectsize,esoepause,lty=2,col='blue',ylim=c(0,1),
ylab='probability',xlab='effect size',typ='l',lwd=2,
cex.axis=2,cex.lab=2)
lines(effectsize,lpdatpause,lty=3,col='red',lwd=2)
legend(0.7,0.6,legend=c('ESOE (n=50)','LPDAT (n=135)'),
lty=c(2,3),col=c('blue','red'),lwd=2,cex=2)
axis(1,at=c(0.2,0.3,0.4,0.5,0.6,0.8),labels=c('0.2','MCID',
'0.4','TV','0.6','0.8'),cex.axis=2)

#plot Stop probabilities
plot(effectsize,tradstop,typ='l',lty=1,col='black',
ylab='probability',xlab='effect size',lwd=2,cex.axis=2,
cex.lab=2)
lines(effectsize,esoestop,lty=2,col='blue',lwd=2)
lines(effectsize,lpdatstop,lty=3,col='red',lwd=2)
lines(effectsize,TVstop,lty=4,col='brown',lwd=2)
lines(effectsize,TVcompstop,lty=5,col='brown',lwd=2)
legend(0.7,0.8,legend=c('Trad (n=175)','ESOE (n=50)',
'LPDAT (n=135)','TV (n=22)',expression(TV[MCID] ~"(n=136)"))
,lty=c(1,2,3,4,5),col=c('black','blue','red','brown',
'brown'),lwd=2,cex=2)
axis(1,at=c(0.2,0.3,0.4,0.5,0.6,0.8),labels=c('0.2','MCID',
'0.4','TV','0.6','0.8'),cex.axis=2)
```

Chapter 7, Tables 7.2 – 7.6

```
#simulate probabilities for Tables 7.2 to 7.6 assessing POC
#designs in chapter 7
#correct decision if positive decision and delta greater
#than or equal to MCID

#set random number seed
set.seed(11684145)
#number of simulations
nsim<-10000
#assumed true sigma
sigma<-1
```

```
#MCID value
MCID<-0.3
#TV value
TV<-0.5
#significance level for traditional test
alphatrad<-0.025

#ESOE error probability for accelerating a compound with no
#effect
ESOEacc0<-0.05
#ESOE probability for killing a compound with no effect
ESOEkill0<-0.80

#confidence for upper confidence limit for lpdat
upplpdat<-0.95
#confidence for lower confidence limit for lpdat
lowlpdat<-0.80

#sample sizes derived as described in chapter
ntrad<-175
nesoe<-50
nlpdat<-135
nTV<-22
nTVMCID<-136

#counters to hold counts of various outcomes for different
#approaches
corrpostrad<-0
incorrpostrad<-0
corrnegtrad<-0
incorrnegtrad<-0

corrposesoe<-0
incorrposesoe<-0
corrnegesoe<-0
incorrnegesoe<-0
pauseesoe_h<-0
pauseesoe_l<-0

corrposlpdat<-0
incorrposlpdat<-0
corrneglpdat<-0
incorrneglpdat<-0
pauselpdat_h<-0
pauselpdat_l<-0

corrposTV<-0
```

```
incorrposTV<-0
corrnegTV<-0
incorrnegTV<-0

corrposTVMCID<-0
incorrposTVMCID<-0
corrnegTVMCID<-0
incorrnegTVMCID<-0

#simulations

for (ss in 1:nsim){
```

```
#simulate from treatment effect prior - start with a
#random number from uniform distribution from 0 to 1
rannum<-runif(1,0,1)

#delta if randum number less than 0.8
if(rannum<0.80)
  delta<-0

#delta if random number greater than or equal to 0.8
if(rannum>=0.80)
  delta<-rnorm(1,0.5,0.17)

#generated sample means for each approach allowing for
#different sample sizes
traddiff<-rnorm(1,delta,sqrt(2*sigma^2/ntrad))
esoediff<-rnorm(1,delta,sqrt(2*sigma^2/nesoe))
lpdatdiff<-rnorm(1,delta, sqrt(2*sigma^2/nlpdat))
TVdiff<-rnorm(1,delta,sqrt(2*sigma^2/nTV))
TVMCIDdiff<-rnorm(1,delta,sqrt(2*sigma^2/nTVMCID))

#correct positive, incorrect positive, incorrect negative and
#correct negative counts by approach
#pause probabilities also captured for ESOE and lpdat
#approaches

if((traddiff/sqrt(2*sigma^2/ntrad)>=qnorm(1-alphatrad))&
(delta>=MCID)){
  corrpostrad<-corrpostrad+1
}else if((traddiff/sqrt(2*sigma^2/ntrad)>=qnorm(1-alphatrad)
)&(delta<MCID)){
  incorrpostrad<-incorrpostrad+1
}else if((traddiff/sqrt(2*sigma^2/ntrad)<qnorm(1-alphatrad))
&(delta>=MCID)){
  incorrnegtrad<-incorrnegtrad+1
}else
  corrnegtrad<-corrnegtrad+1

if((esoediff/sqrt(2*sigma^2/nesoe)>=qnorm(1-ESOEacc0))&
(delta>=MCID)){
```

```
    corrposesoe<-corrposesoe+1
  }else if((esoediff/sqrt(2*sigma^2/nesoe)>=qnorm(1-
ESOEacc0))&(delta<MCID)){
    incorrposesoe<-incorrposesoe+1
  }else if((esoediff/sqrt(2*sigma^2/nesoe)<qnorm(ESOEkill0)
)&(delta>=MCID)){
    incorrnegesoe<-incorrnegesoe+1
  }else if((esoediff/sqrt(2*sigma^2/nesoe)<qnorm(ESOEkill0)
)&(delta<MCID)){
    corrnegesoe<-corrnegesoe+1

  }else if (delta>=MCID){
   pauseesoe_h<-pauseesoe_h+1
  }else
   pauseesoe_l<-pauseesoe_l+1


if((lpdatdiff+qnorm(upplpdat)*sqrt(2*sigma^2/nlpdat)>=TV)
&(lpdatdiff-qnorm(lowlpdat)*sqrt(2*sigma^2/nlpdat)>MCID)&
(delta>=MCID)){
   corrposlpdat<-corrposlpdat+1
 }else if((lpdatdiff+qnorm(upplpdat)*sqrt(2*sigma^2/nlpdat
)>=TV)&(lpdatdiff-qnorm(lowlpdat)*sqrt(2*sigma^2/nlpdat)>
MCID)&(delta<MCID)){
   incorrposlpdat<-incorrposlpdat+1
 }else if((lpdatdiff+qnorm(upplpdat)*sqrt(2*sigma^2/nlpdat
)<TV)&(delta>=MCID)){
   incorrneglpdat<-incorrneglpdat+1
 }else if((lpdatdiff+qnorm(upplpdat)*sqrt(2*sigma^2/nlpdat)
<TV)&(delta<MCID)){
   corrneglpdat<-corrneglpdat+1
 }else if (delta>=MCID){
  pauselpdat_h<-pauselpdat_h+1
 }else
   pauselpdat_l<-pauselpdat_l+1
```

```
if((TVdiff>=TV)&(delta>=MCID)){
  corrposTV<-corrposTV+1
}else if((TVdiff>=TV)&(delta<MCID)){
  incorrposTV<-incorrposTV+1
}else if((TVdiff<TV)&(delta>=MCID)){
  incorrnegTV<-incorrnegTV+1
}else
  corrnegTV<-corrnegTV+1

if((TVMCIDdiff>=TV)&(delta>=MCID)){
  corrposTVMCID<-corrposTVMCID+1
}else if((TVMCIDdiff>=TV)&(delta<MCID)){
  incorrposTVMCID<-incorrposTVMCID+1
}else if((TVMCIDdiff<TV)&(delta>=MCID)){
  incorrnegTVMCID<-incorrnegTVMCID+1
}else
  corrnegTVMCID<-corrnegTVMCID+1
}


#convert counts to probabilities for each approach by
#dividing by nsim
#print correct positive, incorrect positive, correct
#negative and incorrect negative decision for each
#approach; print positive predictive value and negative
#predictive value for each approach
#print pause probabilities by whether true difference >=
#MCID or not

corrpostrad<-corrpostrad/nsim
incorrpostrad<-incorrpostrad/nsim
corrnegtrad<-corrnegtrad/nsim
incorrnegtrad<-incorrnegtrad/nsim
print(cbind(corrpostrad,incorrpostrad,corrnegtrad,
incorrnegtrad))

tradPPV<-corrpostrad/(corrpostrad+incorrpostrad)
tradNPV<-corrnegtrad/(corrnegtrad+incorrnegtrad)
print(cbind(tradPPV,tradNPV))

corrposesoe<-corrposesoe/nsim
incorrposesoe<-incorrposesoe/nsim
corrnegesoe<-corrnegesoe/nsim
incorrnegesoe<-incorrnegesoe/nsim
print(cbind(corrposesoe,incorrposesoe,corrnegesoe,
incorrnegesoe))
```

```
esoePPV<-corrposesoe/(corrposesoe+incorrposesoe)
esoeNPV<-corrnegesoe/(corrnegesoe+incorrnegesoe)
print(cbind(esoePPV,esoeNPV))
print(cbind(pauseesoe_h/nsim,pauseesoe_l/nsim))

corrposlpdat<-corrposlpdat/nsim
incorrposlpdat<-incorrposlpdat/nsim
corrneglpdat<-corrneglpdat/nsim
incorrneglpdat<-incorrneglpdat/nsim
print(cbind(corrposlpdat,incorrposlpdat,corrneglpdat,
incorrneglpdat))
lpdatPPV<-corrposlpdat/(corrposlpdat+incorrposlpdat)
lpdatNPV<-corrneglpdat/(corrneglpdat+incorrneglpdat)
print(cbind(lpdatPPV,lpdatNPV))
print(cbind(pauselpdat_h/nsim,pauselpdat_l/nsim))

corrposTV<-corrposTV/nsim
incorrposTV<-incorrposTV/nsim
corrnegTV<-corrnegTV/nsim
incorrnegTV<-incorrnegTV/nsim
print(cbind(corrposTV,incorrposTV,corrnegTV,incorrnegTV))
TVPPV<-corrposTV/(corrposTV+incorrposTV)
TVNPV<-corrnegTV/(corrnegTV+incorrnegTV)
print(cbind(TVPPV,TVNPV))

corrposTVMCID<-corrposTVMCID/nsim
incorrposTVMCID<-incorrposTVMCID/nsim
corrnegTVMCID<-corrnegTVMCID/nsim
incorrnegTVMCID<-incorrnegTVMCID/nsim
print(cbind(corrposTVMCID,incorrposTVMCID,corrnegTVMCID,
incorrnegTVMCID))
TVMCIDPPV<-corrposTVMCID/(corrposTVMCID+incorrposTVMCID)
TVMCIDNPV<-corrnegTVMCID/(corrnegTVMCID+incorrnegTVMCID)
print(cbind(TVMCIDPPV,TVMCIDNPV))
```

Chapter 7, Figures 7.5 – 7.7

```
#first set of plot commands give Go probabilities
#second set of plot commands give Pause probabilities
#third set of plot commands give Stop probabilities
#placebo response
plaresp<-0.3
#minimum clinically important difference
MCID<-0.2
#target value
TV<-0.3
```

```
#vector of effect sizes with increment of 0.01, from 0 to TV
effectsize<-c(seq(0,TV,0.01))

#sample size per group under Trad approach (one-sided 2.5%
#significance level and 80% power)
vardiff<-(plaresp+MCID)*(1-plaresp-MCID)+plaresp*(1-plaresp)
tradn<-ceiling(((qnorm(0.975)+qnorm(0.8))^2*vardiff)/MCID^2)

#vectors to store Go and Stop probabilities for the Trad
#approach
tradgo<-NA
tradstop<-NA

#index for vectors to hold Trad results
index<-0

#calculate Trad Go and Stop probabilities for vector of
#effect sizes
for (ee in effectsize){

            index<-index+1
            vardiff<-(plaresp+ee)*(1-plaresp-ee)+(plaresp)*
            (1-plaresp)
            tradgo[index]<-pnorm(sqrt(tradn*ee^2/vardiff)-
            qnorm(0.975))
            tradstop[index]<-1-tradgo[index]
        }

#sample size per group for the ESOE approach
#set to 0.5*tradn if > 0.5*tradn
vardiff<-(plaresp+TV)*(1-plaresp-TV)+plaresp*(1-plaresp)
esoen<-ceiling(((qnorm(0.95)+qnorm(0.80))^2*vardiff)/TV^2)
halftradn<-floor(tradn/2)
if(esoen>halftradn)

            esoen<-halftradn

#vectors to store Go, Stop and Pause probabilities for ESOE
esoego<-NA
esoestop<-NA
esoepause<-NA
#index for vectors to hold results
index<-0
```

```
#calculate ESOE Go, Stop and Pause probabilities for vector
#of effect sizes
for (ee in effectsize){


        index<-index+1
        vardiff<-(plaresp+ee)*(1-plaresp-ee)+(1-plaresp)*plaresp
        esoego[index]<-pnorm(sqrt(esoen*ee^2/vardiff)
        -qnorm(0.95))
        esoestop[index]<-1-pnorm(sqrt(esoen*ee^2/vardiff)
        -qnorm(0.80))
        esoepause[index]<-1-esoego[index]-esoestop[index]
}


#number supplied from a separate sample size calculation for
#LPDAT
lpdatn<-124

#vectors to store Go, Stop and Pause probabilities for LPDAT
lpdatgo<-NA
lpdatstop<-NA
lpdatpause<-NA
#index for vectors to hold results
index<-0

#calculate LPDAT Go, Stop and Pause probabilities for vector
#of effect sizes
#NB Go probability can be calculated as below because
#requirement that lower confidence interval limit exceeds
#MCID dominates requirement that upper confidence interval
#limit exceeds TV for this example
for (ee in effectsize){


        index<-index+1
        vardiff<-(plaresp+ee)*(1-plaresp-ee)+(1-plaresp)*plaresp
        lpdatgo[index]<-1-pnorm(MCID,ee-qnorm(0.80)*
        sqrt(vardiff/lpdatn),sqrt(vardiff/lpdatn))
        lpdatstop[index]<-pnorm(TV,ee+qnorm(0.95)*
        sqrt(vardiff/lpdatn),sqrt(vardiff/lpdatn))
        lpdatpause[index]<-(1-lpdatgo[index]-lpdatstop[index])
}


#sample size per group for TV
vardiff<-(plaresp+TV)*(1-plaresp-TV)+(1-plaresp)*plaresp
```

```
TVn<-ceiling(vardiff*qnorm(0.95)^2/TV^2)

#vectors to store Go and Stop probabilities for TV
TVgo<-NA
TVstop<-NA

#index for vectors to hold results
index<-0

#calculate TV Go and Stop probabilities for vector of effect
#sizes
#NB Go probability can be calculated as below because
#precision requirement satisfied if observed
#effect >= TV
for (ee in effectsize){


        index<-index+1
        vardiff<-(plaresp+ee)*(1-plaresp-ee)+(1-plaresp)*plaresp
        TVgo[index]<-(1-pnorm(TV,ee,sqrt(vardiff/TVn)))
        TVstop[index]<-1-TVgo[index]
    }

#sample size per group for TVMCID
vardiff<-(plaresp+TV)*(1-plaresp-TV)+plaresp*(1-plaresp)
TVncomp<-ceiling(vardiff*qnorm(0.95)^2/(TV-MCID)^2)

#vector to store Go and Stop probabilities for TVMCID
TVcompgo<-NA
TVcompstop<-NA

#index for vectors to hold results
#NB Go probability can be calculated as below because
#precision requirement is satisfied if observed effect >= TV
index<-0

#calculate Go and Stop probabilities for TVMCID
for (ee in effectsize){


    index<-index+1
    vardiff<-(plaresp+ee)*(1-plaresp-ee)+(1-plaresp)*plaresp
    TVcompgo[index]<-(1-pnorm(TV,ee,sqrt(vardiff/TVncomp)))
    TVcompstop[index]<-1-TVcompgo[index]
  }
```

```
#plot Go probabilities
plot(effectsize,tradgo,typ='l',lty=1,col='black',
ylab='probability',xlab='effect size',lwd=2,cex.axis=2,
cex.lab=2,xaxt='n',ylim=c(0,1))
lines(effectsize,esoego,lty=2,col='blue',lwd=2)
lines(effectsize,lpdatgo,lty=3,col='red',lwd=2)
lines(effectsize,TVgo,lty=4,col='brown',lwd=2)
lines(effectsize,TVcompgo,lty=5,col='brown',lwd=2)
legend('topleft',legend=c('Trad (n=91)','ESOE (n=31)',
'LPDAT (n=124)','TV (n=14)',expression(TV[MCID] ~"(n=122)"))
,lty=c(1,2,3,4,5),
col=c('black','blue','red','brown','brown'),
lwd=1.5,cex=1.5)
axis(1,at=c(0,0.1,0.2,0.3),labels=c('0','0.1','0.2','0.3'),
cex.axis=2)

#plot Pause probabilities
plot(effectsize,esoepause,lty=2,col='blue',ylim=c(0,1),
ylab='probability',xlab='effect size',typ='l',lwd=2,
cex.axis=2,cex.lab=2,xaxt='n')
lines(effectsize,lpdatpause,lty=3,col='red',lwd=2)
legend('topleft',legend=c('ESOE (n=31)','LPDAT (n=124)'),
lty=c(2,3),col=c('blue','red'),lwd=1.5,cex=1.5)
axis(1,at=c(0.2,0.3),labels=c('0.2','0.3'),cex.axis=2)

#plot Stop probabilities
plot(effectsize,tradstop,typ='l',lty=1,col='black',
ylab='probability',xlab='effect size',lwd=2,cex.axis=2,
cex.lab=2,ylim=c(0,1),xaxt='n')
lines(effectsize,esoestop,lty=2,col='blue',lwd=2)
lines(effectsize,lpdatstop,lty=3,col='red',lwd=2)
lines(effectsize,TVstop,lty=4,col='brown',lwd=2)
lines(effectsize,TVcompstop,lty=5,col='brown',lwd=2)
legend('bottomleft',legend=c('Trad (n=91)','ESOE (n=31)',
'LPDAT (n=124)','TV (n=14)',expression(TV[MCID] ~"(n=122)"))
,lty=c(1,2,3,4,5),col=c('black','blue','red','brown',
'brown'),lwd=1.5,cex=1.5)
axis(1,at=c(0.2,0.3),labels=c('0.2','0.3'),cex.axis=2)
```

Chapter 8, Tables 8.2 – 8.5

```
#for table 8.2
#width=0.1
#dose<-c(rep(0,30),rep(2,30),rep(4,30),rep(6,30),rep(8,30))
#alldose<-c(0,2,4,6,8)
#Emax varied as -1.2, -1.5 and -1.8
```

#seeds used for random numbers
#pessimistic 66558519
#base 215551
#optimistic 4665132

#For table 8.3
#width=0.1
#dose<-c(rep(0,60),rep(2,60),rep(4,60),rep(6,60),rep(8,60))
#alldose<-c(0,2,4,6,8)
#Emax varied as -1.2, -1.5 and -1.8
#seeds used for random numbers
#pessimistic 61213048
#base 72937763
#optimistic 33979873

#For table 8.4
#width=0.15, 0.20, 0.25 or 0.30
#dose<-c(rep(0,30),rep(2,30),rep(4,30),rep(6,30),rep(8,30))
#alldose<-c(0,2,4,6,8)
#Emax varied as -1.2, -1.5 and -1.8
#seeds used for random numbers
#0.15 width, pessimistic 69002499
#0.15 width, base 73928088
#0.15 width, optimistic 55318173
#0.20 width, pessimistic 6915962
#0.20 width, base 83966698
#0.20 width, optimistic 70845545
#0.25 width, pessimistic 20776442
#0.25 width, base 11384123
#0.25 width, optimistic 86133592
#0.30 width, pessimistic 59115048
#0.30 width, base 36608344
#0.30 width, optimistic 73736949

#For table 8.5
#width=0.1
#dose<-c(rep(0,40),rep(1,40),rep(2,15),rep(5,15),rep(8,40))
#alldose<-c(0,1,2,5,8)
#Emax varied as -1.2, -1.5 and -1.8
#seeds used for random numbers
#pessimistic 89681883
#base 53257519
#optimistic 28034564

#settings for a particular (width, dose, sample size, Emax)
#combination

```
width<-0.10
dose<-c(rep(0,40),rep(1,40),rep(2,15),rep(5,15),rep(8,40))
#available doses
alldose<-c(0,1,2,5,8)
trueEmax<-(-1.8)
rand<-28034564

set.seed(rand)

#number of simulations
nsim<-10000

#true variance
sigmasq<-4.5

#true values of parameters
trueE0<-0
trueED50<-0.79
truelogED50<-log(trueED50)

#target efficacy
target<-(-1)

#target value interval from lowtarget to hightarget allowing
#for width difference from target value
lowtarget<-target*(1-width)
hightarget<-target*(1+width)

#true doses satisfying lowtarget and hightarget values
#if hightarget value not achieveable then dose set to a
#large value
lowtargetdose<-trueED50/(trueEmax/lowtarget-1)
hightargetdose<-trueED50/(trueEmax/hightarget-1)
if(trueEmax>=hightarget){

                    hightargetdose<-1000000
                    }

#bounds for parameter values

lower.E0<-(-1000000)
upper.E0<-1000000

lower.Emax<-(-1000000)
upper.Emax<-1000000

lower.logED50<-(-10)
```

```
upper.logED50<-10

#number of doses
ndose<-length(alldose)
#counter for trend test
trendcount<-0
#counter for estimated dose being in target dose interval
targetdosecount<-0
#sum of average prediction error
sumAPE<-0
#sum of relative average prediction error
sumpAPE<-0

#true response for all available doses under the 3-parameter
#Emax model with ED50=0.79.
truealldose<-trueEmax*alldose/(0.79+alldose)

targetdosecount<-0

#for loop for simulations
for(ss in 1:nsim){
```

```
#simulate errors
errorsim<-rnorm(150,0,sqrt(4.5))

#add errors to true response
ysim<-trueEmax*dose/(trueED50+dose)+errorsim

#fit linear regression on dose
fit2<-lm(ysim~dose)
#t test for slope coefficient
ttest<-summary(fit2)$coef[,"t value"][2]
pval<-pt(ttest,fit2$df.residual)

#assess significance of trend test
if(pval<0.05){
  trendyes<-1
  trendcount<-trendcount+trendyes
}else{
  trendyes<-0
}

#nls fit
fit<-nls(ysim ~ E0+Emax*dose/(exp(logED50)+dose),
start=list(E0=0,Emax=trueEmax,logED50=truelogED50),
alg="port",lower=c(lower.E0,lower.Emax,lower.logED50),
upper=c(upper.E0,upper.Emax,upper.logED50),
trace=FALSE,control=nls.control(tol=1e-05,warnOnly=TRUE))

#estimated parameters
estparams<-coef(fit)

#fit for all available doses
allfit<-estparams[1]+estparams[2]*alldose/(exp(estparams[3])
+alldose)
```

```
        #if estimated Emax < target value of -1 then calculated dose
        #estimated to give target effect
        #otherwise set estimated dose to 0
        if(estparams[2]<target){
          estdose<-exp(estparams[3])/(estparams[2]/target-1)
        }else{
          estdose<-0
        }

        #increment targetdosecount if trend test significant and
        #estimated dose in target dose interval
        if((estdose>=lowtargetdose)&(estdose<=hightargetdose)&
        (trendyes==1))
          targetdosecount<-targetdosecount+1

        #average prediction error
        APE<-(sum(abs(allfit-truealldose))/ndose)
        #sum average prediction error
        sumAPE<-sumAPE+APE
        #relative average prediction error
        pAPE<-APE/abs(target)
        #sum relative average prediction error
        sumpAPE<-sumpAPE+pAPE
      }

#probability of trend test being significant
trendcount/nsim
#trend test significant
targetdosecount/trendcount
#mean of the average prediction error
sumAPE/nsim
#mean of the relative average prediction error
sumpAPE/nsim
```

Chapter 8, Table 8.6

```
#Priors for the parameters
#N(0, 0.1^2) for E0
#N(-1.5, 0.2^2) for Emax
#t distn with 3 df with scale parameter = 0.6 and
#mean = 0.79 for log(ED50/P50)
#P50 (coincidentally) set equal to 0.79
#beta distribution with parameters 3.03 and 18.15 scaled to
#the interval (0, 6) for lambda
```

```
#number of simulations
nsim<-10000
#P50<-0.79
#available non-zero doses
dose<-c(1,2,3,4,5,6,7,8)
#random number used for seed 7546193
rand<-7546193
set.seed(rand)

#simulate E0
rE0<-rnorm(nsim,0,0.1)
#simulate Emax
rEmax<-rnorm(nsim,-1.5,0.2)
#simulate ED50
tval<-rt(nsim,3)
rED50<-exp(tval*0.6+0.79)*P50
#simulate lambda
rlambda<-rbeta(nsim,3.03,18.15)*6

#repeat dose sequence for each simulation
alldose<-c(rep(dose,nsim))

#repeat each simulated parameter by number of doses
allrE0<-rep(rE0,each=8)
allrEmax<-rep(rEmax,each=8)
allrED50<-rep(rED50, each=8)
allrlambda<-rep(rlambda, each=8)
#effect versus placebo for simulated parameters
effect<-(allrEmax*alldose^allrlambda)/(allrED50^allrlambda+
alldose^allrlambda)

#summary statistics of effects at different doses
summary(effect[alldose==1])
summary(effect[alldose==2])
summary(effect[alldose==3])
summary(effect[alldose==4])
summary(effect[alldose==5])
summary(effect[alldose==6])
summary(effect[alldose==7])
summary(effect[alldose==8])
```

Chapter 8, Tables 8.8 to 8.9

```
#For table 8.8
#dose<-c(rep(0,30),rep(2,30),rep(4,30),rep(6,30),rep(8,30))
#alldose<-c(0,2,4,6,8)
#random number used for seed
```

```
#72320230

#For table 8.9
#dose<-c(rep(0,40),rep(1,40),rep(2,15),rep(5,15),rep(8,40))
#alldose<-c(0,1,2,5,8)
#random number used for seed
#33254623

#settings for a particular program run (e.g., Table 8.9)
dose<-c(rep(0,40),rep(1,40),rep(2,15),rep(5,15),rep(8,40))
#available doses
alldose<-c(0,1,2,5,8)
rand<-33254623

set.seed(rand)

#Priors for the parameters in the 4-parameter Emax model
#N(0, 0.1^2) for E0
#N(-1.5, 0.2^2) for Emax
#t distn with 3 df with scale parameter = 0.6 and
#mean = 0.79 for log(ED50/P50)
#P50 (coincidentally) set equal to 0.79
#beta with parameters 3.03 and 18.15 scaled by 6 for lambda

#number of simulations
nsim<-10000
#true variance
sigmasq<-4.5
P50<-0.79
#target efficacy
target<-(-1)
#bounds for parameter values
lower.E0<-(-1000000)
upper.E0<-1000000
lower.Emax<-(-1000000)
upper.Emax<-1000000
lower.logED50<-(-10)
upper.logED50<-10
lower.lambda<-0.01
upper.lambda<-5

#number of doses
ndose<-length(alldose)
#counter for trend test
trendcounttrue<-0
trendcountfalse<-0
#counter for estimated dose in target dose interval
```

```
targetdosetrue<-0
targetdosefalse<-0
#sum of average prediction error
sumAPE<-0
#sum of relative average prediction error
sumpAPE<-0
sumpAPEtrue<-0
sumpAPEfalse<-0
ntrue<-0
nfalse<-0

#for loop for simulations
for(ss in 1:nsim){
```

```
#simulate E0
rE0<-rnorm(1,0,0.1)

#simulate Emax
rEmax<-rnorm(1,-1.5,0.2)

#simulate ED50
tval<-rt(1,3)
rED50<-exp(tval*0.6+0.79)*P50

#log simulated ED50 for R fit
logrED50<-log(rED50)

#simulate lambda
rlambda<-rbeta(1,3.03,18.15)*6

#true mean responses
truealldose<-rE0+rEmax*alldose^rlambda/(rED50^rlambda+
alldose^rlambda)
truealleffect<-rEmax*alldose^rlambda/(rED50^rlambda+
alldose^rlambda)

#low and high targets for allowed target interval
lowtarget<-target*0.9
hightarget<-target*1.1


#true doses giving lowtarget and hightarget values

#if lowtarget achieveable determine true dose giving
#lowtarget else set this dose to a large value
if(rEmax<lowtarget){
  lowtargetdose<-rED50/((rEmax/lowtarget-1)^(1/rlambda))
}else{
  lowtargetdose<-1000000
}
```

```
#if hightarget achieveable determine true dose giving
#hightarget else set this dose to a large value
if(rEmax<hightarget){
  hightargetdose<-rED50/((rEmax/hightarget-1)^
(1/rlambda))
}else{
  hightargetdose<-1000000
}

#whether top dose achieves target efficacy, initially set
#to 0 for no
topdoseokay<-0

if(truealleffect[ndose]<=-1)
  topdoseokay<-1

#simulate errors
errorsim<-rnorm(150,0,sqrt(sigmasq))

#add errors to model
ysim<-rE0+rEmax*dose^rlambda/(rED50^rlambda+dose^rlambda)
+errorsim

#fit linear regression on dose
fit2<-lm(ysim~dose)

# t test for slope coefficient
ttest<-summary(fit2)$coef[,"t value"][2]
pval<-pt(ttest,fit2$df.residual)

trendyes<-0

#assess significance of trend test
if((pval<0.05)&(topdoseokay==1)){
  trendcounttrue<-trendcounttrue+1
  trendyes<-1
}else if((pval<0.05)){
  trendcountfalse<-trendcountfalse+1
  trendyes<-1
}
```

```
#nls fit
fit<-nls(ysim ~ E0+Emax*dose^lambda/(exp(logED50)^lambda+
dose^lambda),
start=list(E0=rE0,Emax=rEmax,logED50=logrED50,
lambda=rlambda),alg="port",lower=c(lower.E0,lower.Emax,
lower.logED50,lower.lambda),upper=c(upper.E0,upper.Emax,
upper.logED50,upper.lambda),trace=FALSE,
control=nls.control(tol=1e-05,warnOnly=TRUE))

#estimated parameters
estparams<-coef(fit)

#fit for all available doses
allfit<-estparams[1]+estparams[2]*alldose^estparams[4]/
(exp(estparams[3])^estparams[4]+alldose^estparams[4])

#if estimated Emax < target of -1 calculate dose giving
#target effect else set estimated dose to 0
if(estparams[2]<target){
  estdose<-exp(estparams[3])/((estparams[2]/target-1)^
  (1/estparams[4]))
}else{
  estdose<-0
}

#if estimated dose in target dose interval and trend test
#significant then increment targetdosetrue or
#targetdosefalse depending if top dose gives a true effect of
#at least 1 compared with placebo
if((estdose>=lowtargetdose)&(estdose<=hightargetdose)&
(trendyes==1)){
  if(topdoseokay==1){
    targetdosetrue<-targetdosetrue+1
  }else{
    targetdosefalse<-targetdosefalse+1
  }
}
```

```
            #average prediction error
            APE<-(sum(abs(allfit-truealldose))/ndose)

            #sum average prediction error
            sumAPE<-sumAPE+APE

            #relative average prediction error
            pAPE<-APE/abs(target)

            #sum relative average prediction error
            if(topdoseokay==1){
              sumpAPEtrue<-sumpAPEtrue+pAPE
              ntrue<-ntrue+1
            }else{
              sumpAPEfalse<-sumpAPEfalse+pAPE
              nfalse<-nfalse+1
            }

            sumpAPE<-sumpAPE+pAPE
          }

#probability of trend test being significant and effect of top
#dose <=-1
trendcounttrue/nsim

#probability of trend dose being significant and effect of
#top dose not <= -1
trendcountfalse/nsim

#probability estimated dose in target dose interval and
#effect of top dose <=-1 given trend test significant
targetdosetrue/(trendcounttrue+trendcountfalse)

#probability estimated dose in target dose interval and
#effect of top dose NOT <=-1 given trend test significant
targetdosefalse/(trendcounttrue+trendcountfalse)

#APE
sumAPE/nsim
#pAPE overall
sumpAPE/nsim
#pAPE when top dose gives at least target effect
sumpAPEtrue/ntrue
#pAPE when top dose does not achieve target effect
sumpAPEfalse/nfalse
```

Chapter 8, Tables 8.10 – 8.11

```
library("R2WinBUGS")

#For Table 8.10
#dose<-c(rep(0,30),rep(2,30),rep(4,30),rep(6,30),rep(8,30))
#alldose<-c(0,2,4,6,8)
#simulations done as 4 sets of 250 with following seeds for
#random numbers
#68162410
#13624885
#62080175
#34180515

#For Table 8.11
#dose<-c(rep(0,40),rep(1,40),rep(2,15),rep(5,15),rep(8,40))
#alldose<-c(0,1,2,5,8)
#simulations done as 4 sets of 250 with following seeds for
#random numbers
#70029005
#84436182
#53321012
#35248536

#settings for a particular program run
dose<-c(rep(0,40),rep(1,40),rep(2,15),rep(5,15),rep(8,40))
#available doses
alldose<-c(0,1,2,5,8)
rand<-35248536

#Bayesian prior for design
#E0 N(0, 0.1^2) for E0
#Emax N(-1.5, 0.2^2) for Emax
#t distn with 3 df with scale parameter = 0.6 and
#mean = 0.79 for log(ED50/P50)
#P50 (coincidentally) set equal to 0.79
#beta with parameters 3.03 and 18.15 scaled by 6 for lambda

set.seed(rand)

#number of simulations
nsim<-250
#true variance
sigmasq<-4.5
P50<-0.79
#target efficacy
target<-(-1)
```

```
#number of subjects
N<-length(dose)
#number of doses
K<-length(alldose)
#counter for Emax test
Emaxcounttrue<-0
Emaxcountfalse<-0
#counter for estimated dose in target dose interval
targetdosetrue<-0
targetdosefalse<-0
#sum of average prediction error
sumAPE<-0
#sum of relative average prediction error
sumpAPE<-0
sumpAPEtrue<-0
sumpAPEfalse<-0
ntrue<-0
nfalse<-0

#initial values to supply to WinBUGS
inits<-list(list(E0=0,Emax=(-1.2),logratio=0.7,lambda=1,
prec=0.01),
list(E0=0,Emax=(-1.5),logratio=0.79,lambda=0.9,prec=0.01),
list(E0=0,Emax=(-1.8),logratio=0.9,lambda=0.8,prec=0.01))

#for loop for simulations
for(ss in 1:nsim){
```

```
#simulate true E0
rE0<-rnorm(1,0,0.1)
#simulate true Emax
rEmax<-rnorm(1,-1.5,0.2)
#simulate true ED50
tval<-rt(1,3)
rED50<-exp(tval*0.6+0.79)*P50
#log of ED50
logrED50<-log(rED50)
#simulate true lambda
rlambda<-rbeta(1,3.03,18.15)*6

truealldose<-rE0+(rEmax*alldose^rlambda)/(rED50^rlambda+
alldose^rlambda)
truealleffect<-(rEmax*alldose^rlambda)/(rED50^rlambda+
alldose^rlambda)

#low and high targets
lowtarget<-target*0.9
hightarget<-target*1.1

#low and high target doses
if(rEmax<lowtarget){
  lowtargetdose<-rED50/((rEmax/lowtarget-1)^(1/rlambda))
}else{
  lowtargetdose<-1000000
}

if(rEmax<hightarget){
  hightargetdose<-rED50/((rEmax/hightarget-1)^(1/rlambda))
}else{
  hightargetdose<-1000000

}

#whether top dose achieves target efficacy
topdoseokay<-0
if(truealleffect[K]<=-1)
  topdoseokay<-1
```

```
#simulate errors
errorsim<-rnorm(150,0,sqrt(4.5))
#add errors to model
ysim<-rE0+(rEmax*dose^rlambda)/(rED50^rlambda+dose^
rlambda)+errorsim

#data for WinBUGS
data<-list(N=N,dose=dose,ysim=ysim,K=K,alldose=alldose,
lowtargetdose=lowtargetdose,
hightargetdose=hightargetdose)

#where WinBUGS file is – replace with file location
filetxt=c(
"M:/book/Chapter 8/programs and outputs/Emax
- 20160916.txt")

#call WinBUGS – replace directory location
emaxfit<-bugs(data,inits,model.file=filetxt,
parameters=c("E0","Emax","logED50","lambda","allfit",
"alleffect","loweffect","higheffect"),n.chains=3,
n.iter=100000,n.burnin=50000,
bugs.directory='C:\\Program Files (x86)\\WinBUGS14',
program='OpenBUGS')

#place simulated Emax values in a vector
emaxsims<-emaxfit$sims.matrix[,2]

#sort simulated Emax values
emaxsort<-sort(emaxsims)

#95th percentile of distribution of simulated Emax values
testper<-quantile(emaxsort,0.95)

#counter for Emax test
Emaxyes<-0
```

```
#if 95th percentile of simulated Emax values less than 0 then
#test is significant
#further if top dose gives at least required effect using
#true parameter values then Emaxcounttrue
#incremented by 1 else Emaxcountfalse
if((testper<0)&(topdoseokay==1)){
   Emaxcounttrue<-Emaxcounttrue+1
   Emaxyes<-1
}else if(testper<0){
   Emaxcountfalse<-Emaxcountfalse+1
   Emaxyes<-1
}
#if posterior mean effect for lowest dose in target dose
#interval > target of -1 and estimated
#posterior mean effect for highest dose in target dose
#interval < target of -1 then dose giving
#posterior mean effect equal to target must be in allowed
#target dose interval
if((emaxfit$mean$loweffect>=target)&
(emaxfit$mean$higheffect<=target)){
   if(topdoseokay==1){
      targetdosetrue<-targetdosetrue+1
   }else{
      targetdosefalse<-targetdosefalse+1
   }
}

#average prediction error
APE<-(sum(abs(emaxfit$mean$allfit-truealldose))/K)
#sum average prediction error
sumAPE<-sumAPE+APE
#relative average prediction error
pAPE<-APE/abs(target)
#sum relative average prediction error
```

```
                    if(topdoseokay==1){
                      sumpAPEtrue<-sumpAPEtrue+pAPE
                      ntrue<-ntrue+1
                    }else{
                      sumpAPEfalse<-sumpAPEfalse+pAPE
                      nfalse<-nfalse+1
                    }

                    sumpAPE<-sumpAPE+pAPE
                  }
```

#probability of Emax test being significant when top dose
#achieves at least target effect using true parameter values
Emaxcounttrue/nsim

#probability of Emax test being significant when top dose
#does not achieve at least the target
Emaxcountfalse/nsim

#probability estimated dose in target dose interval given a
#significant Emax test when top dose achieves target
#efficacy using true #parameter values
targetdosetrue/(Emaxcounttrue+Emaxcountfalse)

#probability estimated dose in target dose interval given a
#significant Emax test when top dose does not achieve at
#least the target effect using true parameter values
targetdosefalse/(Emaxcounttrue+Emaxcountfalse)

#APE
sumAPE/nsim
#pAPE
sumpAPE/nsim

#pAPE when top dose does achieve target efficacy using true
#parameter values
sumpAPEtrue/ntrue
#pAPE when top dose does not achieve target efficacy using
#true parameter values
sumpAPEfalse/nfalse

WinBUGS program for Tables 8.10–8.11

#WinBUGS code for fit of Emax model with informative prior
#prior for E0 Normal with mean 0 and variance 0.1^2
#prior for Emax Normal with mean -1.5 and variance 0.2^2
#prior for log(ED50/P50) t with 3 degrees of freedom,

#location = 0.79 and scale 0.6, P50 set equal to 0.79

```
model{

        for (i in 1:N)
          {
            #distribution for individual observation
            ysim[i] ~ dnorm(mean[i],prec)

            #model mean
            mean[i]<-E0+(Emax*pow(dose[i],slambda))/
            (pow(exp(logED50),slambda)+
            pow(dose[i],slambda))
          }

        #placebo fit
        allfit[1]<-E0

        #fit and effects for all doses
        for (i in 2:K)
          {
            allfit[i]<-E0+(Emax*pow(alldose[i],slambda)
             )/(pow(exp(logED50),slambda)
            +pow(alldose[i],slambda))
            alleffect[i]<-(Emax*pow(alldose[i],slambda)
             )/(pow(exp(logED50),slambda)+
            pow(alldose[i],slambda))
          }

        #effect for lowest dose in target dose interval
        loweffect<-(Emax*pow(lowtargetdose,slambda))/
        (pow(exp(logED50),slambda)
        +pow(lowtargetdose,slambda))
        #effect for highest dose in target dose interval
        higheffect<-(Emax*pow(hightargetdose,slambda)
         )/(pow(exp(logED50),slambda)+
        pow(hightargetdose,slambda))
```

```
                              #priors
                              E0~dnorm(0,100)
                              Emax~dnorm(-1.5,25)
                              logratio~dt(0.79,2.78,3)
                              logED50<-logratio+log(0.79)
                              lambda~dbeta(3.03,18.15)
                              slambda<-lambda*6

                              prec~dgamma(0.001,0.001)
                  }
```

Chapter 9, Table 9.1

```
#values at which power is to be calculated
powerpts<-c(0.35,0.45,0.55,0.65,0.75,0.85,0.95,1.05)

#set prob to NA so prob recognised by R
prob<-NA

#probabilities of required intervals
prob[1]<-pnorm(log(0.4),-0.34,0.24)
prob[2]<-pnorm(log(0.5),-0.34,0.24)-
pnorm(log(0.4),-0.34,0.24)
prob[3]<-pnorm(log(0.6),-0.34,0.24)-
pnorm(log(0.5),-0.34,0.24)
prob[4]<-pnorm(log(0.7),-0.34,0.24)-
pnorm(log(0.6),-0.34,0.24)
prob[5]<-pnorm(log(0.8),-0.34,0.24)-
pnorm(log(0.7),-0.34,0.24)
prob[6]<-pnorm(log(0.9),-0.34,0.24)-
pnorm(log(0.8),-0.34,0.24)
prob[7]<-pnorm(log(1),-0.34,0.24)-
pnorm(log(0.9),-0.34,0.24)
prob[8]<-1-pnorm(log(1),-0.34,0.24)

#print vector of probabilities
prob

#power at required values
power<-pnorm(-qnorm(0.975)-log(powerpts)/sqrt(4/460))
power

#components of probability of success
pos<-power*prob
pos

#overall probability of success
```

sum(pos)

Chapter 9, Table 9.2

```
#set random number seed
set.seed(38683166)

#number of simulations
nsim<-10000

#counters for correct positive, incorrect negative,
#incorrect positive and correct negative decisions
#when a true positive decision is defined by the true log
#hazard ratio is less than or equal to 0.75 and the
#one-sided p-value <=0.025
correctpos<-0
incorrneg<-0
incorrpos<-0
correctneg<-0

for(ss in 1:nsim){


              #simulate true log hazard
              loghazard<-rnorm(1,-0.34,0.24)
              #simulate observed log hazard
              estloghazard<-rnorm(1,loghazard,sqrt(4/460))

              #one-sided p-value for test of log hazard
              pval<-1-pnorm(0,estloghazard,sqrt(4/460))

              if((exp(loghazard)<=0.75)&(pval<=0.025)){
                correctpos<-correctpos+1
              }else if((exp(loghazard)<=0.75)&(pval>0.025)){
                incorrneg<-incorrneg+1
              }else if((exp(loghazard)>0.75)&(pval<=0.025)){
                incorrpos<-incorrpos+1
              }else
                correctneg<-correctneg+1


}

#proportions of correct positive, incorrect negative,
#incorrect positive and correct negative results
correctpos/nsim
incorrneg/nsim
```

incorrpos/nsim
correctneg/nsim

Chapter 10, Tables 10.4 – 10.5

```
#sample size = 191 for Table 10.4
#sample size varied for Table 10.5
#random number seed for Table 10.4
#17041253
#random number seeds for Table 10.5
#n=250 27777393
#n=400 27709135
#n=600 79130894
#n=800 74768143
#n=1000 5562509

#codes for when sample size is set at 1000
sampsize<-1000

#set seed
rand<-5562509
set.seed(rand)

#number of simulations
nsim<-10000

#counters for true positive, false positive, true negative
#and false negative results
#positive decision is defined by significance at the
#one-sided 2.5% level
truepos<-0
falsepos<-0
trueneg<-0
falseneg<-0

#critical value for one-sided test
critval<-qnorm(0.975)
#assumed variance
var<-1

#simulations
for(ss in 1:nsim){
```

```
#simulate delta
simdelta<-rnorm(1,0.287,0.2504)
#simulate difference using simulated delta
simdiff<-rnorm(1,simdelta,sqrt(2/sampsize))
#standard error
se<-sqrt(2*var/sampsize)
#test statistic
zval<-simdiff/se

if((zval>=critval)&(simdelta>0)){
   truepos<-truepos+1
}else if((zval>=critval)&(simdelta<=0)){
   falsepos<-falsepos+1
}else if((zval<critval)&(simdelta>0)){
   falseneg<-falseneg+1
}else
   trueneg<-trueneg+1
}
```

```
#proportions of true positive, false positive,
#false negative and true negative results
truepos/nsim
falsepos/nsim
falseneg/nsim
trueneg/nsim

#probability of study success poss
poss<-(truepos+falsepos)/nsim
poss

#positive predictive value

ppv<-truepos/(truepos+falsepos)
ppv
#print sample size, probability of study success and
#positive predictive value
cbind(sampsize,poss,ppv)
```

Chapter 12, Figure 12.3

```
#prior as used for pain example in chapter 2
#use discretized grid to calculate
#theta value for first component
theta1<-0
#density for first component
```

```
prior1<-0.2
#theta values for second component
theta2<-c(seq(0.01,5,0.01))
#density for second component
prior2<-dnorm(theta2,2.5,0.8)*0.8

#observed effects for plotting
yval<-c(seq(1.94,5,0.01))
#counter for indexing vector of posterior expected values
count<-0
#vector to hold posterior expected values
expect<-NA

for(yy in yval){

        count<-count+1
        #sum over theta of prior times likelihood for first
        #component
        sumy1<-sum(dnorm(yy,theta1,sqrt(2*49/100))*prior1)
        #sum over theta of prior times likelihood for second
        #component
        sumy2<-sum(dnorm(yy,theta2,sqrt(2*49/100))*prior2)
        #probability of data
        proby<-sumy1+sumy2

        #prior times likelihood divided by probability of data
        # - first component
        post1<-prior1*dnorm(yy,theta1,sqrt(2*49/100))/proby
        #prior times likelihood divided by probability of data
        # - second component
        post2<-prior2*dnorm(yy,theta2,sqrt(2*49/100))/proby
        #posterior expected value
        expect[count]<-sum(c(post1,post2)*c(theta1,theta2))
        #print observed difference and posterior expected value
        print(cbind(yy,expect[count]))
}

#plot observed difference versus posterior expected value
plot(yval,expect,xlim=c(1.94,5),ylim=c(1.94,5),typ='l',
xlab='observed Phase 2 treatment effect',
ylab='posterior expected effect',lwd=2,cex=2,cex.lab=2,
cex.axis=2,col='blue')
```

```
#observed values greater than 2.5
resyval<-yval[yval>2.5]
#reverse order of observed values
resyval<-rev(resyval)

#posterior expected values for observed values greater
#than 2.5
resexp<-expect[yval>2.5]
#reverse order of expected values
resexp<-rev(resexp)

#shade in area between 45 degree line and plot of observed
#versus posterior expected value
polygon(x=c(2.5,5,resyval),y=c(2.5,5,resexp),density=5)

#add 45 degree line
abline(a=0,b=1)
```

Chapter 12, Figure 12.4

```
#prior as used for pain example in chapter 2
#use discretized grid to calculate
#theta values for first component
theta1<-0

#density for first component
prior1<-0.2

#theta values for second component
theta2<-c(seq(0.01,5,0.01))

#density for second component
prior2<-dnorm(theta2,2.5,0.8)*0.8
#observed effects for plotting
yval<-c(seq(1.94,5,0.01))

#index for vector of posterior expected values
count<-0
#vector for posterior expected values
expect<-NA
#vector for difference between observed and posterior
#expected value
diff<-NA
#vector for difference between observed and posterior
#expected value as percentage of observed value
per<-NA
for(yy in yval){
```

```
    count<-count+1
    #sum over theta of prior times likelihood for first
    #component
    sumy1<-sum(dnorm(yy,theta1,sqrt(2*49/100))*prior1)
    #sum over theta of prior times likelihood for second
    # component
    sumy2<-sum(dnorm(yy,theta2,sqrt(2*49/100))*prior2)
    #probability of data
    proby<-sumy1+sumy2

    #prior times likelihood divided by probability of data
    # - first component
    post1<-prior1*dnorm(yy,theta1,sqrt(2*49/100))/proby
    #prior times likelihood divided by probability of data
    # - second component
    post2<-prior2*dnorm(yy,theta2,sqrt(2*49/100))/proby
    #posterior expected value
    expect[count]<-sum(c(post1,post2)*c(theta1,theta2))
    #print observed difference and posterior expected value
    print(cbind(yy,expect[count]))
    #difference between observed and posterior expected value
    diff[count]<-(yy-expect[count])
    #difference as percentage of observed value
    per[count]<-diff[count]/yy*100
  }

#plot of observed value versus difference as percentage of
#observed
plot(yval,per,xlim=c(2.5,5),ylim=c(0,35),typ='l',
xlab='observed Phase 2 treatment effect',
ylab='difference (as %)',lwd=2,cex=2,cex.lab=2,cex.axis=2)
```

Chapter 13, Tables 13.5 - 13.6 and 13.9

```
#program to calculate metrics for fixed design for

#two Scenarios

#load library MASS to be able to use mvrnorm function
library(MASS)

#seed for scenario 1
set.seed(4516891)

#seed for scenario 2
```

```
#set.seed(5714783)

#all doses used in original study
alldose<-c(0.1,0.3,0.5,1,0,2.5,4,10)

#all log doses - log dose for enoxaparin set equal to 0
alllogdose<-log(c(0.1,0.3,0.5,1,1,2.5,4,10))

#Factor Xa VTE results in original study

#number of patients with VTEs in original study
responders<-c(13,33,30,23,34,16,1,3)

#number of patients assessed for VTE in original study
denom<-c(35,89,104,120,188,112,74,27)

#factor distinguishing enoxaparin from doses of Pfizer drug
allenoxfac<-factor(x=c(1,1,1,1,2,1,1,1))

#0/1 vector picking out enoxaparin result
allenoxselect<-c(0,0,0,0,1,0,0,0)

#number of patients without a VTE in original study
nonresponders<-denom-responders

#combined vector for number of subjects with
#and without a VTE
y<-cbind(responders,nonresponders)

#fit logistic model
fit<-glm(y ~ allenoxfac+alllogdose,family=binomial)
#save coefficients
mu<-fit$coefficients[1]
alpha<-fit$coefficients[2]
beta<-fit$coefficients[3]
vcov<-vcov(fit)

#save linear predictor
linpred<-fit$linear.predictors

#obtain stand errors for linear predictor
predout<-predict.glm(fit,se.fit=TRUE)
selinpred<-predout$se.fit
#transformed lower 99.9% confidence interval for prediction
lcllin<-linpred-qnorm(0.999)*selinpred
lcllin<-exp(lcllin)/(1+exp(lcllin))

#transformed upper 99.9% confidence interval for prediction
ucllin<-linpred+qnorm(0.999)*selinpred
```

```
ucllin<-exp(ucllin)/(1+exp(ucllin))

#transformed prediction
pred<-exp(linpred)/(1+exp(linpred))

#vector to pick out Pfizer drug doses
doseselect<-c(1,2,3,4,6,7,8)

#frame for 2 graphs in one row
par(mfrow=c(1,2))

#plot transformed predictions and 99.9% confidence intervals
plot(exp(alllogdose[doseselect]),pred[doseselect],typ='l',
xlim=c(0,10),ylim=c(0,1),
xlab='dose mg',ylab='proportion of patients with VTE')
lines(exp(alllogdose[doseselect]),ucllin[doseselect],lty=2)
lines(exp(alllogdose[doseselect]),lcllin[doseselect],lty=2)
title(main=
'Transformed fit\n and 99.9% confidence interval')

#mu and alpha parameters for perturbed fit for VTE
#for scenario 2
mu2<-(-0.43)
alpha2<-(-1.08)

#linear predictor for changed linear predictor
linpred<-mu2+alpha2*allenoxselect+beta*alllogdose

#lower and upper confidence limits assuming same
#standard error
lcllin<-linpred-qnorm(0.999)*selinpred
lcllin<-exp(lcllin)/(1+exp(lcllin))
ucllin<-linpred+qnorm(0.999)*selinpred
ucllin<-exp(ucllin)/(1+exp(ucllin))

pred<-exp(linpred)/(1+exp(linpred))

plot(exp(alllogdose[doseselect]),pred[doseselect],typ='l',
xlim=c(0,10),ylim=c(0,1),
xlab='dose mg',ylab='proportion of patients with VTE')
lines(exp(alllogdose[doseselect]),ucllin[doseselect],lty=2)
lines(exp(alllogdose[doseselect]),lcllin[doseselect],lty=2)
title(main=
'Transformed perturbed fit\n and 99.9% confidence interval')

#Factor Xa TB results in original study

#number of patients with bleeds in original study
```

```
responders<-c(3,8,19,16,25,16,15,9)

#number of patients assessed for bleeds in original study
denom<-c(61,141,183,202,397,200,140,65)

#number of patients without bleeds in original study
nonresponders<-denom-responders

y<-cbind(responders,nonresponders)

#fit logistic model
tbfit<-glm(y ~ allenoxfac+alldose,family=binomial)

#save coefficients
tbmu<-tbfit$coefficients[1]
tbalpha<-tbfit$coefficients[2]
tbbeta<-tbfit$coefficients[3]
tbvcov<-vcov(tbfit)

tblinpred<-tbfit$linear.predictors

predout<-predict.glm(fit,se.fit=TRUE)

tbselinpred<-predout$se.fit

tblcllin<-tblinpred-qnorm(0.999)*tbselinpred
tblcllin<-exp(tblcllin)/(1+exp(tblcllin))
tbucllin<-tblinpred+qnorm(0.999)*tbselinpred
tbucllin<-exp(tbucllin)/(1+exp(tbucllin))

tbpred<-exp(tblinpred)/(1+exp(tblinpred))

plot(alldose[doseselect],tbpred[doseselect],typ='l
,xlim=c(0,10),ylim=c(0,1),
xlab='dose mg',
ylab='proportion of patients with bleeds')
lines(alldose[doseselect],tbucllin[doseselect],lty=2)
lines(alldose[doseselect],tblcllin[doseselect],lty=2)
title(main=
'Transformed fit\n and 99.9% confidence interval')


#mu and alpha parameters for perturbed fit for scenario 2
tbmu2<-(-3.47)
tbalpha2<-(0.77)

tblinpred<-tbmu2+tbalpha2*allenoxselect++tbbeta*alldose
tblcllin<-tblinpred-3.09*tbselinpred
```

```
tblcllin<-exp(tblcllin)/(1+exp(tblcllin))
tbucllin<-tblinpred+3.09*tbselinpred
tbucllin<-exp(tbucllin)/(1+exp(tbucllin))

tblinpred<-exp(tblinpred)/(1+exp(tblinpred))
plot(alldose[doseselect],tblinpred[doseselect],typ='l',
xlim=c(0,10),ylim=c(0,1),
xlab='dose mg',
ylab='proportion of patients with bleeds')
lines(alldose[doseselect],tbucllin[doseselect],lty=2)
lines(alldose[doseselect],tblcllin[doseselect],lty=2)
title(main=
'Transformed perturbed fit\n and 99.9% confidence interval')

#change parameter values for Scenario 2
#mu<-mu2
#alpha<-alpha2
#tbmu<-tbmu2
#tbalpha<-tbalpha2

#generate VTE parameters for selected scenario

#doses used in fixed dose study
fixeddose<-c(0.1,0.3,0.5,1,0,2.5)

#factor distinguishing enoxaparin treatment
fixedenoxfac<-factor(x=c(1,1,1,1,2,1))

#0/1 vector picking out enoxaparin result
fixedenoxselect<-c(0,0,0,0,1,0)

#log of doses used with log dose for enoxaparin set to 0
fixedlogdose<-log(c(0.1,0.3,0.5,1,1,2.5))

#vector giving position of Pfizer dose results
fixeddoseselect<-c(1,2,3,4,6)

#sample size
denom<-c(106,106,106,106,210,106)

#number of simulations
nsim<-10000

#count for number of times a dose is correctly selected
total<-0

#vector to hold counts of doses selected
finaldose<-c(0,0,0,0,0,0)
```

```
#count for number of times VTE criterion not satisfied
vteneg<-0

#count for number of times criterion for total bleeds
#not satisfied
tbneg<-0

#count for number of times one or both criteria
#not satisfied
totneg<-c(0,0)

#simulations
for(nn in 1:nsim){
```

```
#generate values for parameters
rparam<-mvrnorm(n=1,mu=c(mu,alpha,beta),Sigma=vcov)
tbrparam<-mvrnorm(n=1,mu=c(tbmu,tbalpha,tbbeta),
Sigma=tbvcov)

#linear predictors for generated parameters
rlogit<-rparam[1]+rparam[2]*fixedenoxselect+rparam[3]*
fixedlogdose
tbrlogit<-tbrparam[1]+tbrparam[2]*fixedenoxselect+
tbrparam[3]*fixeddose

#proportions using generated parameters
rprop<-exp(rlogit)/(1+exp(rlogit))
tbrprop<-exp(tbrlogit)/(1+exp(tbrlogit))

#generate VTE responses
rresp1<-rbinom(length(fixeddose),denom,rprop)

rnonresp1<-denom-rresp1

y<-cbind(rresp1,rnonresp1)

#fit logistic model to generated VTE data
fixedfit<-glm(y ~ fixedenoxfac+fixedlogdose,
family=binomial)

#dose estimated to give equivalent VTE response to enoxaparin
eqlogdose<-fixedfit$coefficients[2]/
fixedfit$coefficients[3]

#value of linear predictor for equivalent dose
eqlinpred<-fixedfit$coefficients[1]+eqlogdose*
fixedfit$coefficients[3]

closest<-999
closedose<-0.1

count<-0
index<-0
```

```
#vector with indices for possible doses
doseselect<-c(1,2,3,4,6)

#find closest dose on logit scale

for(dd in fixeddose[doseselect]){
  count<-count+1
  linpred<-
  fixedfit$linear.predictors[doseselect[count]]
  diff<-abs(eqlinpred-linpred)
  if(diff<closest){
      index<-doseselect[count]
      closedose<-dd
      closest<-diff
    }
}

#true VTE ratio relative to enoxaparin
truevte<-rparam[1]+rparam[2]*fixedenoxselect+rparam[3]
*fixedlogdose
truevte<-exp(truevte)/(1+exp(truevte))
truevteratio<-truevte[index]/truevte[5]

#true TB ratio relative to enoxaparin
truetb<-tbrparam[1]+tbrparam[2]*fixedenoxselect+
tbrparam[3]*fixeddose
truetb<-exp(truetb)/(1+exp(truetb))

truetbratio<-truetb[index]/truetb[5]

#count number of times dose correctly selected
#and reasons for failure
```

```
            if((truevteratio<=1.3)&(truetbratio<=1.5)){
                total<-total+1
            } else {
              countneg<-0
              if(truevteratio>1.3){
                vteneg<-vteneg+1
                countneg<-countneg+1
              }
              if(truetbratio>1.5){
                tbneg<-tbneg+1
                countneg<-countneg+1
              }
              totneg[countneg]<-totneg[countneg]+1
            }

            finaldose[index]<-finaldose[index]+1
        }
```

```
#proportion of times a correct dose is selected
total/nsim
```

```
#proportion of times VTE criterion not satisfied
vteneg/nsim
```

```
#proportion of times criterion for total number of bleeds
#not satisfied
tbneg/nsim
```

```
#proportion of times one or both criteria not satisfied
Totneg
```

Chapter 13, Tables 13.7 - 13.8 and 13.10

```
#program to calculate metrics for adaptive design for
#two scenarios
```

```
#load MASS library to be able to use mvrnorm function
library(MASS)
#seed for scenario 1
set.seed(4516891)
```

```
#seed for scenario 2
```

```
#set.seed(5649288)
```

```
#all doses used in original study
alldose<-c(0.1,0.3,0.5,1,0,2.5,4,10)
```

```
#log of all doses used in original study
#- enoxaparin dose set equal to 1
alllogdose<-log(c(0.1,0.3,0.5,1,1,2.5,4,10))

#Factor Xa VTE results in original study

#number of patients with VTEs in original study
responders<-c(13,33,30,23,34,16,1,3)

#number of patients assessed for VTEs in original study
denom<-c(35,89,104,120,188,112,74,27)

#factor distinguishing enoxaparin from doses of Pfizer drug
allenoxfac<-factor(x=c(1,1,1,1,2,1,1,1))

#0/1 vector picking out enoxaparin treatment
allenoxselect<-c(0,0,0,0,1,0,0,0)

#number of patients without a VTE in original study
nonresponders<-denom-responders

#combined vector for number of subjects with
#and without a VTE
y<-cbind(responders,nonresponders)

#fit logistic model
fit<-glm(y ~ allenoxfac+alllogdose,family=binomial)

#save coefficients
mu<-fit$coefficients[1]
alpha<-fit$coefficients[2]
beta<-fit$coefficients[3]
vcov<-vcov(fit)

#mu and alpha parameters for perturbed fit for VTE for
#scenario 2
mu2<-(-0.43)
alpha2<-(-1.08)

#Factor Xa TB results in original study

#number of patients with bleeds in original study
responders<-c(3,8,19,16,25,16,15,9)

#number of patients assessed for bleeds in original study
denom<-c(61,141,183,202,397,200,140,65)

#number of patients without bleeds in original study
nonresponders<-denom-responders
```

```
y<-cbind(responders,nonresponders)

#fit logistic model
tbfit<-glm(y ~ allenoxfac+alldose,family=binomial)

#save coefficients
tbmu<-tbfit$coefficients[1]
tbalpha<-tbfit$coefficients[2]
tbbeta<-tbfit$coefficients[3]
tbvcov<-vcov(tbfit)

#mu and alpha parameters for perturbed fit for total bleeds
#for scenario 2
tbmu2<-(-3.47)
tbalpha2<-(0.77)

#change mu and alpha parameters for perturbed fits for
#scenario 2
#mu<-mu2
#alpha<-alpha2
#tbmu<-tbmu2
#tbalpha<-tbalpha2

#generate VTE parameters for selected scenario

#doses for part 1 of adaptive trial

part1dose<-c(0.1,0.3,0.5,1,0,2.5)

part1enoxfac<-factor(x=c(1,1,1,1,2,1))

part1enoxselect<-c(0,0,0,0,1,0)

part1logdose<-log(c(0.1,0.3,0.5,1,1,2.5))
part1doseselect<-c(1,2,3,4,6)

#maximum possible trial sample sizes for doses
#initially used
denom<-c(106,106,106,106,210,106)

#sample sizes for doses in part 1 of trial
part1denom<-denom/2
#number of simulations
nsim<-10000

#count for number of times a dose is correctly selected
total<-0

#vector to hold counts of doses selected
```

```
finaldose<-c(0,0,0,0,0,0,0,0)

#count for number of times VTE criterion not satisfied
vteneg<-0

#count for number of times criterion for total bleeds
#not satisfied
tbneg<-0

#counts for number of times one or both criteria
#not satisfied
totneg<-c(0,0)

#safety criterion for TB rate
tbcrit<-0.12

#simulations

for(nn in 1:nsim){
```

```
#generate values for parameters
rparam<-mvrnorm(n=1,mu=c(mu,alpha,beta),Sigma=vcov)
tbrparam<-mvrnorm(n=1,mu=c(tbmu,tbalpha,tbbeta),
Sigma=tbvcov)

#linear predictors for generated parameters
rlogit<-rparam[1]+rparam[2]*part1enoxselect+rparam[3]*
part1logdose
tbrlogit<-tbrparam[1]+tbrparam[2]*part1enoxselect+
tbrparam[3]*part1dose

#proportions using generated parameters
rprop<-exp(rlogit)/(1+exp(rlogit))
tbrprop<-exp(tbrlogit)/(1+exp(tbrlogit))

#generate responses
rresp1<-rbinom(length(part1dose),part1denom,rprop)
tbrresp1<-rbinom(length(part1dose),part1denom,tbrprop)

rnonresp1<-part1denom-rresp1
tbrnonresp1<-part1denom-tbrresp1

y<-cbind(rresp1,rnonresp1)
tby<-cbind(tbrresp1,tbrnonresp1)

#fit logistic models to generated VTE and TB data
#set vteslope to 0

vteslope<-0
part1fit<-glm(y ~ part1enoxfac+part1logdose,
family=binomial)
#if slope unexpectedly positive drop log dose from fit
#and set vteslope equal to 1
if(part1fit$coefficients[3]>0){
   part1fit<-glm(y ~ part1enoxfac,family=binomial)
   vteslope<-1
}
```

```
#set tbslope to 0
tbslope<-0
part1tbfit<-glm(tby ~ part1enoxfac+part1dose,
family=binomial)
#if slope unexpectedly negative drop dose from fit
#and set tbslope to 1
if(part1tbfit$coefficients[3]<0){
   part1tbfit<-glm(tby ~ part1enoxfac, family=binomial)
   tbslope<-1
}


#covariance matrix for VTE fit
part1vcov<-vcov(part1fit)

#odds ratio for VTE for each dose versus enoxaparin
#if slope positive
if(vteslope==0){
   lnoddsratio<-part1fit$coefficients[3]*part1logdose-
   part1fit$coefficients[2]
   ucl<-lnoddsratio+qnorm(0.9)*sqrt(part1vcov[3,3]*
   part1logdose^2+part1vcov[2,2]-
   2*part1vcov[2,3]*part1logdose)
   ucl<-exp(ucl)
}

#odds ratio for VTE for each dose versus enoxaparin
#if term for log dose dropped
if(vteslope==1){
   lnoddsratio<-(-1)*part1fit$coefficients[2]*
   c(1,1,1,1,1,1)
   ucl<-lnoddsratio+qnorm(0.9)*sqrt(part1vcov[2,2])
}

#fitted values for TB fit
predtb<-part1tbfit$fitted.values

#vector for extra possible doses
extradosettb<-vector(length=2)
```

```
#predicted TB rates for extra doses
if(tbslope==0){
  extradosetb<-part1tbfit$coefficients[1]+
  part1tbfit$coefficients[3]*c(4,10)
}

if(tbslope==1){
  extradosetb<-part1tbfit$coefficients[1]*c(1,1)
}
extradosetb<-exp(extradosetb)/(1+exp(extradosetb))

#set selected doses initially to part 1 doses
#- 0 indicates dose not chosen
doseselect<-c(1,2,3,4,5,6,0,0)

#drop doses if TB criterion exceeded
for(dd in part1doseselect){
  if(predtb[dd]>tbcrit)
    doseselect[dd]<-0
}

#drop lowest doses if VTE criterion exceeded
if(ucl[1]>1.5)
  doseselect[1]<-0

if(ucl[2]>1.5)
  doseselect[2]<-0

#add one or both extra doses if one or both lowest doses
#dropped and TB criterion satisfied
if((doseselect[1]==0)&(extradosetb[1]<=tbcrit))
  doseselect[7]<-7

if((doseselect[2]==0)&(extradosetb[2]<=tbcrit))
  doseselect[8]<-8

#vector of potential part 2 sample sizes for all doses
allpart2denom<-c(rep(53,4),105,rep(53,3))
```

```
#vectors to hold total responses and total sample sizes
totresp<-c(rep(0,8))
totdenom<-c(rep(0,8))

#set part2denom to vector of sample sizes
#for selected doses
part2denom<-allpart2denom[doseselect]
```

```
#part 2 doses
newdose<-alldose[doseselect]
#part 2 log doses
lognewdose<-alllogdose[doseselect]
#part 2 vector to pick out enoxaparin result
enoxselect<-allenoxselect[doseselect]
```

```
#generate part 2 VTE responses
rlogit<-rparam[1]+rparam[2]*enoxselect+rparam[3]*
lognewdose
rprop<-exp(rlogit)/(1+exp(rlogit))
rresp2<-rbinom(length(part2denom),part2denom,rprop)
```

```
#add in part 2 responses and sample sizes to vectors
```

```
#for totals
totresp[doseselect]<-rresp2
totdenom[doseselect]<-allpart2denom[doseselect]

#add part 1 responses and sample sizes
totresp<-c(rresp1,0,0)+totresp
totdenom<-c(part1denom,0,0)+totdenom

y<-cbind(totresp,totdenom-totresp)


#fit logistic model to total VTE data set
finalfit<-glm(y ~ allenoxfac+alllogdose,
family=binomial)

#dose estimated to give equivalent VTE response
#to enoxaparin
eqlogdose<-finalfit$coefficients[2]/
finalfit$coefficients[3]

#value of linear predictor for equivalent dose
eqlinpred<-finalfit$coefficients[1]+eqlogdose*
finalfit$coefficients[3]

closest<-999
closedose<-0.1

count<-0
index<-0

#vector with indices for possible doses
doseselect<-c(1,2,3,4,6,7,8)
```

```
#find closest dose on logit scale
for(dd in alldose[doseselect]){
  count<-count+1
  linpred<-
  finalfit$linear.predictors[doseselect[count]]
  diff<-abs(eqlinpred-linpred)
  if(diff<closest){
    index<-doseselect[count]
    closedose<-dd
    closest<-diff
  }
}

#true VTE ratio relative to enoxaparin
truevte<-rparam[1]+rparam[2]*allenoxselect+rparam[3]*
alllogdose
truevte<-exp(truevte)/(1+exp(truevte))
truevteratio<-truevte[index]/truevte[5]

#true TB ratio relative to enoxaparin
truetb<-tbrparam[1]+tbrparam[2]*allenoxselect+
tbrparam[3]*alldose
truetb<-exp(truetb)/(1+exp(truetb))
truetbratio<-truetb[index]/truetb[5]

#count number of times dose correctly selected and
#reasons for failure
if((truevteratio<=1.3)&(truetbratio<=1.5)){
    total<-total+1
} else {
  countneg<-0
  if(truevteratio>1.3){
    vteneg<-vteneg+1
    countneg<-countneg+1
```

```
        }
        if(truetbratio>1.5){
          tbneg<-tbneg+1
          countneg<-countneg+1
        }
        totneg[countneg]<-totneg[countneg]+1

      }
        finaldose[index]<-finaldose[index]+1
    }
```

#proportion of times a correct dose is selected
total/nsim

#proportion of times each dose selected
finaldose

#proportion of times VTE criterion not satisfied
vteneg/nsim

#proportion of times criterion for total number of bleeds

#not satisfied
tbneg/nsim

#proportion of times one or both criteria not satisfied
totneg

Chapter 14, Section 14.1

set.seed(58974593)

#library for simulating from a multivariate
#normal distribution
library(mvtnorm)

#Part A
#derive mean and variability for placebo induction from
#Table 14.1

#placebo induction rates from previous trials
pirate<-c(0.092,0.093,0.15,0.06,0.05,0.08,0.04,0.10)

#sample sizes for placebo induction rates
pisampsize<-c(130,246,121,123,149,122,112,50)

#weighted mean placebo induction rate
pimean<-sum(pisampsize*pirate/sum(pisampsize))

```
print('weighted placebo induction rate')
print(pimean)

#weighted variance of placebo induction rates
wtpivar<-sum(pisampsize*(pirate-pimean)^2/sum(pisampsize))

print('square root of weighted placebo induction variance')
pisd<-sqrt(wtpivar)

print(pisd)

#Part B
#derive mean and variability for placebo maintenance trials
#from Table 14.2

#placebo maintenance rates from previous trials
pmrate<-c(0.11,0.16,0.13)

#sample sizes for placebo maintenance rates
pmsampsize<-c(198,126,50)

#weighted mean placebo maintenanmce rate
pmmean<-sum(pmsampsize*pmrate/sum(pmsampsize))

print('weighted placebo maintenance rate')
print(pmmean)

#weighted variance of placebo maintenance rates
wtpmvar<-sum(pmsampsize*(pmrate-pmmean)^2/sum(pmsampsize))

pmsd<-sqrt(wtpmvar)

print(
'square root of weighted placebo maintenance variance')
print(pmsd)

#Part C
#derive variability for induction effect

#induction effect
indeffect<-0.14
print('induction effect')
print(indeffect)

#placebo rate assumed to be 0.10
varindeffect<-(0.24*0.76/50)+(0.1*0.9/50)

sdindeffect<-sqrt(varindeffect)

print('standard deviation of induction effect')
```

```
print(sdindeffect)

#Part D
#derive variability for maintenance effect

#maintenance effect
maineffect<-0.27

print('maintenance effect')
print(maineffect)

#placebo rate assumed to be 0.13
varmaineffect<-(0.4*0.6/50)+(0.13*0.87/50)

sdmaineffect<-sqrt(varmaineffect)

print('standard deviation of maintenance effect')
print(sdmaineffect)

#Part E
#derive correlation between induction and maintenance
#effects from Table 14.3

#induction effects from previous trials
indeffectvec<-c(0.115,0.12,0.14)

#associated maintenance effects
maineffectvec<-c(0.23,0.26,0.27)

print('correlation of maintenance and induction effects')
coreffect<-cor(indeffectvec,maineffectvec)

#option of setting correlation to 0 to obtain result when
#correlation of zero assumed
#coreffect<-0

#covariance of induction and maintenance effects
coveffect<-coreffect*sdindeffect*sdmaineffect

#covraiance matrix
covmat<-matrix(c(sdindeffect^2,coveffect,coveffect,
sdmaineffect^2),nrow=2,ncol=2)

#Part F
#calculate Probability of Success
indsampsize<-130
mainsampsize<-150

#number of simulations
nsim<-100000
```

```
#number of positive results - all 3 one-sided p-values less
#than 0.025
sumpos<-0

#number of rates set to zero because of use of Normal
#approximation
sumniratezero<-0
sumnmratezero<-0

#derive shape parameters for beta distribution for placebo
#induction rate
pialpha<-((1-pimean)/(pisd^2)-1/pimean)*pimean^2
pibeta<-pialpha*(1/pimean-1)

#derive shape parameters for beta distribution for placebo
#maintenance rate
pmalpha<-((1-pmmean)/(pmsd^2)-1/pmmean)*pmmean^2
pmbeta<-pmalpha*(1/pmmean-1)

for(nn in 1:nsim){
```

```
#sample placebo induction rate
pirate<-rbeta(1,pialpha,pibeta)

#sample placebo maintenance rate
pmrate<-rbeta(1,pmalpha,pmbeta)

#sample effects from bivariate Normal distribution
effectsim<-rmvnorm(1,mean=c(indeffect,maineffect),
sigma=covmat)

#derive sampled new drug induction rate
nirate<-pirate+effectsim[1]
if(nirate<0){
  nirate<-0
  sumniratezero<-sumniratezero+1
}

#derive sampled new drug maintenance rate
nmrate<-pmrate+effectsim[2]
if(nmrate<0){
  nmrate<-0
  sumnmratezero<-sumnmratezero+1
}

#simulate placebo responses in induction trials
pisim1<-rbinom(1,indsampsize,pirate)
pisim2<-rbinom(1,indsampsize,pirate)

#simulate new drug responses in induction trials
nisim1<-rbinom(1,indsampsize,nirate)
nisim2<-rbinom(1,indsampsize,nirate)

#simulate placebo responses in maintenance trial
pmsim<-rbinom(1,mainsampsize,pmrate)
#simulate new drug responses in maintenance trial
nmsim<-rbinom(1,mainsampsize,nmrate)
```

```
#calculate observed rates for induction trials
piprop1<-pisim1/indsampsize
piprop2<-pisim2/indsampsize
niprop1<-nisim1/indsampsize
niprop2<-nisim2/indsampsize

#test statistic for first induction trial
test1<-(niprop1-piprop1)/sqrt(niprop1*(1-niprop1)/
indsampsize+piprop1*(1-piprop1)/indsampsize)
#associated p-value
pval1<-1-pnorm(test1)

#test statistic for second induction trial
test2<-(niprop2-piprop2)/sqrt(niprop2*(1-niprop2)/
indsampsize+piprop2*(1-piprop2)/indsampsize)
#associated p-value
pval2<-1-pnorm(test2)

#calculate observed rates for maintenance trial
pmprop<-pmsim/mainsampsize
nmprop<-nmsim/mainsampsize

#test statistic for maintenance trial
test3<-(nmprop-pmprop)/sqrt(nmprop*(1-nmprop)/
mainsampsize+pmprop*(1-pmprop)/mainsampsize)
#associated p-value
pval3<-1-pnorm(test3)

if((pval1<=0.025)&(pval2<=0.025)&(pval3<=0.025))
  sumpos<-sumpos+1

}

print('proportion of positive results')
print(sumpos/nsim,digits=6)

print('proportion of times new drug induction rate <0')
print(sumniratezero/nsim,digits=6)

print('proportion of times new drug maintenance rate <0')
print(sumnmratezero/nsim,digits=6)
```

Index

A

Accelerated approval, 9–11
Accelerate decision, 101, 118
Acceptance region, 24
ACR20, 117, 118
Actual power, 197, 200–202, 216
Adaptive design, 13, 14, 16, 225–227, 229, 230, 233, 235, 237–240, 243, 245, 248, 249
Adaptive dose-ranging design, 234, 235, 238, 239
Adaptive enrichment, 227, 229
Adaptive randomization, 230
Akaike Information Criterion, 259
Alternative hypothesis, 24–33
Animal studies, 260, 261, 265
Antagonism, 172
ASAS20, 122
Assurance probability, 59, 61–64
Average power, 217–220
Average replication probability, 52–56

B

Base, Pessimistic and Optimistic scenarios, 131
Bayesian decision rule, 122
Bayesian inference, 59, 60
Bayesian latent relationship modelling, 254
Bayesian optimal design, 130
Bayes' Rule, 42
Benefit-cost efficiency score, 178, 193
Beta distribution, 123, 124
Binary endpoint, 100, 117, 121
Binomial distribution, 23–25
Bivariate Normal nonlinear model, 259

B

Bonferroni adjustment, 34
Breakthrough therapy, 10

C

Calibrated optimal γ conservative strategy, 218
'clinDR' R package, 141
Clinical development, 2, 3, 8, 13, 18, 19
Clinical utility index, 194, 195
Closed testing principle, 242
Comparative effectiveness, 163, 168
Complex innovative trial designs, 15
Composite hypothesis, 24
Concurrent control, 72, 74–76
Conditional evaluation, 109, 124, 125
Conditional likelihood weighted bias method, 219
Conditional power, 156–159
Conditional probability of study success, 148, 159, 160
Conditional replication probability, 50–52, 54
Confidence intervals, 23, 35, 36
Critical region, 24
Cumulative logistic distribution, 129, 141
Cumulative Normal distribution, 129

D

Data Monitoring Committee, 233, 240, 246
DcoD adaptive design, 145
(Design) Optimality criteria, 129, 130
Diagnostic test, 39–43, 46
Direct comparisons, 163, 164, 166, 170

Printed in the United States
by Baker & Taylor Publisher Services